# A GLOBAL HISTORY OF BUDDHISM AND MEDICINE

# *A* GLOBAL HISTORY *of* BUDDHISM *and* MEDICINE

C. Pierce Salguero

Columbia University Press *New York*

Columbia University Press
*Publishers Since 1893*
New York Chichester, West Sussex
cup.columbia.edu



Library of Congress Cataloging-in-Publication Data
Names: Salguero, C. Pierce, author.
Title: A global history of Buddhism and medicine /
C. Pierce Salguero.
Description: New York : Columbia University Press, 2022. |
Includes bibliographical references and index.
Identifiers: LCCN 2021015087 (print) | LCCN 2021015088 (ebook) |
ISBN 9780231185264 (hardback) | ISBN 9780231185271
(trade paperback) | ISBN 9780231546072 (ebook)
Subjects: LCSH: Medicine—Religious aspects—Buddhism.
Classification: LCC BQ4570.M4 S25 2022 (print) |
LCC BQ4570.M4 (ebook) | DDC 294.3/3661—dc23
LC record available at https://lccn.loc.gov/2021015087
LC ebook record available at https://lccn.loc.gov/2021015088

Cover image: Statue of Bhaiṣajyaguru from Unified Silla, late 9th–early 10th century
(photo by the author, used with permission from Gyeongju National Museum)

Cover design: Lisa Hamm

# *Contents*

*Acknowledgments* *vii*

Introduction 1

PART I: PRACTICES AND DOCTRINAL PERSPECTIVES

1 Nikāya Buddhism 17

2 Mahāyāna Buddhism 33

3 Tantric Buddhism 48

4 Common Questions 68

PART II: HISTORICAL CURRENTS AND TRANSFORMATIONS

5 Circulations 89

6 Translations 105

7 Localizations 124

8 Modernizations 144

9 Contemporary Buddhist Medicine 159

Conclusion 177

*Notes* *183*

*References* *205*

*Index* *245*

# *Acknowledgments*

It may be a cliché to say that scholarship is a collaborative endeavor, but this book, and the project of which it is a part, literally could not exist if it were not for my colleagues. The purpose of this project has been to forge a new subfield of study that is collaborative and interdisciplinary from the ground up. The two anthology volumes that preceded this book included works by eighty-eight contributors, who have taught me much about various aspects of Buddhist medicine as the project came together over the course of seven years. The present volume, the final one in this series, represents my attempt to synthesize those contributions and conversations. It is a vision of how these various pieces fit together and speak to one another. My intention here is to introduce an overarching narrative that connects my colleagues' contributions to the anthologies with their specialized publications elsewhere, and with as much of the academic work on Buddhist medicine that has been produced by other scholars as possible. Of course, I have also integrated into this story my own scholarship, which primarily concerns Buddhist medicine in medieval China, modern Thailand, and contemporary United States. However, the primary purpose is to highlight the connections between all of our work. I am extremely grateful to all of the participants in this endeavor for their collaboration. And also to Wendy Lochner at Columbia University Press for believing in the project and supporting it all along.

My thinking about Buddhist medicine has been fundamentally shaped by frequent conversations about various aspects of this subject with both Michael Stanley-Baker and Bill McGrath, who continually have both challenged and educated me and for whose friendship I am deeply appreciative. I am additionally indebted to Bill as well as Ronit Yoeli-Tlalim for reading through full drafts of this manuscript, at which time they made many substantial and insightful suggestions. David Carpenter and Amy Langenberg also provided comments on significant portions of the manuscript. I am also thankful for the many other project contributors who read portions and made comments and corrections that have improved this book. These include Anna Andreeva, James Bae, Don Baker, Kin Cheung, Clark Chilson, Céline Coderey, Jo Cook, Susannah Deane, Ed Drott, Douglas Duckworth, Ann Heirman, Alex Hsu, Assunta Hunter, Anthony Irwin, Ben Joffe, Dhivan Jones, Benedetta Lomi, Dan Lusthaus, Andrew Macomber, Alex McKinley, Nathan Michon, Jonathan Pettit, Volker Scheid, Gregory Scott, Nathan Sivin, Michael Slouber, Dominic Steavu, Michele Thompson, Robban Toleno, and Katja Triplett. Other people who contributed at various points in the making of this book—whether knowingly or not—include Ann Gleig, Ira Helderman, and Dominik Wujastyk. To all of you, I am grateful.

# A GLOBAL HISTORY OF BUDDHISM AND MEDICINE

# Introduction

The health benefits of Buddhism are being talked about everywhere. Thanks to the meteoric rise in the global popularity of mindfulness meditation as a stress-reduction technique, it now seems entirely normal to associate Buddhism with better mental health. The English-language popular media report breathlessly on how it helps you to navigate the anxieties of modern life. Regular attendance at classes, workshops, and retreats is now de rigueur among the high-powered economic and cultural global elite.[1] Bolstered by brain scans and other modern medical evidence of efficacy, authoritative voices all over the world now are promoting these activities as necessary to optimize one's potential and well-being.[2]

It is not just meditation, however: a whole spectrum of Buddhist therapies are ubiquitous parts of primary health care in traditionally Buddhist cultures in Asia. These include the therapeutic herbs prescribed by a Buddhist healer in a mountain village in Bhutan, for example, the prayers for health and longevity offered by a group of devotees in a temple in downtown Tokyo, and the protective talisman worn by an expectant mother in Thailand. Countless other healing and health-seeking behaviors such as these are being performed by many of the estimated 400 to 600 million Buddhists alive today around the world.[3] Many non-Buddhists have also been touched by Buddhist approaches and ideas, including both through exposure to Buddhism as well as via hybrid practices such as Christian mindfulness, Japanese New Religious movements, Falun Gong, New Age healing, Reiki, Tibetan singing bowl therapy, and a cacophony of self-help books, podcasts, workshops, and other wares that have flooded the global health and wellness marketplace.[4] Even as I write these words in mid-2020, Buddhist institutions and spokespeople around the world are calling for meditation, charity, prayer, ritual, vegetarianism, and compassion in response to the novel coronavirus (COVID-19) pandemic, finding solace and solutions in the Dharma for this global catastrophe. If we look at the history of Buddhist engagements with health and healing, we will discover even more practices, ideas, and connections with health over the past twenty-four centuries or so that Buddhism has been on the planet.

The primary motivation of this book is to situate our contemporary fascination with therapeutic meditation within this larger global and historical context. I will show that the interconnections between Buddhism and medicine have a fascinating history as old as Buddhism itself. As we will see, Buddhism and medicine have been closely intertwined since the very beginning of the tradition and have continued to develop together over the course of nearly two and a half millennia leading up to the present moment. But, as we will also learn, this relationship has undergone considerable change over that time.

Owing to the constraints of space, it is not possible to tell every detail of the entire history here. (Indeed, that story is so immense that it would actually be impossible to portray in a book of any length.) Rather, the idea here is to make a useful, if reductive, summary of the larger patterns, major themes, and broad strokes of the study of Buddhist engagements with medicine. Because it is a very general map of the territory, this book is not intended to be read in isolation. Rather, it is intended to provide an entry point for the rich, more detailed materials in its two companion volumes: *Buddhism and Medicine: An Anthology of Premodern Sources* and *Buddhism and Medicine: An Anthology of Modern and Contemporary Sources*, published by Columbia University Press in 2017 and 2019, respectively.

The current book refers to those two volumes on a frequent basis (abbreviated as {1} or {2}, followed by a chapter number and optional subsection number). It does so particularly when a translation of a text or an interview with a practitioner is illustrative, adds depth, or brings nuance to the general overview provided here. The anthologies also provide essential context from the history of Buddhism, the history of medicine, and the many cultures and traditions mentioned in passing in this volume. Even more detail is provided in reading recommendations and endnotes appearing after each chapter throughout the three-volume series. All of these materials are intended to work together to provide readers with a comprehensive understanding of the subject matter.

If one were to design a course around these materials, whether for a college or graduate class or just for one's own edification, I would suggest reading a chapter in this book in tandem with the *Anthology* chapters it cites, following up with the further readings and endnotes where more detail and deeper context is desirable. Of course, I will not give here anything resembling a complete history of Buddhism, or of Asian medicine more generally, so readers should consider branching out into these adjacent fields as well.

## "BUDDHIST MEDICINE"

Perhaps the most central assertion of this book, and of the larger project of which it is a part, is that there is a discrete historical phenomenon that we can loosely refer to as "Buddhist medicine." I have written about my use of this term in the introductions to both volumes of the *Anthology*, among other places, but it is worth taking up the question again here in more detail.

Is there such a thing as Buddhist medicine? Whether or not you agree may in the end come down to a question of taste. Certainly, some valid reasons exist for resisting the term.[5] Some scholars prefer not to use it on the grounds that it is almost never used in Buddhist sources. Although equivalent terms have been used in distinct times and places—"insider medicine" (*nangpé men*) in Bhutan, for example—the specific phrase "Buddhist medicine" seems to have become widespread only in the middle of the twentieth century, and only in particular places.[6] So, if we choose to use it to discuss broader concepts, we have to be clear that this is a second-order scholarly category, not a term native to the traditions we are studying.

Further, in an expansive project like this one, there is danger in using any single overarching term as it may mislead readers into overlooking the complexities of the relationship between Buddhism and medicine in different times and places.[7] In the discussion throughout this book, it will become clear that there has never been a fixed or monolithic Buddhist approach to health and healing. On the contrary, the most dominant theme in this three-volume project is the diversity of local variations of Buddhist engagements with medicine across time and space. Buddhist notions of health and illness have always depended on a combination of ancient tradition and new innovations. They have always been products of both external stimuli from cross-cultural exchanges and local and idiosyncratic factors that emerge in specific times and places. My aim here is not to boil all of this down into a cohesive unitary tradition called "Buddhist medicine." It is precisely the tension and interplay between the ancient and the contemporary, the global and the local, that is my primary focus.

While acknowledging these concerns, I find that "Buddhist medicine" nevertheless is useful as a fuzzy term of convenience that facilitates a particular kind of scholarly analysis. I use the term similarly to how scholars use "Buddhist art." That term, which also is not an actor's category and has the danger of being treated reductively, is nevertheless generally acknowledged to be quite useful. It can bring together objects as disparate as a monumental stupa from ancient India, a sculpture from an oasis town on the Silk Road, a poem written in brush-painted calligraphy in early modern Korea, and a contemporary Vietnamese graphic novel about a group of Buddhist superheroes. At first glance, these items appear to have little in common. Given that they differ from one another aesthetically and technologically, they can and should be studied and contextualized within the separate currents of Indian, Central Asian, Korean, and Vietnamese art respectively. Each can and should be understood and examined alongside other architectural, sculptural, calligraphic, and print arts of the eras in which they were produced. Of course, much of those contexts have nothing to do with Buddhism.

However, at the same time that these art forms clearly are the products of local customs, practices, and material cultures, they just as assuredly are also related to one another via their connections with Buddhism, and ignoring the opportunity to compare and contrast them on that basis would be a mistake. That is to say, while focusing on these artworks in relation to their specific local contexts reveals what is unique about them, grouping them together using an invented category like "Buddhist art" allows us to see how they all are shaped by shared Buddhist motifs, the similarity in the practices involved in their production, and the convergences in the social contexts or intellectual milieux of the artists.[8]

As with "Buddhist art," we also have to weigh the advantages of lumping versus splitting in our use of "Buddhist architecture," "Buddhist poetry," "Buddhist aesthetics," and all kinds of other similar fuzzy categories. None of these is native to the Buddhist tradition, but all are used widely by scholars as terms of convenience. None of these is an actual "thing" with the power to influence history in its own right. However, when used loosely, these terms can be helpful in focusing our attention on particular traditions, currents, streams, or approaches that were influential and placing these in transnational and transhistorical perspective.

Examining these as examples of a broader category makes visible the cross-cultural exchange of shared elements across geographic distances, as well as the development and transformation of those shared elements over time. It allows us to better understand how they form a whole larger than the sum of its parts.

If we are going to use the term "Buddhist medicine," it is essential to cast a wide net. While the term draws our attention to similarities across time and space, it also attunes us to sites of disagreement and negotiation. As I have written elsewhere, "Buddhist medicine" refers to the totality of the different intersections and relations between Buddhism and medicine, in whatever shape those may have taken. Indeed, to study this topic means not only to study how bridges have been built to connect Buddhism and medicine in some times or places but also how lines have been drawn to separate them into two distinct fields of knowledge in others.[9]

Furthermore, we must resist defining Buddhist medicine on the basis of our preconceived notions or any particular tradition of therapeutic practice. The English word "medicine" has a wide range of meanings. When used on its own, these days, it often refers to modern scientific medicine, and some readers may immediately equate the word with that. However, it is quite acceptable to combine the word with an adjective—as in the case of "folk medicine," "alternative medicine," "traditional medicine," or "domestic medicine"—to refer to therapeutic practices from radically different contexts, which operate on completely different social and cultural logics. In this book, I intend my use of "Buddhist medicine" to be as inclusive as possible, employing it to refer to just about any form of therapy as long as it was understood by practitioners to be an expression of Buddhist values, commitments, or traditions. Drawing firm distinctions between "medicine," "healing," "folk practice," and other categories—relevant as they may be for other projects—is not our concern here.

All of that is to say that my job here is not to police the boundaries of what counts as "Buddhist medicine" but rather to use the category to orient readers to the richness of the human experience it is pointing to. Again, my position is clarified by making a parallel with art: If, say, a graffiti artist understood her work to be an expression of her Buddha Nature, a scholar would be wrong to exclude her oeuvre from the category of Buddhist art on the basis that it is not the "right kind" of artistic practice, as predetermined by us. Similarly, whether they be monastics, yogis, shamans, spirit mediums, physicians, neurosurgeons, psychiatrists, or anyone else, a certain subset of practitioners of all kinds of medical systems across the millennia has understood their practice of healing to fit into their practice of Buddhism. They may feel their therapies are empowered by a Buddhist deity, or they may consider their medical career as an integral part of their personal Buddhist path. Even if there is nothing special or different about the therapeutic technique these practitioners employ in contrast to their non-Buddhist contemporaries—and even if no other Buddhist in history has practiced that technique—we still will want to consider their practice to be an example of Buddhist medicine.

With such a broad remit, can we say anything concrete about Buddhist medicine? Just as it would be difficult to come up with a definitive list of the characteristics of Buddhist art, it is difficult to do so for this new category. There is a huge amount of variability in how Buddhist ideas and practices of health and healing have been expressed in different times, places, languages, and cultural contexts. A cavernous gulf separates ancient Indian scriptural depictions of the Buddha nursing a sick monk (chapter 1), a group of medieval Tibetan yogis doing subtle body manipulations (chapter 3), and a neurological scan of a meditator's brain taken as part of a clinical trial (chapter 9). We do not have a checklist of epistemological, ontological, or metaphysical considerations that must be satisfied before something is considered Buddhist medicine.

Nevertheless, we can see some common orientations, perspectives, concerns, and approaches emerge from the diverse examples presented throughout this book. These shared sensibilities allow us to place items side by side in order to investigate them as connected and intertwined phenomena. For example, regardless of the specifics of their practice, practitioners who have understood themselves to be participating in a specifically Buddhist tradition of healing have often named Buddhist figures (such as Jīvaka, Bhaiṣajyaguru, Yutok,[10] the Buddha himself, and others who are discussed in the chapters to come) as the sources of particularly efficacious medical insights or techniques. Practitioners have often considered these heroes to be exemplary and their methods to be distinct from and superior to other therapies. Such practitioners have also often identified themselves as members of formal lineages or schools of medicine founded by these figures and frequently differentiate themselves as a special class of healers on those grounds.

In many Buddhist societies, these lineages have also been closely connected with Buddhist institutions and power structures. Practitioners may proffer their medical arts within an institution that is explicitly Buddhist, such as a monastic hospital, temple clinic, or charitable organization. As we will see, monastic

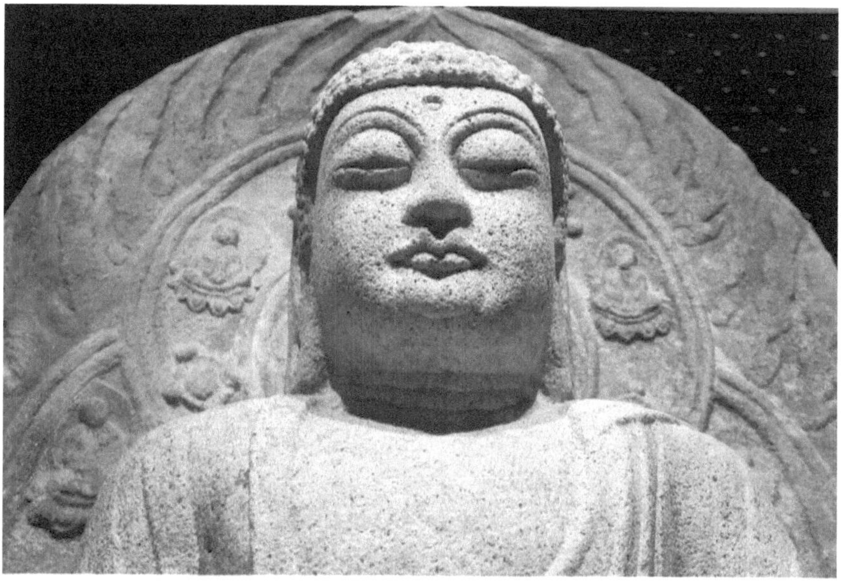

**INT.1** Statue of Bhaiṣajyaguru from the Unified Silla kingdom, ninth century.
Photo by the author, with permission from the National Museum of Korea, Seoul, and the National Research Foundation of Korea.

communities have historically played a major role in documenting, promulgating, systematizing, and preserving Buddhist medical knowledge.

The category "Buddhist medicine" helps bring into focus general patterns such as these and gives us the opportunity to compare and contrast how they have manifested in local historical contexts. By collecting so many disparate examples into a common field of study, this book brings together scholarship on radically different medical theories, practices, social contexts, and understandings into the dialogue of a shared project. This book shows that when we do this, "Buddhist medicine" opens up previously hidden vistas that change the way we understand the history of medicine and the history of Buddhism alike.

## AN EMERGENT FIELD

The clinical study of meditation has been a prolific area of scientific research, and research on mindfulness in particular has exploded in the twenty-first century. I will summarize the history of therapeutic meditation, and how this came to be seen as a legitimate object of scientific inquiry, in chapter 8. However, this book will neither take up the specifically scientific questions of how meditation affects the brain or the physiology of the body, nor discuss specific mental or physical health outcomes. Readers interested in the medical efficacy of meditation should consult published meta-studies, which represent the most accessible starting points for the scientific literature.[11] Several edited volumes discussing various aspects of these practices from the clinician's perspective have also recently been published.[12]

In contrast, this book will focus on bringing together historical and anthropological scholarship. Despite having been initiated by Buddhologists in the early twentieth century (Paul Demiéville's 1937 essay "Byō" was the birth of this field in the West), the academic study of Buddhist medicine by humanists and social scientists has garnered nowhere near the same amount of attention as the scientific research.[13] Because scholars from these fields have not yet seen themselves as part of a common field of inquiry, the currently existing work on disparate traditions of Buddhist medicine is grounded in a variety of conflicting literatures that have not yet gelled into a coherent research agenda.

Nevertheless, by examining the various publications on the topic, several "centers of gravity" can be detected. One is the ethnographic investigation of the nexus of Buddhism, medicine, modern biomedical power structures, and globalization in Tibetan communities. Studies in this arena have tended to focus on how both practitioners and patients understand, navigate, and balance these competing forces.[14] Another growing area of research concerns the overlap of Buddhist medicine and gender studies. Scholars working in this area have examined the historical development and circulation of Buddhist models of embryology, obstetrics, and women's medicine, as well as the role of women as healers in various forms of Buddhism.[15] Finally, a third cluster of articles and books has concentrated on the history of Buddhist medicine in medieval East Asia. These works have prioritized the transmission and translation of Indian knowledge in China and Japan, as well as local social and political contexts affecting how Buddhist medicine was adapted to fit with East Asian cultural norms.[16]

As the discussion so far suggests, the existing literature on Buddhist medicine is largely fractured and unsynthesized. Most scientists studying the health benefits of Buddhist-influenced meditation, for example, lack the linguistic or disciplinary training to seriously investigate the Asian cultural contexts that gave rise to these practices. Anthropologists studying Asia, on the other hand, approach contemporary practice by deeply analyzing one location, without necessarily having an awareness of the connected history of that practice in different cultures or historical periods. Scholars trained in the history of Buddhism likewise tend to relate aspects of Buddhist medicine to a limited range of historical issues within their own field, perhaps totally unaware that the same practices are highly relevant in many parts of the world today. Meanwhile, historians of science, medicine, and technology have only rarely paid attention to Buddhism at all, often overlooking altogether the importance of the religion as a catalyst for global medical exchange.

In the past decade or so, several academic conferences have raised the profile of research on Buddhist medicine and encouraged communication across disciplinary divides.[17] In addition, several recently published edited volumes and special journal issues have aimed to unite scholars from across the spectrum to foster a more comparative and collaborative investigation of Buddhist medicine.[18] With all of this activity, it might be fair to say that Buddhist medicine is now emerging as a cohesive field of research. Part of the purpose of the current book, and the series of which it is a part, is to encourage this emergence. By drawing the various existing pieces of scholarship into conversation, these works intend to provide a framework for the future interdisciplinary study of this topic.

Moving forward, I hope that the newly forming field outlined here will continue to attract interest and receive support from an increasingly diverse scholarly community. I also hope that in the near future some of the glaring omissions that so far have marked this nascent field will begin to be addressed. While a lot of research has been done on South Asia, East Asia, and Tibet, numerous Buddhist communities remain vastly underrepresented in the literature, including most notably Korea, Laos, Nepal, and Vietnam, as well as contemporary Asian diasporic communities around the world. Another purpose of the current volume is to show where the holes are and provide the impetus for further research in these areas.

Even with the gaps and omissions in the new field of Buddhist medicine, however, it is already clear that it is making important contributions to scholars' understanding of history. One of the goals of this book is to draw out these contributions and make them more explicit. Many of these new insights have great relevance for scholars of Buddhism. In particular, scholars have definitively demonstrated that health and medicine were central topics of concern in virtually all forms of Buddhism throughout history. Buddhist studies scholars may previously have thought of health as a "worldly" matter tangential to the larger Buddhist project of liberation or that medicine is simply a metaphor that sometimes has been useful for illustrating Buddhist doctrine. Although medicine was never Buddhism's main concern, the emerging research has conclusively shown that, from its inception, the Dharma usually has been understood quite literally to be a vital source of healing knowledge.

This emergent field also has begun making an important intervention into the history of medicine. All too often, Buddhism has been written out of the history of medicine because scholars in that field have considered it to be a religion and therefore outside their purview. Buddhism's importance has even been overlooked by many scholars who study the history of medicine in China, Japan, and India—some of the places where historical records on Buddhist medicine are voluminous. This book and the scholarship it cites definitively overturn the assumption that the history of religion is divorced from the history of medicine. On the contrary, it reveals that Buddhism has been one of the most important global contexts for cross-cultural medical exchange in human history and that historians of medicine must start taking this fact into account in their scholarship.

Even among the minority of scholars who have appreciated Buddhism's influence on Asian medical traditions, its role in stimulating cross-cultural exchange has all too frequently been overlooked. Owing to hyper-specialization, scholars of Chinese medicine tend to look at sources written only in Chinese, scholars of Indian medicine solely at Indic languages, scholars of Tibetan medicine only at Tibetan, and so forth, and it is relatively rare for anyone to seriously integrate more than one region.[19] This book and its related anthologies, in contrast, focus on global interconnectivity. They place different traditions of Asian religion and medicine usually studied in separate silos within a single cross-cultural framework. In so doing, they seek to break down the walls that have kept scholars from interacting and engaging with one other's work.

Aside from these major interventions in history and anthropology, I hope that this project also will stimulate some important conversations among readers in the health sciences. As mentioned, a large number of researchers are now interested in the effectiveness of Buddhist interventions. These individuals come from a variety of fields, including but not limited to cognitive science, medicine, neuroscience, psychiatry, and psychology. For readers from these disciplines, the way that this project decenters Western scientific research on meditation in the story of Buddhism's intersections with health is particularly salient. They may gain an appreciation for how much Buddhist traditions historically have had to say about health and medicine, going far beyond the narrow scope of the current clinical research. I hope that such readers find that this book hints at possibilities for new lines of research into previously uninvestigated Buddhist healing practices. I also imagine they will find that many Buddhist ideas discussed here do not fit so well with current scientific models or methodologies and hope this realization may inspire new research agendas and methodologies that challenge the status quo.[20]

Finally, another goal of this book is to digest and introduce a wide array of scholarly work to students and nonspecialist readers curious about Buddhism, Asian medicine, meditation, and other Buddhist-influenced and Buddhist-inspired therapies. I anticipate that the majority of readers who pick up this book will come from the Anglosphere (i.e., the English-speaking world) and will already be familiar with the current discourse on meditation in the popular media. For such readers, I hope that this book will open up a much wider world beyond the buzzwords of the current day. By amplifying diverse voices, both historical and contemporary, in an accessible way, I hope to help readers gain an appreciation for the wide range of perspectives that have been prevalent in the global conversation about Buddhism and health and the rich multicultural roots of that millennia-old dialogue.

## CONTENTS OF THIS BOOK

This book is organized into two parts. Part 1 mainly focuses on outlining the repertoire of Buddhist ideas, practices, and texts related to health and medicine. Chapters 1 to 3, which comprise the bulk of this section, give an overview of Buddhist medicine according to the three traditional divisions of Buddhism, here called Nikāya, Mahayana, and Tantric Buddhism. Each chapter provides a thematic introduction to Buddhist healing practices, organized under topical subheadings. These chapters presume that readers may not have much prior knowledge of Buddhism or Asian medicine and thus lay the groundwork for the second half of the book. Chapter 4 concludes the section by providing a summary of some common doctrinal questions that have characterized multiple strands of Buddhist medicine over the centuries.

In part 2, our attention shifts from the thematic to the historical, tracing the development and transformation of Buddhist medicine as it spread across Asia and eventually globally. Unlike part 1, this part gives a chronological account of specific historical actors, events, and contexts. Chapter 5 discusses how Buddhist medicine spread through Asia in the first millennium CE. Instead of trying to comprehensively catalog every example of cross-cultural exchange in history, it outlines the networks, nodes, and patterns of movement that shaped this exchange overall. In chapter 6, I focus on the circulation of texts, with emphasis on how Buddhist knowledge from India was refracted through indigenous knowledge systems when translated into new cultures. Chapter 7 turns to a discussion of three divergent long-term trajectories that characterized the history of Buddhist medicine in different parts of Asia, drawing attention to patterns of "displacement," "domestication," and "translocation." Picking up the story in the early modern period, chapter 8 highlights the transformation of Buddhist medicine through the processes of colonialism and the increasing hegemony of scientific biomedicine in the twentieth century. Chapter 9 focuses on the contemporary situation, in particular how globalization and the Information Age have continued to fundamentally transform the way that Buddhists engage with health. Finally, a brief conclusion provides an update on how Buddhist medicine is playing a role in the global response to the COVID-19 pandemic.

Following each chapter, I provide a few recommended titles for readers looking for more information pertaining to the major topics covered. The readings recommended at the end of this introduction, for example, represent general reference materials for learning more about Buddhism, as well as the two anthology volumes that accompany this text. With few exceptions, these further reading lists are limited to English-language books. Because they omit many valuable articles, chapters, dissertations, and non-English publications, these suggestions should be thought of as accessible starting points rather than comprehensive bibliographies. Readers are highly encouraged to consult the endnotes for more information than can be provided in the lists of further readings.

## FURTHER READING

Buswell, Robert E, ed. 2004. *Encyclopedia of Buddhism*. 2 vols. New York: MacMillan. A general reference for all matters pertaining to Buddhism.

Jackson, Mark, ed. 2018. *A Global History of Medicine*. New York: Oxford University Press. A collection of essays introducing the history of medicine on a global scale.

Powers, John. 2016. *The Buddhist World*. Abingdon: Routledge. A collection of essays presenting a wide-ranging introduction to Buddhist history, philosophy, social formations, and individuals.

Salguero, C. Pierce. 2014 (last updated 2018). "Medicine." *Oxford Bibliographies.* https://doi.org/10.1093/obo/9780195393521-0140. A continually updated bibliography of major academic writing and translation efforts related to Buddhist medicine.

Salguero, C. Pierce, ed. 2017. *Buddhism and Medicine: An Anthology of Premodern Sources.* New York: Columbia University Press. A collection of sixty-two chapters by fifty-seven contributors introducing translations of texts about Buddhism and medicine covering much of premodern Asia. Abbreviated throughout this book as {1}.

Salguero, C. Pierce, ed. 2019. *Buddhism and Medicine: An Anthology of Modern and Contemporary Sources.* New York: Columbia University Press. A collection of thirty-five chapters by thirty-one contributors introducing translations of texts and ethnographic transcripts about Buddhist healing in the modern era. Abbreviated throughout this book as {2}.

# PART I

## *Practices and Doctrinal Perspectives*

## CHAPTER 1

# *Nikāya Buddhism*

Illness lies at the very foundation of the story Buddhism tells about itself. Its central protagonist, Siddhārtha Gautama (also called Śākyamuni Buddha), is thought to have lived in an area of India called Magadha, in the eastern part of the Gangetic plain, from around 450 to 350 BCE.[1] Stories about his life say he was a prince raised in confinement within the royal palace to shield him from the pains and inconveniences of life. In an episode commonly known as the "Four Signs" or the "Four Sights," however, the adult Siddhārtha finally ventures beyond the palace only to confront four realities that shock him to his core: an old person, a sick person, a dead person, and a serene ascetic who had renounced the world for a life of religious cultivation. Overcome by feelings of dismay and urgency at this new understanding of the realities of the human condition, Siddhārtha is propelled onto the epic quest that ultimately results in his becoming the "Awakened One," the Buddha. Illness, as one of these four signs, is thus an essential starting point for his spiritual path.

Scholars are virtually unanimous in thinking that this account of Siddhārtha Gautama's life is legendary.[2] We know very little about the historical founder of Buddhism—and what he and his followers may or may not have taught, practiced, or believed—other than what we can glean from texts written down several centuries after his lifetime. However, the earliest extant texts confirm that seeking freedom from illness did indeed play a major role in early Buddhist thought and practice. Early Buddhists were intensely interested in exploring the relationship between mind and body, and they attempted to address the discomforts of both mental and physical illness through a range of philosophical, religious, and practical means. Throughout the centuries these concerns continued to be developed in Buddhist circles, eventually coming to be expressed in a wide range of texts across the Buddhist world. This chapter and the two that follow explore those developments, organized according to the traditional model of the "vehicles" (Skt. *yānas*), which are the principal sectarian divisions of Buddhism. These chapters discuss how the topics of health and medicine were dealt with in the Nikāya (sometimes pejoratively labeled "Hīnayāna," meaning the "Lesser Vehicle"), Mahāyāna (the "Great Vehicle"), and Tantric traditions (also called Esoteric Buddhism or Vajrayāna).

Although the chronology of the development of these three vehicles was not always a clear linear progression, these traditions loosely correspond to successive phases in the historical development of Buddhism in Asia. Thus, in a way, the discussion over the next three chapters is also a timeline of the emergence of certain features of Buddhist thought and practice. Eventually, the three traditions became so different from one another that some scholars prefer to refer to them not as different sects or schools but rather as three separate Buddhist religions.[3] This book, however, finds that there are many commonalities among the vehicles in how they approach illness and health. Successive forms of Buddhist medicine did not wholly replace, but rather built upon, what came before. Today, all three vehicles continue to thrive around the world, and all contribute equally to contemporary global trends. Therefore, these chapters are better understood as a topical introduction to the principal themes of Buddhist medicine, rather than a history of those developments per se.

## MEDICINE IN THE MONASTIC DISCIPLINARY LITERATURE

The earliest extant Buddhist texts were set down in the first century BCE in Sri Lanka.[4] Written in Pāli, a language related to Sanskrit that tradition holds to be the original language of the Buddha, these texts ostensibly preserved an oral tradition that had been in circulation since the death of the Buddha in northeastern India some centuries earlier. While this Pāli textual tradition was developing in Sri Lanka, other Buddhist groups also began producing texts in Sanskrit and various other Sanskrit-like local languages (called Prakrits) in other parts of India. These schools of early Buddhism traditionally numbered eighteen but in reality represented many more sectarian divisions.[5] Geographically, they were spread out over the whole of the subcontinent, from modern-day Afghanistan in the north to Sri Lanka in the south.

Aside from the Pāli sources, only a small portion of this early layer of Buddhist literature is still extant in the original Indic languages. However, a collection of first-century CE birch-bark manuscripts has been archaeologically recovered at Gandhāra, located in the Peshawar Basin on the border of modern-day Pakistan and Afghanistan. Additional early Indian material now lost in the original languages is also recoverable from Chinese and Tibetan translations. These translations often preserve the flavor and content of the earlier Buddhist corpus and therefore are generally used by scholars as a window into early Buddhist thought and practice in India. (For further discussion of texts and translations, see chapter 6.)

Across this corpus of early texts, the balance of evidence suggests that medicine was a recurring theme in Nikāya Buddhist thought. However, that is not to say that these early texts give us an unambiguously positive assessment of medicine. In fact, the extant monastic disciplinary codes, the *vinayas*, of several of the early Indian schools, composed between the first and fourth centuries CE, insist that the practice of healing is a "worldly art" that is unbecoming for members of the Buddhist sangha (Skt. *saṃgha*, i.e., the ordained monastics) to practice.[6]

Such proclamations are based on an important Buddhist doctrine that differentiates between the "worldly" or "mundane" (Skt. *laukika*) activities of ordinary unenlightened society and the "otherworldly" or "supramundane" (Skt. *lokottara*) activities associated with the pursuit of enlightenment or Nirvana (Skt. *nirvāṇa*).[7] Ascetics or renunciates ordained into the Buddhist monastic order were supposed to be exclusively focused on the latter. Thus, members of the sangha who engaged in healing were chastised for pursuing a "deviant" or "wrong livelihood" (Skt. *mithyājīva*)—particularly if they accepted payment or special favors in exchange {1: 10}. Female monastics (Skt. *bhikṣuṇī*), who often found themselves under additional scrutiny when it came to monastic discipline, were subject to harsher penalties if caught providing healing services {1: 11}.[8] Of course, the presence of such strictures in the monastic disciplinary literature is very likely an indication that Buddhist monastics (and probably nuns in particular) were habitually involved in healing activities, or else why would such rules be necessary?

Whereas there are some texts that suggest that it was healing per se that was problematic, most of these disciplinary texts seem to focus on the social implications—in particular, they seem concerned with how members of society outside the monastery perceived the sangha. Forbidding monks and nuns to engage in healing activities as a means of livelihood served to demonstrate publicly the

Buddhist sangha's single-minded commitment to liberation. It also was intended to visibly separate the sangha from other contemporary groups of renunciates and practitioners who were not as restrictive {1: 10§2}.

Such prohibitions notwithstanding, depictions of medicine and healing one finds across the monastic disciplinary literature are mainly positive. On the whole, one has the impression that medical knowledge—at least when practiced within the confines of the monastery and not done for the purpose of personal gain—was typically highly valued within the sangha.[9] Narratives of the Buddha or close disciples caring for sick members of the community suggest that healing or nursing one another was a laudable, even noble, undertaking {1: 18–20}. The *vinayas* list the traits of an ideal patient and an ideal nurse; they also often provide some leeway for monastics to heal or medically advise members of the laity, including their parents, other family members, patrons, and various assistants or residents within the monastery.[10]

Perhaps the most well-known Buddhist healing narrative is a story from the *vinaya* in which the Buddha cares for a monk stricken with dysentery {1: 1§3}.[11] Left alone in the monastery while the others go on almsrounds, the sick monk lies in his own excrement until the Buddha finds him. With the help of his attendant, the Buddha then cleans the monk's body, clothing, and residence and arranges his bed for him. When the rest of the monks return, the Buddha addresses them, mandating that they care for one another just as they would care for him. This story is told numerous times in the various extant *vinayas* and, with variations, circulated widely in other literary contexts {1: 21§3}. In China in later times, this story became an important precedent authorizing the sangha's involvement in healing activities and is still invoked today in modern medical settings.[12]

The Buddha not only condones nursing the sick; he also allows monks to obtain, store, and use a range of medicinal substances. Indeed, medicines were counted among the fundamental requisites that sustain the peripatetic lifestyle of the sangha, alongside the robe, almsfood, and shelter. Some texts specify that the allowable medicines should be limited to the urine and dung of animals, particularly cows. There is evidence from medieval Chinese writings that Buddhist communities did indeed use the excrement of several animals as medicine {1: 16, 46}.[13] However, the majority of Buddhist texts allow for a wider range of more conventional medicinal substances. Many mention ghee, butter, curdled milk products, oil, animal fats, honey, and various types of sugar as the "principal" or "great" medicines, which are to be used to treat a variety of ailments. While those

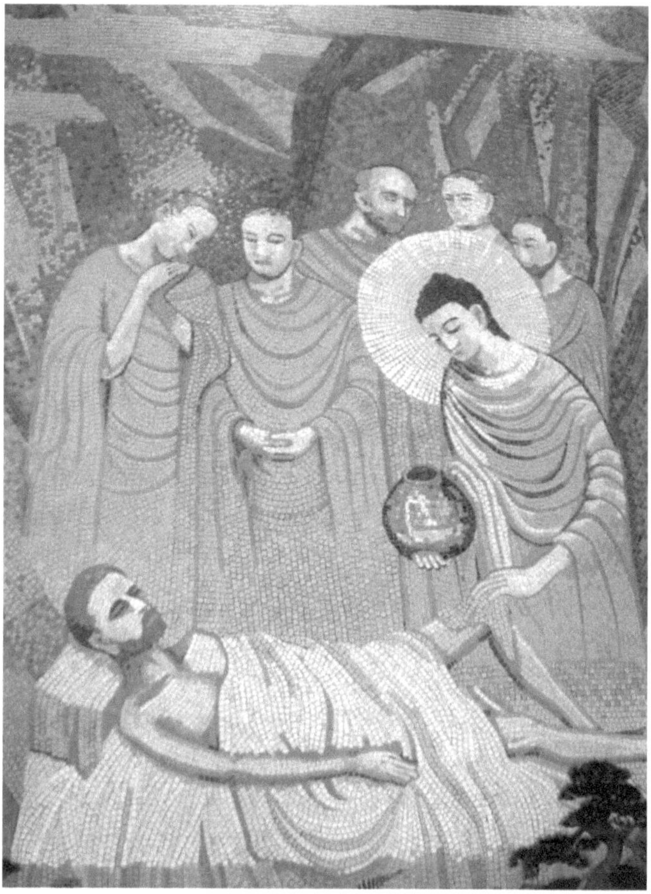

**1.1** Mosaic from the Tzu Chi Foundation hospital in Hualien, Taiwan, illustrating a famous story from the early Buddhist tradition, wherein the Buddha nurses a monk sick with dysentery.

Photo by the author, with permission from the Tzu Chi Foundation.

substances are the most frequently cited, the extant *vinayas* also list many other foods, drinks, minerals, animal parts, and other substances that monastics were allowed to collect, make, or consume for purposes of healing.[14]

The largest concentration of references to therapeutic substances appears in the sections of the *vinayas* dedicated to rules pertaining to medicine {1: 13}.[15] These sections are typically structured in a repetitive format: a monk falls sick with an illness, his fellow monks ask the Buddha for permission to give him a particular medicine or treatment, and the Buddha almost always gives his consent. Because each section on medicine might introduce dozens of such scenarios, these texts provide a rundown of the illnesses, medicinal substances, and procedures that likely were common in the times and places where the texts were written.

A comparison of the medical sections of the *vinayas* reveals diversity in terms of the medicinal substances they include.[16] While the reason for this remains unclear at present, perhaps the variation suggests divergences in the medical cultures of different parts of India or in different Buddhist sectarian contexts, or perhaps simply indicates different local nomenclatures for a similar range of medicines. While the list of medicinal substances mentioned in the extant *vinayas* numbers well into the hundreds, the substances were typically divided into four basic categories, depending on when they were allowed to be consumed and for how long they could be stored. "Mealtime medicines" could be taken during the monastic mealtime (from dawn until midday), "non-mealtime medicines" could be taken outside of that time, "seven-day medicines" were prescribed for a period of seven days only, and "lifelong medicines" could be taken at any time for any duration {1: 14}.

Though they are informative sources on the consumption of medicinals, the *vinayas* offer little information about how illnesses were to be diagnosed. Rather, they routinely suggest that sick monks should consult physicians, who represented a distinct occupational category.[17] In contrast to monastics, physicians are never criticized for pursuing a "worldly" livelihood. Although they are sometimes characterized as charlatans, they also are celebrated for their diagnostic skills and held up as model lay patrons of the Buddhist order.[18]

Several physicians are mentioned by name in the early Indian literature, the most notable being Jīvaka Kumārabhṛta {1: 1§4, 20}, often referred to as the "Royal Physician" or "King of Physicians."[19] He is famed as a generous supporter of the sangha and celebrated as being particularly well versed in the healing arts. Jīvaka's biography is embedded in the *vinayas*, although surprisingly not in the sections on medicine. This text not only gives us interesting details about the social station of early Indian physicians and other aspects of contemporary society but also contains much material relevant to the history of medical practice. The various versions of Jīvaka's biography detail his performance of abdominal and cranial surgeries, the administration of medicines via oral and nasal routes, and his use of a therapy evoking specific emotions to cure illness.

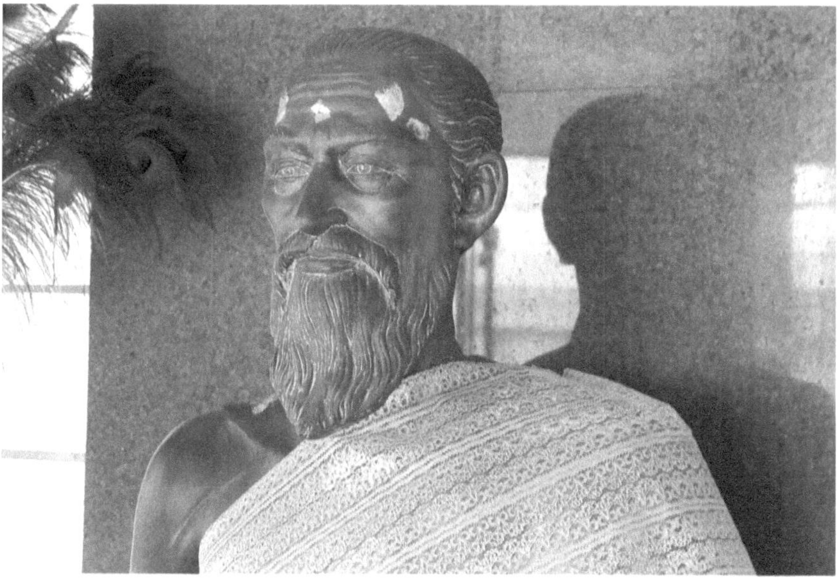

**1.2** Statue of Jīvaka Kumārabhṛta, the model Buddhist physician, from Chiang Mai, Thailand, where he is honored by practitioners as the forefather of traditional medicine. Wat Phra Singh temple, Chiang Mai.
Photo by the author.

Such details notwithstanding, the main function of Jīvaka's biography seems not to have been to relate the healing techniques of a particular historical person but rather to construct the image of an idealized doctor.[20] Although Jīvaka's healing techniques sometimes involve trickery, lies, and other behaviors that would be considered ethically questionable if committed by monks, he is always celebrated for his unfailing medical insight and the efficacy of the remedies he employs.

One passage in the *vinaya* even identifies Jīvaka's fame as an effective physician as the cause of an unmanageable upsurge in the number of sick candidates seeking ordination into the sangha.[21] The situation became so dire, we are told, that the Buddha had to make a rule that the sick were not permitted to be ordained until they had recovered. While likely fictional, this narrative suggests that the opportunity to receive competent medical care may in fact have been a motivating factor behind ordination for some—or, at least, that such a motivation would have seemed plausible to contemporary audiences. Like the anxiety over "wrong livelihoods" and the episode of the monk with dysentery discussed earlier, this narrative suggests an ongoing tension between the supposed exclusively otherworldly focus of the sangha and their pursuit of the worldly benefit of health.

## EARLY INDIAN MEDICAL CONCEPTS

Medical knowledge does not appear only in the context of monastic disciplinary texts. Anatomical and physiological terminology is frequently found in the scriptures (Pāli *sutta*; Skt. *sūtra*), including in descriptions of many of the most common Buddhist doctrines and practices.[22] These ideas seem to have played an important role in how Buddhist practitioners understood and worked with the body. For example, ascetically oriented texts from the earlier layers of Buddhist literature tend to describe the physical body as an amalgamation of the "Four Great Elements" (Skt. *mahābhūta* or *dhātu*): Earth, Water, Fire, and Wind.[23] This doctrine is also foundational in Āyurveda (literally "knowledge of life"), the predominant secular medical tradition of early India.[24] (It also reminds us of the core principles of Greco-Roman or Hippocratic medicine, and some scholars have speculated that ancient Greek ideas may have been a source of influence for the emergence of this feature of Indian medical thought.)[25]

A common convention in early Buddhist and Āyurvedic medical sources alike is to relate the Elements to specific parts of the physical body and specific physiological functions.[26] Normally in such lists, the solid parts of the body correspond with the Earth Element, the liquids with Water, body heat and the processes of digestion with Fire, and the movement and breath of the body with Wind. Many texts add to the list Space or Void (Skt. *ākāśa*) as a sort of fifth Element, indicating those areas of the body that are empty spaces devoid of the others (the orifices and cavities, for example). A sixth Element, consciousness (Skt. *vijñāna*), is sometimes additionally present in Buddhist sources, especially when the purpose of the text is to underscore mind-body interrelation.

The Elements that make up the body are also the components of the entire physical world. Because of this interconnection, the body is constantly subject to the influences of the foods we eat, the activities we engage in, the effects of the seasons, and other environmental and behavioral factors. As there is never any respite from these fluctuations, the natural state of the physical body is one of turmoil and instability. As one common metaphor aptly puts it, it is like a basket containing four poisonous snakes.[27]

The fluctuations of the Elements are not just unpredictable but also dangerous to one's health. The Elements can become "imbalanced" (Skt. *saṃkṣobha*) or "coarse" (Skt. *karkaśa*). They also can give rise to the *tridoṣa*, the fundamental disease factors in early Indian medicine.[28] This term is sometimes translated as "three humors," though literally it means "three defects" or "three faults." These defects are Wind, Bile, and Phlegm (*vāta*, *pitta*, and *śleṣman* or *kapha*): Wind illnesses refer to disorders characterized by mobility, instability, and agitation; Bile illnesses are characterized by heat, infection, and vomiting; and Phlegm illnesses are characterized by cold, mucus, and stagnation. The *tridoṣa* are mentioned in many Buddhist writings, either individually or as a set. According to several texts, when directly asked to name the major causes of illness that afflicted humankind, the Buddha gave a list that included these three defects as well as their combination {1: 1§1}.[29]

Many of the passages discussing the Elements and *tridoṣa* in early Buddhist texts closely mirror the Āyurvedic medical classics *Caraka's Compendium* (*Caraka saṃhitā*, compiled between 100 BCE and 200 CE) and *Suśruta's Compendium* (*Suśruta saṃhitā*, compiled by the fifth century CE).[30] However, what sets Buddhist descriptions apart from others is that they tend to use these concepts to highlight Buddhism's basic position that one should avoid thinking of the corporeal body as a "self."[31] Because of the impermanent, constructed, and unreliable nature of the Elements, the body is constantly in flux and unpredictable. We should therefore disidentify with it and learn to see it as impermanent, non-self (Skt. *anātman*), and a source of suffering.

Connections between basic Buddhist ideas and medicine are established not only through doctrines such as the Elements and *tridoṣa* but also through the use of a rich assortment of metaphors, similes, and parables. Honorifics such as "Great Physician" and "King of Physicians" are routinely applied to the Buddha {1: 17§1}.[32] He is also called "Remover of Arrows," likening him to a surgeon treating a person who had been shot with an arrow. In the same vein, Buddhist texts frequently refer to the Dharma as the "Great Medicine." They often draw parallels between how an efficacious doctor would use a handful of key medicines (such as oil, butter, ghee, sugar, and honey) to manage the *tridoṣa* and how the Buddha prescribes a handful of key practices to overcome mental afflictions {1: 17§2}.[33]

The frequent use of medical doctrines, metaphors, and similes in Buddhist texts confirm that early Buddhists were aware of the medical currents of their time. Indeed, some scholars have argued that the principal ideas and methods of Āyurvedic medicine likely originated in the same circles of ascetics and yogis (Skt. *śramana*) from which Buddhism itself emerged.[34] Freed from the strict Brahmanical religious taboos guarding against pollution or contamination, the argument goes, practitioners in these circles were able to innovate and experiment with methods of working with the human body that eventually resulted in the development of a more empirical approach to medicine.

In truth, it is difficult to say where or when such parallels between Buddhism and medicine first appeared. It is unclear whether Buddhist authors were inspired to mimic medical authors or vice versa. However, it is clear that such equivalencies are not merely ornamental ways of speaking. Rather, the metaphorical linkage between the Dharma and medicine is a deeply ingrained pattern that has structured both Buddhist discourses on medicine and the most basic principles of the Dharma for millennia.[35]

## HEALING AND PROTECTION

In addition to the *tridoṣa*, spirits were also widely considered one of the principal causes of disease in early India, representing a major concern in both Āyurvedic and Buddhist healing.[36] Buddhist texts often differentiate "natural" causes of disease, such as food, climate, karma, and other factors that affect the bodily Elements, from "unnatural" causes, such as attack by humans, animals, or evil spirits {2: 31}.

Unseen sources of danger were thought to be everywhere. The early Indian cosmos was populated by spirits of various classes, including *devas* (gods and demigods), *gandharvas* (angelic musicians), *nāgas* and *mahoragas* (serpent spirits), *garuḍas* (bird spirits), and *kimṇaras* (chimeric beings whose bodies are made of human and animal parts).[37] While these entities could be helpful, harmful, or ambiguous depending on the circumstances, other beings were much more dangerous. *Yakṣas*, *rākṣasas*, and *piśācas* were demonic ogres or goblins that roamed the earth seeking to cause illness and mayhem. *Vetālas* were zombielike figures controlled by sorcerers who animated them through black magic to cause harm. *Kumbhaṇḍas* were demons with huge testicles who sapped one's vitality and

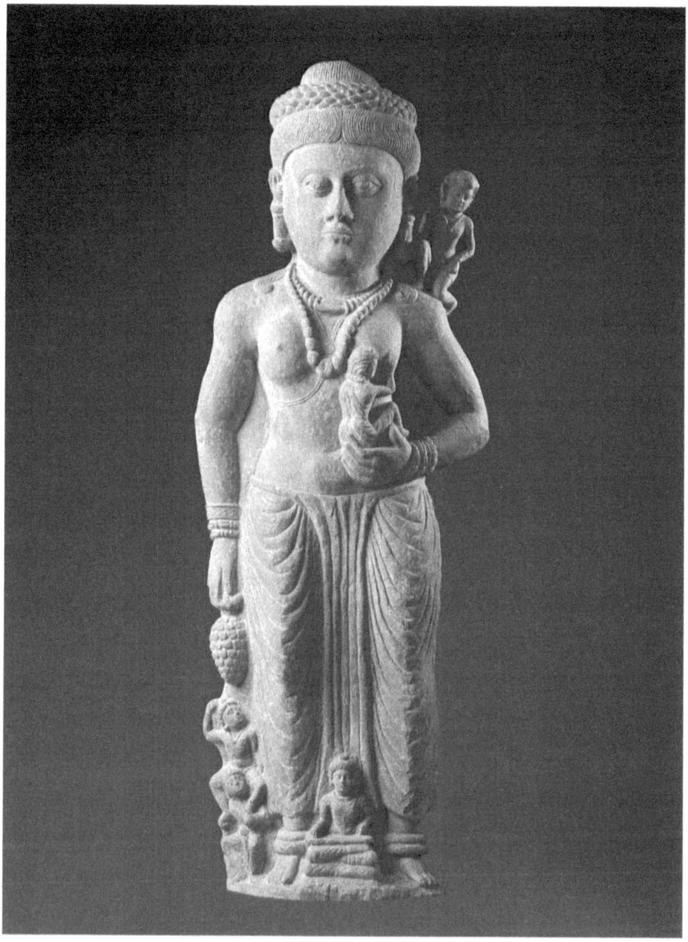

**1.3** Statue of the demoness Hāritī with her children and the Buddha, from the Gandhara region, first century BCE.

From the Los Angeles County Museum of Art. Image courtesy of Wikimedia Commons, public domain.

shortened one's life span. *Grahas*, or "seizers," accosted infants and children in the night, causing severe illness and death. Such entities lurked all around and were a constant menace unless one had powerful protectors.

The Buddha, the great protector against all evils, was thought to be able to transform such dangerous entities into beneficial agents.[38] Many Buddhist texts tell stories about demons that once had menaced humankind but had been converted by the Buddha into protectors and now guarded against the very ailments they used to cause. A prominent example of this conversion is the story of the demoness Hārītī, who had previously taken the lives of young children and was greatly feared.[39] One day, the Buddha hid one of Hārītī's own children under his begging bowl to teach her a lesson about the pain she was causing others. When she became distraught, she realized the effects of her previous actions. Thus "tamed" by the Buddha, Hārītī became a protector of children and mothers to be, as well as a guardian over the process of childbirth.

Images of Hārītī, the goat-headed deity Naigamesha, and several other converted demons have been found in archaeological sites around India, demonstrating that these helper spirits were part of the cultic life of Indian monasteries.[40] Their origin narratives, iconography, and rituals were further transported across cultural and geographic divides as Buddhism spread to new areas.[41] To this day, visitors to temples across the Buddhist world are greeted by an array of *nāgas* and other ferocious-looking beings who protect the grounds and the devotees.

Aside from the Buddha's power over demons, Buddhist narratives make clear that he was considered a source of great healing power in his own right. In healing narratives, the Buddha usually does not resort to conventional medicines or procedures.[42] If he does administer medicines, he often gets *devas* or other deities to fetch them from faraway places or gives them to the patient along with instructions on meditations or other ritual practices. More typically, it is his glance, his touch, his fragrance, his ability to summon protective spirits, the transformative power of his wisdom, or other such wondrous factors that heal the patient. The Buddha's corpse and relics also are characterized as having special healing potency.[43]

Narratives also frequently detail the Buddha's healing exploits during his innumerable previous incarnations. Stories about his past lives appear in collections of *jātakas* and *avadānas* (literally "births" and "legends," respectively). In many of these tales, the Buddha performs repeated compassionate acts of self-sacrifice in order to heal people. For example, in one lifetime in which he was a king, he realized that the only way to save his people from a deadly plague was to obtain the meat of the rare *rohita* fish. Unable to find that fish, he killed himself, reincarnated as one, and then fed his body to the people to save them. In the text that frames this narrative, the Buddha links good karma with good health. He explains that the karmic merit he received from this sacrifice is the reason that now, in his present life, he is "endowed with a stomach whose digestion is regular"

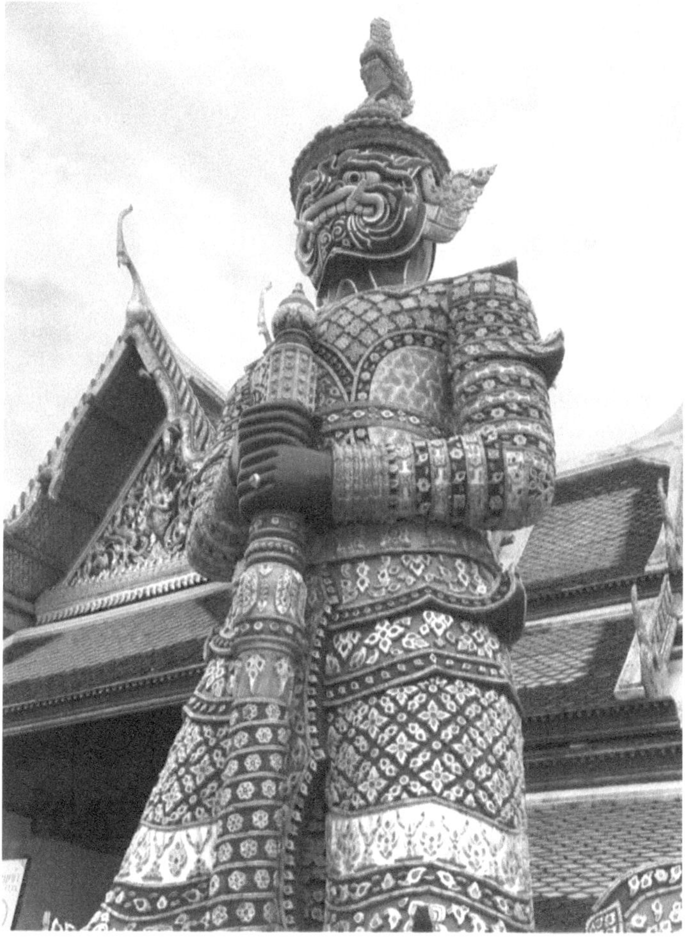

**1.4** Demons, once converted to Buddhism, serve to protect the Dharma and its adherents from all calamities, including illness. This demon is a *yakṣa* overlooking the grounds of the Wat Phra Chetuphon temple in Bangkok, Thailand.
Photo by the author.

and "free of disease."[44] (A fuller discussion of the connections between karma and health, which represent important common ground among many Buddhist traditions, is presented in chapter 4.)

Another story with a similar plotline involves the Buddha's reincarnation as an enormous dog, whose medicinal flesh is violently carved up and eaten by desperate people suffering from an epidemic {1: 18§3}. Equally illustrative are stories about the Buddha's previous life as a doctor {1: 19}. Such stories about the healing exploits and powers of the Buddha circulated widely in India. While they are particularly Buddhist in many of their details, they share a number of features with contemporary narratives told by Jains and authors from other Indian religions, suggesting that healing was an exciting or interesting narrative element that readily crossed doctrinal lines.[45]

Like the Buddha, his close disciples were endowed with healing powers. The *Discourse to Angulimāla* (*Angulimāla sutta*), for example, focuses on the conversion of Angulimāla from a murderer to an accomplished monk. In one scene, which takes place after he has converted, he comes across a mother laboring with a breech birth. The Buddha instructs him to bless the mother and her unborn child through the power of a truth statement. Angulimāla goes to her and recites, "Sister, since I was born in the noble birth [i.e., since becoming a monk], I do not recall intentionally killing a living being. Through this may there be well-being for you, well-being for your fetus."[46] The text tells us that through the power of this truth statement, both mother and child were saved. The story illustrates both Angulimāla's complete reformation and the power of ritualized speech as an agent of healing.[47]

Buddhist tradition came to use texts that depict such healing events as *parittas*, recitations for protective or beneficial effect {1: 34}. To this day, the *Discourse to Angulimāla*, for example, is chanted in Southeast Asia to cure disease, ameliorate symptoms, or lessen the pain or anguish one is experiencing because of illness.[48] Other *paritta* texts include narratives in which preaching the Dharma results in a cure. In one story that appears in several Pāli variations and also circulated widely in other languages, the Buddha heals a sick disciple by preaching to him on the Awakening Factors {1: 2}.[49] Roused by thoughts of mindfulness, investigation, energy, joy, tranquility, concentration, and equanimity, the patient delights in the Dharma and spontaneously recovers his health. In one version of the story {1: 2§3}, the Buddha himself is the patient, and he beseeches his disciple Ānanda to proclaim the Factors for his own benefit. The logic behind the use of this text as a *paritta* is that by hearing this story chanted aloud, patients may also experience spontaneous healing.

Before we move on, it is interesting to note, given our contemporary fascination with meditation, that the earliest forms of Buddhism did not emphasize the power of formal meditation techniques to promote health or overcome disease. The account of the healing powers of hearing the Awakening Factors certainly suggests that mental agitation was thought to be closely linked to physical illness and that positive mental states were thought to be able to reverse the condition. However, the protagonists in these stories are not explicitly depicted meditating.

Another variation on this theme is the *Discourse to Girimānanda* (*Girimānanda sutta*).[50] Again a monk is sick, and this time the Buddha recommends that his attendant Ānanda visit the monk to try to alleviate his condition. He instructs Ānanda to recite the "ten perceptions," which include impermanence, non-self, detachment, and a number of other doctrinal points, concluding with the perception of mindfulness of the breath. As Girimānanda hears these perceptions spoken, his illness is spontaneously cured. While some modern interpreters have read this text as an example of the use of meditation to cure, again no one in the story is explicitly depicted doing anything other than explaining or listening to doctrine. This is as close as we get to a depiction of the healing benefits of contemplative practice in early Buddhist literature.

* * *

Based on this chapter's discussion, it is difficult to conclude that early Buddhism presents a coherent viewpoint on health and healing, never mind a medical system per se. Early Buddhist texts discuss some subjects in detail. These include the ethics of the practice of nursing and medical care by the sangha, the monastic rules governing the storage and use of medicinal substances, the body's Elemental constituents, protection from disease-causing demons, and enlightened people's power to heal. Some discussion about etiology (the causes of disease) and nosology (the categorization of disease) is found, principally in relation to the doctrines of the Elements, *tridoṣa*, and karma. The biography of Jīvaka gives us both a notion of how an ideal healer should be trained and some guiding principles for medical ethics. Other subjects are not elaborated. Glaring omissions include instructions on how to diagnose patients and precisely how to administer therapeutics. It is impossible to know whether these omissions result from the fact that these subjects were not discussed in Buddhist circles or whether they simply were not written down in texts available to us today.

Surveying the extant material and weighing the evidence, it is apparent that members of the sangha would not have thought of themselves as medical specialists. They may have been valued as healers of ailments of demonic or mental origin, which were important categories of disease in the ancient period. But, they would not necessarily have viewed themselves as participating in a discrete tradition of therapeutics comparable to (or in competition with) that of the physicians of the era. While occasionally engaging with physicians on an ad hoc basis, monastics most likely would have considered them to be practitioners of worldly arts and would have described themselves in contrast as focused on the otherworldly goal of attaining Nirvana.

Nevertheless, based on the available evidence, it is also fair to say that contemporary Indian medical doctrines closely informed the ways that early Buddhists thought of their bodies. Likewise, mutual nursing care, self-medication with commonly available foodstuffs, and ready access to physicians were common features of daily communal life within the monastery. Rites of healing and protection were widespread, used for the benefit of both the monastic residents and their lay patrons.

Finally, from the vantage point of the modern scholar, it is important to note that the corpus of early Buddhist materials discussed in this chapter are among the earliest sources of the history of medicine in ancient India. These texts are roughly contemporaneous with (and some may even predate) the extant Āyurvedic treatises and originate from areas dispersed across the Indian subcontinent. These diverse materials thus offer an important window onto the medical ideas and practices of a wide swath of ancient Indian society. Of course, these texts also are important in that they form the basis for all future developments of Buddhist thinking about health and medicine, which we will explore in the chapters to come.

## FURTHER READING

Anālayo. 2016. *Mindfully Facing Disease and Death: Compassionate Advice from Early Buddhist Texts.* Cambridge: Windhorse. Translations of passages from Nikāya Buddhist texts related to illness and death. Covers many of the subjects raised in this chapter.

Gethin, Rupert. 1998. *The Foundations of Buddhism.* Oxford and New York: Oxford University Press. A classic introduction to early Indian Buddhism and the central Buddhist doctrines that influenced later traditions.

Gombrich, Richard. 2006. *Theravada Buddhism: A Social History from Ancient Benares to Modern Colombo.* 2nd ed. London and New York: Routledge. An introduction to the history of the only remaining Nikāya school of Buddhism, from the time of the Buddha to present-day Sri Lanka.

Mitra, Jyotir. 1985. *A Critical Appraisal of Ayurvedic Material in Buddhist Literature with Special Reference to Tripitaka.* Varanasi: Jyotiralok Prakashan. A useful general overview of the medical materials in the Pāli canon, comparing them with historical Āyurvedic materials.

Zysk, Kenneth. 1998. *Asceticism and Healing in Ancient India: Medicine in the Buddhist Monastery.* Delhi: Motilal Banarsidass. A brief, readable introduction to some of the connections between Buddhism and medicine in early India.

## CHAPTER 2

# *Mahāyāna Buddhism*

Mahāyāna (the "Great Vehicle"), which was beginning to take shape in India by the first century CE, represented a significant departure from Nikāya Buddhism.[1] Originating among forest-dwelling ascetics and spreading to urban monastics and lay practitioners, the Mahāyāna movement became increasingly influential in India in the second half of the first millennium. Even before that time, the tradition had already become established as the predominant form of Buddhism in East Asia. It is still the most widely practiced form today in China, Korea, Japan, and Vietnam. As the Tantric style of Buddhism discussed in the next chapter considers itself an advanced form of Mahāyāna, one may also wish to include Tibet, the Himalayan region, Mongolia, and other parts of Central Asia on this list.

The basic doctrines introduced in early texts continued to be relevant in this new context. Mahāyāna writings discuss Indian medical theories, demonology, healing powers, karma, and other topics discussed in the previous chapter. However, the movement embraced an ethos that strongly emphasized compassion and selfless service toward all beings. It introduced new expressions of devotionalism toward an expanded pantheon of deities and a new repertoire of ritual activities. Influential new scriptures introduced reformulated philosophical perspectives on illness and healing. All of these innovations impacted Mahāyāna Buddhists' individual and collective engagements with healing and significantly strengthened the relationship between Buddhism and medicine in practice.

While only a small number of Mahāyāna texts related to health and healing are extant from India, from the second century CE through the end of the first millennium, teams of Chinese translators produced hundreds of scriptures and commentaries, many of which are directly relevant to this topic.[2] Tibetan translations commenced in the seventh century, also resulting in the preservation in that language of much material subsequently lost in India. The translation and transmission of Buddhist texts throughout Asia will be discussed in more detail in chapter 6. For the purposes of our discussion here, we will focus on the main ideas and practices introduced in these texts, which unambiguously demonstrate that medicine was a major concern in this form of Buddhism.

## HEALING AND THE BODHISATTVA PATH

Among the innovations that Mahāyāna Buddhism offered was a new ideal for aspiring practitioners. Nikāya Buddhism taught serious practitioners to pursue the goal of becoming an *arhat*, a liberated individual who escaped the cycles of birth and death by virtue of their meditation along the lines pioneered by Siddhārta Gautama. Ideal Mahāyāna practitioners aimed instead at becoming bodhisattvas.[3] The term "bodhisattva" had existed in pre-Mahāyānic Buddhism, but its use had been limited to referring to the few individuals destined to become buddhas, including, most notably, Siddhārtha Gautama in his previous incarnations. In the Mahāyāna use of the term, a bodhisattva was reinterpreted as any devotee who took vows committing him- or herself to seeking enlightenment in the service of others. Rather than work toward attaining Nirvana for personal salvation, a bodhisattva planned to spend an endless number of lifetimes doing the arduous work of liberating all sentient beings throughout the cosmos from all forms of suffering.

This change in perspective resulted in the reconfiguration of the relationship between healing and the Dharma.[4] Whereas Nikāya Buddhist texts critique the worldly nature of healing, Mahāyāna texts generally view ameliorating the suffering of illness as an integral part of the bodhisattva's mission of compassionate care for all sentient beings. Healing activities are characterized as examples of the bodhisattva's "skillful means," "expedient means," or "tactical skill" (*upāyakauśalya*). The Mahāyāna use of this term most often describes the pursuit of this-worldly gains in the service of what is ultimately a transcendent goal.[5] That is to say, while not necessarily directly resulting in liberation, skillful means are ways of alleviating suffering or inspiring beings that are conducive to achieving the long-term goal of total universal liberation.

Thanks to the concept of skillful means, the gap between worldly and otherworldly activities could be closed, the former absorbed into the latter.[6] It is on the grounds of skillful means that Mahāyāna texts advocate that bodhisattvas seek out and freely employ medical knowledge to help others. Healing not only alleviates the suffering of other beings but also extends their lives so that they can continue to progress on the Dharmic path. If they are not yet practitioners of the Dharma, then relief from illness provides the necessary conditions of comfort or ease that people require to begin to practice. In addition, helping the sick or contributing to the maintenance of their health earns the healer immense karmic merits {1: 8}. Thus, in the end, engaging in healing also helps the serious practitioner along their path.[7]

With such benefits to be gained, Mahāyāna practitioners began to prioritize healing activities. New texts were composed that superseded the *vinayas*, providing both the authorization and the motivation for giving medical care. Authors of these texts enjoined monastics and lay devotees alike to care for the sick without reservation. For example, the influential fifth-century Chinese disciplinary manual for monastic and lay devotees, the *Brahmā's Net Sūtra* (*Fanwang jing*), decreed that caring for the sick was a requirement for disciples of the Buddha and even established disciplinary penalties for not doing so.[8]

While any occupation dedicated to healing others could be identified as a beneficial and worthwhile livelihood, physicians, pharmacists, and herbalists were particularly viewed as role models for aspiring bodhisattvas. Mahāyāna *sūtras* introduced exemplars, including Jalavāhana, a physician's son who appears in the *Sūtra of Golden Light* (*Suvarnṇaprabhāsa sūtra*). Actually the Buddha in a previous lifetime, he learns the craft from his aged father and becomes a great healer {1: 4}. Another example is Samantanetra, a compounder of aromatic medicines, whose medical teachings take center stage in a chapter of the *Sūtra of the Entry Into the Realm of Reality* (*Gaṇḍavyūha sūtra*) {1: 9}.

Across the Mahāyāna world, monastics and laypeople alike heeded the call to become involved in medical care. They organized charitable initiatives for this purpose, established bathhouses {1: 8}, funded hospitals {1: 24}, and inscribed medicinal recipes in stone at Buddhist pilgrimage sites as a resource for the public {1: 46}. In East Asia, Mahāyāna monks earned fame for spreading medical knowledge, offering healing services to the sick, and controlling epidemics with protection rituals {1: 21}. Nuns were celebrated for loyally and skillfully providing medical assistance to patrons {1: 21§5}. Exegetes wrote treatises synthesizing and systematizing the medical information within the *sūtras*, *vinayas*, and other genres {1: 3, 5, 7, 14, 37, 38}.

Mahāyāna narratives presented the ideal practitioner as a selfless individual for whom no step—no matter how distasteful or personally inconvenient—went too far in the quest to alleviate the suffering of illness {1: 22}. Across all of these texts, the Mahāyāna ethos called for bodhisattvas to cast aside their personal preferences, feelings, and reticence and wholeheartedly commit to assisting the sick with genuine compassion. Occasionally, conservative exegetes voiced concerns about healing activities and tried to limit their practice by monastics.[9] But this seems to have been a minority position in most of the Mahāyāna world. The new consensus was that contributing to the health of all sentient beings was inseparable from the practice of the Dharma itself. With the Mahāyāna, healing became an essential part of the practice of Buddhism.

## BUDDHIST MEDICINE VERSUS ĀYURVEDA

In Mahāyāna discourses, knowledge of medicine is counted as one of the "Five Sciences" (*pañcavidyā*), the spheres of secular knowledge most beneficial to bodhisattvas as expedient means. (The traditional list of the five includes linguistics, logic, medicine, technical arts or mathematics, and philosophy.) Reframed in this way, medical knowledge became acceptable for study by ordained monastics. The great monastic universities of the premodern period, such as Nālandā in northeastern India, included medicine in the monastic curriculum (see chapter 5).

The frequency with which Āyurvedic theories appear in Mahāyāna treatises suggests that Buddhist authors and thinkers were continuing to closely follow developments in medicine.[10] Like the Nikāya Buddhist texts before them, Mahāyāna writings described the body and disease in terms of the Great Elements and *tridoṣa*. Other well-known Āyurvedic anatomical and physiological concepts—such as the seven bodily constituents (*saptadhātu*), vital points (*marman*), the power of particular flavors (*rasa*) to treat disease, and the correlation of both the onset of disease and the efficacy of the medicinal flavors with particular seasons of the Indian year (*ṛtu*)—also make frequent appearances in Mahāyāna literature.[11] There is a whole category of texts dedicated to matters of fertility, the processes of conception, and stages of fetal development (e.g., *kalala, arbuda, peśi*) that has close parallels with the medical literature on these matters.[12]

As mentioned, the *Sūtra of Golden Light* {1: 4} and the *Sūtra of the Entry Into the Realm of Reality* (*Gaṇḍavyūha sūtra*) {1: 9} were important sources of a new ideal of the bodhisattva physician. Both narratives include detailed passages on etiology, diagnosis, and nosology that present obvious parallels with Āyurvedic ideas. The presentation in the *Sūtra of Golden Light*, for example, hinges on the categorization of medicinals by flavor (*rasa*) and quality (*guna*). The elderly physician teaches his son to prescribe Oily, Salty, Sour, and Hot foods in the summer for conditions of the Wind *doṣa*; Cold and Sweet in the autumn for conditions of Bile; Oily, Pungent, and Hot in the spring for conditions of Phlegm; and Sweet, Sour, and Oily in the winter for combinations of the three *doṣa*. Other techniques mentioned in this *sūtra* include *tridoṣa* constitutional diagnosis (i.e., discerning the patient's propensity toward illness according to their personality traits, physical characteristics, and dreams) and prognosis according to the "death signs" (i.e., physical indicators of impending mortality).

Aside from incorporating specific medical doctrines, there also continued to be a close affinity between the ways that Āyurveda and the Dharma were conceived structurally. Both realms of knowledge were divided into eight domains of practice: the Eightfold Noble Path of the Buddha (Skt. *āryāṣṭāṅga-mārga*) and the eightfold Āyurvedic medical tradition (*aṣṭāṅga-āyurveda*).[13] Extending the parallelism further, Buddhist authors often noted that the four essential skills at the core of the Buddha's teaching were parallel to those exhibited by a good physician: just as an effective doctor must have a thorough understanding of disease, its cause, its cure, and how to prevent it, the Buddha similarly exhibits a thorough understanding of suffering, how it accumulates, how it can be eliminated, and the path that leads to its end {1: 17§2}.[14]

Despite all of these connections, however, it is an oversimplification to simply say that Buddhist texts are promulgating Āyurvedic medicine. Buddhist treatises typically reframe the medical ideas they borrow to emphasize patently Buddhist concerns such as emptiness (*śūnyatā*), suffering, and karma. For example, it is common in Mahāyāna texts to make parallels between the *tridoṣa* and the three mental "afflictions" or "poisons" of *rāga*, *dveṣa*, and *moha* (often translated as greed/craving, anger/avarice, and delusion/ignorance, respectively). In this model, greed is typically linked with Wind, anger with Bile, and delusion with Phlegm.[15] Thus, caring for one's mental health becomes intimately linked with caring for one's physical health as well. Put another way, we might say that Buddhists borrowed the *tridoṣa* as a means of organizing their knowledge about mental health.

Aside from the propensity of Mahāyāna texts to reinterpret Āyurvedic doctrines, it is also telling that these texts do not refer to the medical ideas and practices they present using the term "Āyurveda." Instead, they typically favor generic words for "medicine" or "healing" such as *cikitsā* or *bhaiṣajya*. Further, a close analysis shows that Mahāyāna texts seldom agree on the details of any medical doctrine, even when it comes to the most basic ones.[16] Some texts focus, for example, on the Four Great Elements (Earth, Water, Fire, and Wind), whereas others describe five or six. Some texts recognize only the standard three *doṣa* (Wind, Bile, and Phlegm), but many treat the combination of the three (Skt. *sannipāta*) as a distinct fourth disease factor. Texts diverge from one another in how they understand the Elements or *doṣa* to be affected by the fluctuations of the seasons, diet, lifestyle, environmental factors, and specific pharmaceutical interventions. They differ from one another in how they understand the efficacy of certain medicinal substances, as well as in how the medicinal flavors correlate with particular therapeutic effects, and even on what the basic flavor categories actually are. Buddhist texts tend to differ not only from the major Āyurvedic classics (at least in the forms available to us today) but also from one another on all of these points.

All of this taken together gives us the distinct impression that Āyurveda was less hegemonic in ancient India than is commonly supposed. The texts suggest instead that multiple related but conflicting transmissions of medical knowledge circulated in different social circles or in different parts of India. These diverse strands were gathered together in one way in the Āyurvedic compendia but combined in various other ways in Buddhist texts. Buddhist writings thus represent separate transmissions of ancient Indian medical ideas: patently Buddhist medical traditions with diverse and unique variations diverging from those formulated in the secular medical literature. This fact makes these texts highly significant for historians of medicine in addition to scholars of religion. Indeed, the serious study of Mahāyāna texts available only in translations from outside the Indian subcontinent might very well revolutionize our understanding of the history of Āyurveda, if only these different bodies of scholarship were brought together.

## HEALING DEITIES

Mahāyāna Buddhism offered a range of new possibilities for devotees to get involved in healing as a means of progressing on the bodhisattva path. It also promised that the most advanced bodhisattvas—celestial beings with great powers accumulated over countless lifetimes of selfless practice—would intervene to assist the faithful in times of crisis. These deities could appear in person, in a vision, or in a dream and could effortlessly eradicate illness and other sources of suffering {1: 21, 25, 26}.

One such advanced bodhisattva was Avalokiteśvara, considered the embodiment of pure compassion. Ever on the lookout for those in peril, he—or, more commonly in China after the twelfth century, *she*—is probably the most popular deity in the Mahāyāna Buddhist pantheon.[17] In male or female form, this bodhisattva empowers the ritual practices of healers, saves victims of injury from serious consequences, and gives succor to those who have experienced emotional trauma or personal disaster.[18]

Certainly, the main texts associated with Avalokiteśvara count among the most popular Buddhist texts of all time. The chapter of the *Lotus Sūtra* that introduces him, which circulated as an independent text in East Asia, promises that he could

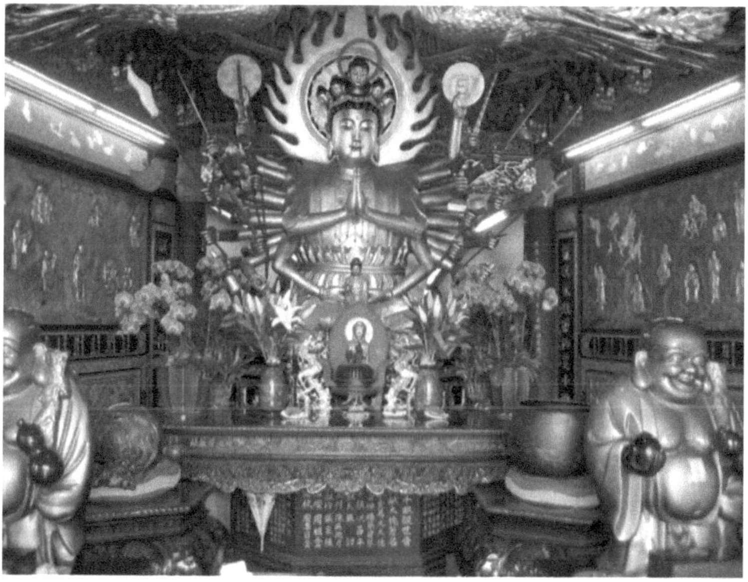

**2.1** Avalokiteśvara, the most widely revered bodhisattva in Mahāyāna Buddhism, is here depicted in the "thousand-arm form" symbolizing omnipotence. This deity is frequently called upon for assistance in dealing with illness, childbirth, untimely death, and other medical emergencies. Guandu Temple, Beitou, Taiwan.
Photo by the author.

be called upon to save a devotee from catastrophe of any kind, including shipwreck, wrongful imprisonment, attack by bandits, and any causes of premature death, in addition to illness. The *Great Compassion Dhāraṇī Sūtra*, the text that contains the principal ritual to invoke Avalokiteśvara's blessings, exists in many editions from across Asia. Some versions include instructions for the ritual blessing of medicinals and other procedures for the treatment of a wide range of ailments {1: 26}.

Other bodhisattvas that could intervene in cases of illness included Medicine King (Skt. *Bhaiṣajyaraja*). In the *Lotus Sūtra*, he is most noted for his demonstration of piety through acts of self-mutilation and self-immolation. However, a separate text dedicated to him and his brother, Supreme Medicine (Skt. *Bhaiṣajyasamudgata*), teaches a number of visualization meditations that could be used for healing disease and eradicating misfortune.[19] Another bodhisattva, Earth Treasury (Skt. *Kṣitigarbha*), was associated with liberating the unfortunate dead from the realms of hell, but his protective talismans also could provide healing benefits in this world {1: 21§11}.

While important, bodhisattvas were not the highest beings with healing powers in the Mahāyāna pantheon. In addition to new conceptions of bodhisattvahood, a new vision of buddhahood also emerged in Mahāyāna. Whereas Nikāya Buddhism tended to see a buddha as an enlightened person who lived and died in a particular time and place in history, Mahāyāna discourses present buddhas as timeless, omniscient, all-powerful deities. Moreover, Buddhas now were thought to populate the cosmos in all directions.[20] Among the new buddhas, Amitābha or Amitāyus ("Infinite Light" or "Infinite Life") was no doubt the most popularly venerated. He lived in the "Land of Bliss" (Skt. *Sukhāvatī*), a paradisiacal Buddha-realm or "Pure Land" far to the west of our world.[21] Reciting his name could result in rebirth within a lotus flower in a pond at his feet, thus ensuring a life of bliss, ease, and freedom from illness. Amitābha became highly influential in Buddhist mortality cults, which attracted wide support from the laity in East Asia.[22] An account from seventh-century China suggests that his worship was also important in monastic hospice practices. The author describes how dying members of the sangha were to be placed in the "Hall of Impermanence," under a statue of Amitābha. Facing westward, the statue was connected to the patients by a cord or string, thus symbolically leading them to Sukhāvatī upon their death. The deity played a similarly central role in Japanese death practices {1: 7}.[23]

Although Amitābha was key in some Mahāyāna narratives involving healing, the so-called Medicine Buddha who lived in a Pure Land to the east was even more significant. This deity is formally named Bhaiṣajyaguru-vaiḍūrya-prabhārāja (literally "He who has the Radiance of the Beryl of the Important [or Best] Medicine"), although he is best known as simply Bhaiṣajyaguru {1: 25}.[24] Scholars have long suspected that this deity may historically have originated in far northwestern India or even Central Asia.[25] Whether or not that is accurate, he seems originally to have been most popular in that area, never having much cultic or iconographic significance in central India.[26] He was known in Southeast Asia but became most important in East Asia and the Himalayas, where he was worshipped as a major healing deity.[27] Many versions of the principle scripture dedicated to Bhaiṣajyaguru are extant from these regions, as are commentaries and devotional texts that describe the use of "cartwheel lamps," banners, and *sūtra* chanting over the course of a multiday ceremony in his honor. Historical records indicate that this ritual was often used both to heal individual patrons and protect the population against epidemics.

It is not only buddhas and advanced bodhisattvas who are associated with the powers to heal and protect in the Mahāyāna. As with Nikāya Buddhism, ritualists also continued to enlist the help of a wide range of protector deities, demigods, and converted demons. Certain high-profile historical people were also elevated to positions of great power and veneration in the pantheon. One such figure is Nāgārjuna. This was the name of a Buddhist philosopher who lived in the early centuries CE, a seventh-century alchemist, and a ninth-century physician who wrote both an important medical treatise (*Yogaśataka*) and an appendix to a major Āyurvedic compendium (the "Uttara Sthānā" from the *Compendium of Suśruta*). In Buddhist lore, these three historical figures were conflated—possibly along with other historical or legendary Nāgārjunas as well—and came to be worshipped as a single bodhisattva.[28] Feats attributed to this composite saintly figure include having compounded an alchemical elixir of longevity that enabled him to live for centuries. He was also attributed with the authorship of a treatise on ophthalmology {1: 54} and esoteric ritual texts on talismans, medicinals, and healing rites {1: 45}.[29] In most Mahāyāna societies today, the bodhisattva Nāgārjuna continues to be venerated as a patron deity of medical, alchemical, and apotropaic knowledge.

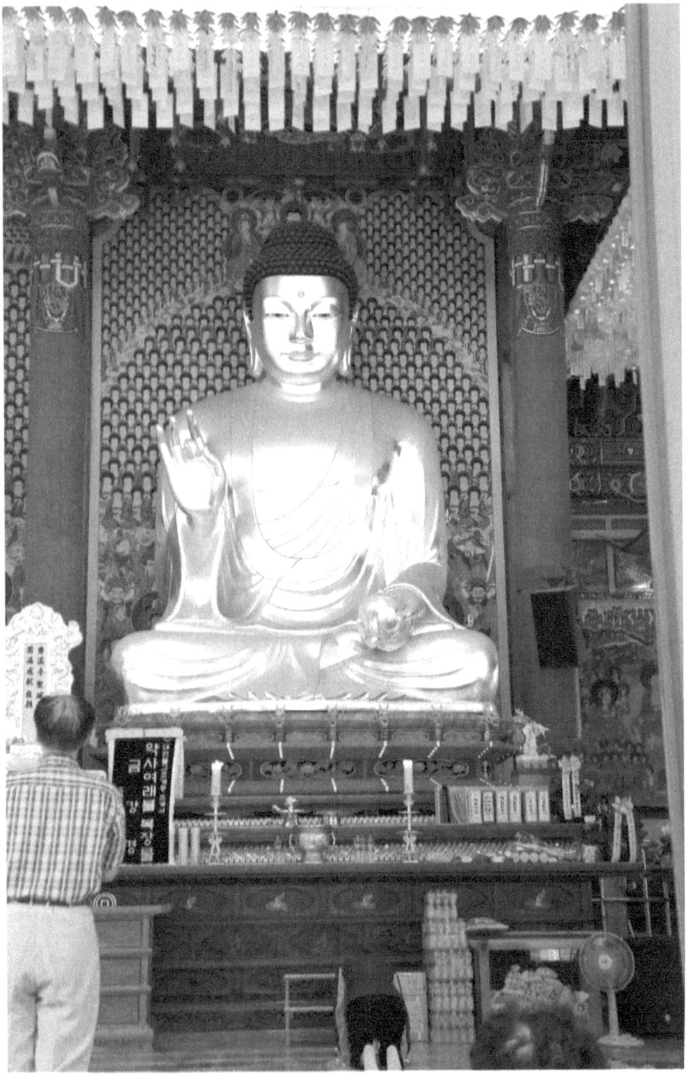


**2.2** Statue of Bhaiṣajyaguru at Jogyesa temple in Seoul, South Korea. Adherents pray and give offerings to the Buddha to be released from suffering and misfortune of all kinds, including illness.
Photo by the author.

## HEALING RITUALS

Mahāyāna Buddhism promised that one could achieve health and longevity by ritually tapping into the awesome power of the buddhas and other deities. As will be discussed in subsequent chapters, the techniques by which this could be accomplished became mainstays of the health-care landscape across most of Asia. Mahāyāna healing rites prominently involved the chanting of scriptures, a practice closely related to the incantation of *paritta* texts mentioned in the previous chapter. Scriptures chanted regularly for health and protection included the aforementioned *Bhaiṣajyaguru Sūtra* {1: 25}, the *Great Compassion Dhāraṇī Sūtra* {1: 26}, and sections of the *Lotus Sūtra* associated with healing deities. Written texts also were thought to have purifying or protective powers, and they were worshipped as material objects and used as protective talismans.

A further innovation in this area was the development of *dhāraṇī*.[30] These were short, powerful utterances or incantations thought to crystallize the powers of the scriptures and the deities with which they were associated into easily memorizable and portable forms. *Dhāraṇī* associated with Bhaiṣajyaguru appear in the *sūtra* that bears his name, with Avalokiteśvara in the *Great Compassion Dhāraṇī Sūtra*, and with a range of other helpful deities in the *Lotus Sūtra*.[31] The latter text, for example, includes an all-purpose spell for protection against harmful spirits taught by none other than Hāritī, the protector demoness discussed in the previous chapter.[32] In this passage, Hāritī lists all of the demonic beings her *dhāraṇī* will protect against, in addition to numerous forms of fever. She and her demonic entourage warn that dangerous spirits must heed this *dhāraṇī* (i.e., must leave the faithful alone), or else they will be destroyed.

As Mahāyāna Buddhism continued to develop, fascination with the power of incantations inspired the creation of a seemingly infinite number of *dhāraṇī* that could be used for virtually any purpose. *Dhāraṇī* exist to control the weather, protect crops, clean laundry, and exterminate vermin. A significant subset of the overall corpus of *dhāraṇī* relates to healing and protection from disease. Among the Buddhist texts compiled in medieval China, for example, one finds incantations to counter seasonal ailments, childhood diseases, eye disorders, toothache, and sores, among other problems, and even some *dhāraṇī* that claim to alleviate all illnesses whatsoever {1: 28, 30}. Such texts frequently provide instructions on how to use the incantations, for example by performing a certain number of oral repetitions, inscribing them, wearing them, or even ingesting them.

On rare occasions, these Chinese incantations were composed in natural language {1: 28§4}, but more often, they were inscrutable jumbles of transliterated Sanskrit or nonsensical pseudo-Sanskrit syllables. For example, a Chinese spell for "seasonal illnesses of *qi*" reads: "A-QU-NI-NI-QU-NI-A-QU-YE-NI-QU-NI-A-PI-LUO-MAN-DUO-LI-BO-CHI-NI-BO-TI-LI" {1: 28§1}. The meaning of this incantation was not necessarily known by practitioners. It was the pronunciation that was paramount, as it was believed that sound encapsulated the powers of protective texts and deities. Typically the exoticism or foreign mystique of the incantations was also a large part of its appeal.

*Dhāraṇī* were only one of many types of ritual practice designed to harness healing powers for use in times of need. A closely related activity was the preparation of talismans or charms. Whether composed of written *dhāraṇī*, passages from *sūtras*, Sanskrit letters written in the *siddhaṃ* or *khom* alphabets or Chinese-style

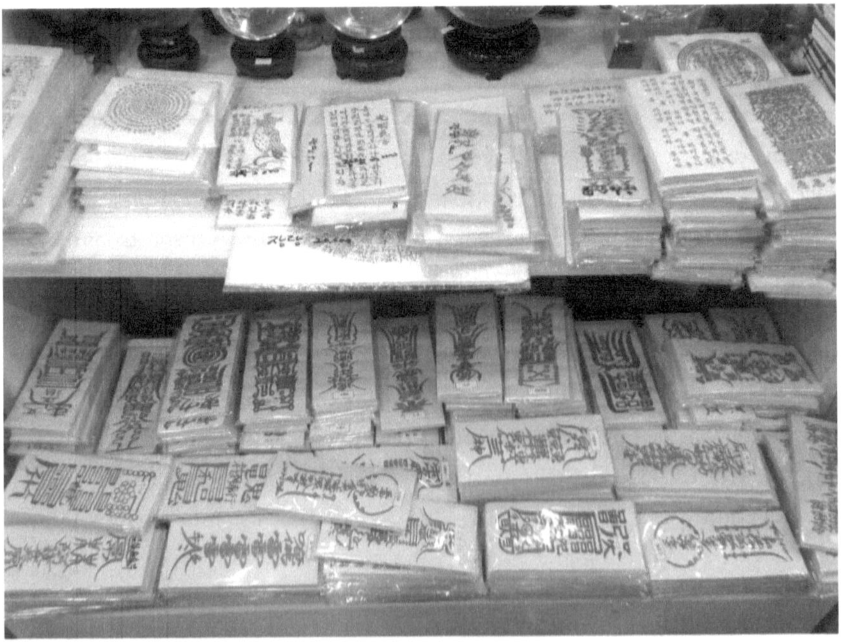

**2.3** Chinese-style talismans for sale outside temple grounds in Seoul, South Korea. Such talismans can be hung, worn, or carried for protection from misfortune and illness. Photo by the author.

scripts, across Asia, talismans might be worn on the body, displayed, or even ingested to harness their purifying influences {1: 21§11, 29, 45; 2: 33}.

All of these Mahāyāna ritual interventions operated on the logic of empowerment (Skt. *adhiṣṭhāna*). Human supplicants performed ceremonial actions and vows and provided offerings to the deities, and they received blessings or assistance in return. Those blessings might come in the form of spontaneous healing of an illness, relief from an impending catastrophe, or alleviation of another form of suffering. Alternatively, blessings could be stored in consecrated objects for later use. Buddhist healing rites thus could involve a wide range of material objects—not only written talismans but also water, string, drawings, effigies, seeds, whisks, bells, musical instruments, and other implements used to capture, preserve, and transport healing powers. A healer consequently might have an armamentarium of rites and objects that they would pull out in the course of treating a patient, calling on a number of divine sources of power until the forces causing the illness are defeated.

Medicinal substances were of particular importance among the material implements used in healing rites, which often call for the use of specific plants, minerals, or animal products. Normally, these are invested with the power of the deities through *dhāraṇīs* and other ritual procedures before being ingested or applied to the body {1: 26, 28§8}. In a chapter in the *Sūtra of Golden Light*, to name but one example, the river goddess Sarasvatī teaches the supplicant (in this case, the king) to soak in a medicinal bath of calamus, coriander, cinnamon, saffron, mustard, spikenard, and a litany of other medicinals to strengthen and protect his body from "oppressions" caused by astrological configurations or various demons.[33] Mahāyāna texts also call for the use of a similar range of medicines as offerings to healing deities, and medicinal substances were also sometimes inserted inside statues of those deities to consecrate or empower them.[34]

The material culture of Buddhist rites varied from place to place in accordance with local customs, and the materia medica were adjusted to account for the availability of plants in different regions. (I will come back to role of materia medica in intercultural exchanges in chapter 5.) Local variance notwithstanding, certain substances emerge from the written and archaeological record as cross-culturally important ingredients for Mahāyāna healing rituals. In particular, aloeswood, bezoar (concretions found in the stomachs of ruminants), cow dung, incense, and sandalwood are mentioned again and again as potent substances in Buddhist writings across Asia {1: 26, 33, 45, 46}.

Over time, ritual protocols, or fixed sequences of ritual actions and tools, came to be developed for healing purposes in particular settings. These could be relatively simple liturgies for use in ceremonies at a local temple. Historical examples of this type of protocol include a set of liturgical documents discovered within a cache of medieval manuscripts in the Mogao Caves at Dunhuang, an oasis town along the Silk Road. These short scripts guide monks through the performance of a ceremony to transfer the karmic merit earned by a supplicant to a sick patient to help with their healing {1: 31}.

On the other hand, rulers could afford to enact much more complex ritual protocols. A description of a royal ritual appears in a liturgy for a Bhaiṣajyaguru "repentance fast" (*zhaichan*) attributed to Emperor Wen (r. 559–566 CE), a ruler of the short-lived Chen dynasty (557–589 CE) in southern China.[35] The recitation of this text accompanied a concentrated period of fasting and repentance by a group of monastics—which may also have included the emperor himself. The text mentions lighting lamps in the shape of cartwheels, knotting cords, burning incense, placing banners, and other elaborate ritual actions and material objects as prescribed in the *Bhaiṣajyaguru Sūtra* {1: 25}.[36]

In addition to Emperor Wen's rite, we are fortunate to have a detailed chronicle of the rituals that took place when a royal consort went into labor in late twelfth-century Japan {1: 32}. Here, a range of officiants and specialists representing both Buddhism and indigenous Japanese traditions engaged in a highly orchestrated, formal series of actions to ritually protect the mother and newborn child. The rites focused on chanting the *Lotus Sūtra* and scriptures related to Bhaiṣajyaguru and Avalokiteśvara, giving gifts to various priests and members of the household, and preparing an ointment made with bezoar. The ritual protocols proceeded strictly according to historical precedent and were logged with precision for future reference. Such liturgical documents are important in that they give us a sense of how the range of Mahāyāna innovations discussed throughout this chapter were combined in practice by devotees in specific historical settings.

* * *

The previous chapter concluded with the observation that Nikāya Buddhist texts do not provide evidence of a coherent or complete medical system. The Mahāyāna literature fills in many of the lacunae. Whereas the earlier texts, at least in the forms available to us now, largely neglect diagnosis, Mahāyāna *sūtras* and commentaries discuss diagnostic practices in detail. Whereas the earlier sources often do not discuss how to administer therapeutics, Mahāyāna ritual texts provide in-depth instructions for the ceremonial preparation and ingestion of medicines for countless ailments. Beyond narratives about a handful of idealized physicians, Mahāyāna texts introduce us to a wide range of healers from all walks of life. The relationships between patients, practitioners, institutions, and society as a whole are articulated much more clearly than in the Nikāya texts.

While the basic medical theories presented in Mahāyāna writings continued to look in large part like those of Nikāya Buddhism and secular Indian medicine, new deities dedicated to healing and new healing rituals added significantly to the repertoire of Buddhist ideas and practices related to managing health and disease. The Mahāyāna notions of compassion and skillful means also provided concrete guidelines for the development of medical ethics. Far from dissuading devotees from the worldly practice of medicine, Mahāyāna texts encouraged—even on occasion explicitly required—them to get involved.

It is not an exaggeration to conclude that the development of the Mahāyāna occasioned a complete reevaluation of the relationship between healing and the Dharma. That is not to say that these positions were not controversial or that they were not debated by exegetes or *vinaya* specialists. However, the overwhelming message of the most important Mahāyāna literature was that medicine was something that all aspiring bodhisattvas could and should integrate into their spiritual paths. If the function of the Mahāyāna was to bring relief from suffering to as many beings as possible, then healing was surely part of its core mission.

## FURTHER READING

Birnbaum, Raoul. 1989. *The Healing Buddha*. Revised ed. Boulder, Colo.: Shambhala. A discussion of the main sources of and practices associated with some of the chief Mahāyāna medical deities: Bhaiṣajyaguru, Bhaiṣajyaraja, and Bhaiṣajyasamudgata.

Faure, Bernard. 2015. *Gods of Medieval Japan*. 2 vols. Honolulu: University of Hawai'i Press. A catalogue-like introduction to the pantheon of Japanese deities, mainly drawn from the Buddhist tradition.

Heirman, Ann, and Mathieu Torck. 2012. *A Pure Mind in a Clean Body: Bodily Care in the Buddhist Monasteries of Ancient India and China*. Ghent, Belgium: Academia. A discussion of monastic practices related to health and hygiene, based on Indian and Chinese sources.

Williams, Paul. 2009. *Mahāyāna Buddhism: The Doctrinal Foundations*. 2nd ed. Abingdon and New York: Routledge. The definitive introduction to Mahāyāna Buddhist thought, covering all major schools.

Yü, Chün-Fang. 2001. *Kuan-Yin: The Chinese Transformation of Avalokitesvara*. New York: Columbia University Press. A seminal book on the origins and history of the most popular deity in the Mahāyāna pantheon.

## CHAPTER 3

# *Tantric Buddhism*

Beginning in the middle of first millennium CE, a third wave of innovation in India gave rise to another major new form of Buddhism.[1] This was closely connected with a broader Indian religious movement known as Tantra. In this period, proponents of Buddhism, Jainism, and various Hindu traditions alike became interested in secret teachings about invisible levels of reality that could be unlocked through new kinds of religious practice.[2] These practices quickly made an indelible mark on all of the major religions in India and also became highly influential in the rest of Asia.

Scholars have disagreed on the range of features that must be present for a tradition properly to be labelled "Tantric," but we will not enter into those debates here.[3] Certain practices discussed in the previous chapter (such as the chanting of incantations and deity invocation) have sometimes been characterized as "proto-Tantric," since they eventually became central practices of the new movement. Given such continuities, there is no universally agreed-upon way to draw a clear line at which ordinary Mahāyāna ends and Tantric Buddhism begins. However, one clear marker of full-blown Tantra is the integration of visualization, deity invocation, mantras (i.e., incantations typically more condensed and powerful than *dhāraṇī*), and mandalas (i.e., cosmic diagrams or sacred symbols with esoteric meanings) into complex rituals designed to increase the spiritual or magical potency of the practitioner.

Another distinctive feature of Tantric Buddhism is the shroud of secrecy in which much of its ritual practice was enveloped. Details of the performance of its carefully orchestrated ritual regimes normally were known only by the initiated and were not meant to be transmitted to the general population. This fact gives

Tantric Buddhism one of its most common appellations, "Esoteric Buddhism" (Ch. *mijiao*; Jp. *mikkyō*), the name by which it is known in East Asia.

In Indian and Tibetan contexts, Tantric Buddhism is commonly referred to as Vajrayāna, literally the "vehicle of the *vajra*." A *vajra* can be a sacred object, a divine king's scepter, an adamantine weapon, a thunderbolt, or a penis depending on the context. The use of this particular symbol of power and spontaneity for the revolutionary reorientations of Buddhism in this period is apt. A unique facet of Tantric Buddhism is that it mobilized an extensive complex of political and military symbols and metaphors. Tantric practitioners (*tāntrikas*) were often initiated with rituals modeled on coronation rites.[4] Fashioning themselves as divine warrior kings, they cultivated an array of spiritual weapons to destroy demons, sorcerers, and other enemies. A new model of the ideal practitioner replaced the Mahāyānic bodhisattva. The *mahāsiddha*, the "great adept," was someone whose Tantric practice led them to acquire immense spiritual, as well as worldly, powers (*siddhi*).[5] This often involved rewriting Buddhist stories; for example, the celebrated hero Nāgārjuna, mentioned in the previous chapter, was recast in Tantric tales as a *mahāsiddha* with great healing abilities.[6]

Tantra went through several phases of development, culminating in what the Tibetans call the Supreme Yoga (*anuttarayoga*) class of *tantras*.[7] (Here, the term "*tantra*," written in lower case and italicized, refers to a genre distinct from *vinayas*, *sūtras*, *jātakas*, *avadānas*, and other types of text previously discussed, which contains written instructions for carrying out Tantric rituals and meditations.) Supreme Yoga involved the internalization of ritual practices and an emphasis on the practice of meditation. It was also characterized by an interest in manipulating the "subtle body," the energies that connect mind and body in order to optimize the potential for transformation. (We will come back to these topics later in this chapter.)

As this book is concerned only with giving an overview of Buddhist medicine, not all Tantric developments are directly relevant to us. However, there is much in this new form of Buddhism worth mentioning here. The Tantric revolution inspired a number of new approaches to health and healing. Like most of the new Tantric practices, these were assembled differently by different lineages. Various texts and teachers organized practices into specific stages, cycles, or systems.[8] These configurations developed over time into divergent sequences and terminology, which have always been hotly contested. Because we are talking in general terms here, I will not present Tantric Buddhist healing innovations within the context of any particular lineage or tradition or within a historical timeline. Rather, I will survey the material in a more thematic fashion.

The Tantric Buddhist healing repertoire includes aspects that both developed upon previous Buddhist traditions and departed significantly from them. Only in Tibet, the Himalayas, and the far northern areas of the Indian subcontinent was the full range of practices adopted. However, many Tantric elements became important in medieval China and Korea, and especially in Japan.[9] Recently, scholars also have been using the word "Tantra" to characterize certain practices within the Southeast Asian Theravāda tradition (such as those described in {1: 43}).[10] Theravādins self-describe as adherents of Nikāya Buddhism and would strongly refute this characterization. Whether or not one agrees with the use of the term "Tantric Theravāda," the larger point is uncontested: the influence of the practices associated with Tantra was wide ranging, affecting in one way or another nearly all forms of Buddhism across Asia.

## CONTINUITIES WITH MAHĀYĀNA HEALING PRACTICES

Tantra offered much that was revolutionary and new, but it was not invented from whole cloth. The movement emerged organically from and maintained significant continuities with what had come before. Many Tantric healing practices represent logical developments of Mahāyāna ritual therapies. Tantric Buddhists inherited the entire Mahāyāna pantheon, with all of its ritual, textual, and iconographic richness. Many of the established Mahāyāna healing deities discussed in the previous chapter—Bhaiṣajyaguru, Avalokiteśvara, and others—thus continued to figure significantly in Tantric practice and be the focal points of healing rituals.

On the other hand, new deities were added to the Buddhist pantheon, and some of those who had previously been minor were elevated in importance. One development in this regard was the emergence of a cult of seven Bhaiṣajyaugurus, as opposed to just one.[11] Also notable was the expansion of the roles of Mahāyāna female bodhisattvas and spirits. The bodhisattva Tārā, considered an emanation of Avalokiteśvara, was known as a source of great compassion and skillful means.[12] Particularly in her white form (Sita Tārā), she was associated with healing, longevity, and fertility. In Tibet, longevity meditations and rituals (*āyuḥsādhana*) often centered on a triad including her, the female bodhisattva Uṣṇīṣavijaya, and Amitāyus (the Buddha of Infinite Life) {1: 40}.[13]

A group of five protector goddesses (Mahāpratisarā, Mahāmāyūrī, Mahāsāhasarapramarddinī, Mahāśitavatī, and Mahāmantrānusāriṇī) became especially important for health.[14] As personifications of protective spells, they guarded against a range of diseases and dangers, such as snakebite, attack by evil spirits, smallpox, and difficult pregnancies. One of these goddesses, the Great Peahen Wisdom Queen (Mahāmāyūrī Vidyārājñī), became known across Asia

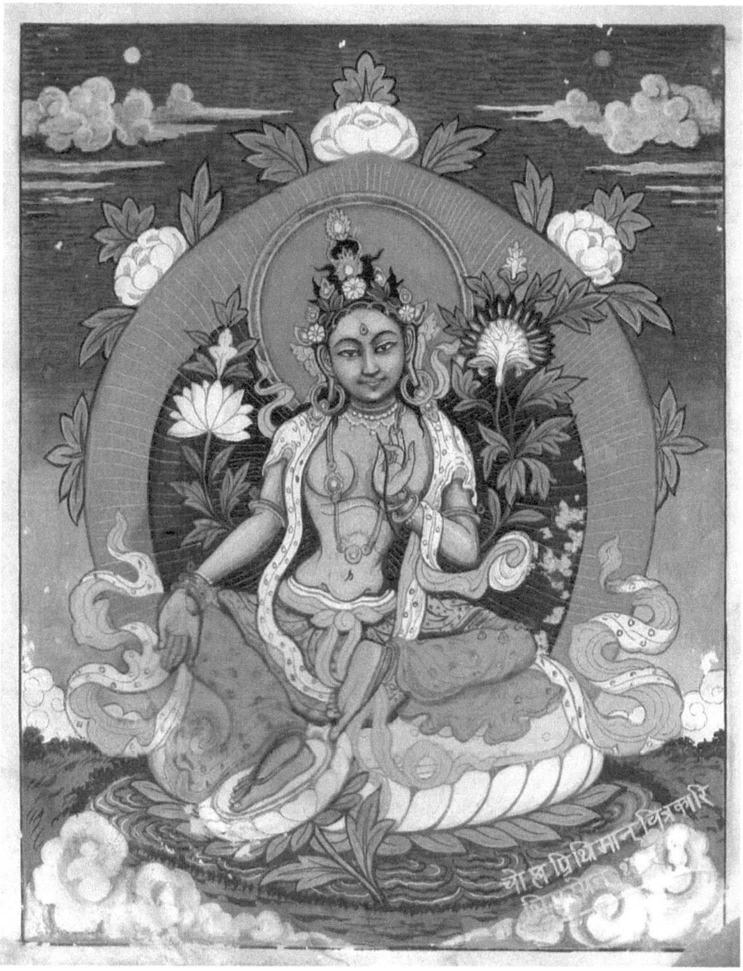

**3.1** The Buddhist goddess Tārā, in her green manifestation. Painting by Prithvi Man Chitrakari, completed in 1947.

Image courtesy of Wikimedia Commons, public domain.

and was important in Japan as the patroness of imperial birth rituals {1: 32, 33}. Other goddesses represented converted demons or "wrathful deities." For example, the "Poison Woman" Jāṅgulī, a frightful demoness whose body was covered with snakes, commanded serpents and *nāga* spirits. Devotees who knew her rituals could use them to nullify the pernicious effects of any poison {1: 47}.[15]

Another continuity with Mahāyāna practice accentuated in Tantric rituals was the practice of visualization. For example, a repertoire of healing visualizations is found in a mid-fifth century Chinese translation of a text from Khotan in Central Asia called *Secret Essential Methods for Curing Meditation Sickness* (*Zhi chanbing miyao fa*). This text contains surprisingly early references to the Tantric subtle body system (see below). The text also introduces extensive visualization sequences for treating various ailments, including errant Winds within the subtle body, imbalances in the Four Elements, attack by demons, madness, and obsessive thoughts that arise from improper meditation. One section, called "The Enveloping Butter Contemplation," calls upon the meditator to visualize a series of nine divinities performing various medical procedures on the meditator's body {1: 36}. These include opening the skull with a golden knife and filling the meditator's body with medicated ghee, applying topical medicines, administering acupuncture, giving massage, and performing irrigations and enemas, among other procedures. Other sections of the text introduce equally complex visualizations that harness or neutralize the Elements, invoke deities bearing medicinal substances, and describe the inner recesses of the human body.[16]

Early Tantric texts from India also emphasized healing visualizations. The *Fundamental Spell Book of Mañjuśrī* (*Mañjuśrī[ya]mūlakalpa*), composed in the late sixth or early seventh century, contains one and a half chapters that focus on healing snakebite.[17] Here, the practitioner is told to visualize the bodhisattva Mañjuśrī atop the snake-killing eagle god Garuḍa, appearing in different colors at different parts of the victim's body. Another snakebite text, the *Tantra of the Buddha's Skull* (*Buddhakapāla tantra*), uses visualizations to battle *nāga* spirits.[18] The practitioner visualizes sending fiery solar rays at the *nāgas*, "burning their hearts," and sending cooling lunar rays toward the victim to neutralize the poison. Another Tantric snakebite therapy in the eighth-century Chinese collection *Sūtra on the Mantras of Garuḍa and Other Gods* (*Jialouluo ji zhutian miyan jing*) involves visualizing the mantra ṬHA (associated with the cooling power of the moon) encircling the heart of the victim.[19] As a set, these texts were in close conversation with various strains of non-Buddhist Tantra in India.

As Tantric Buddhism developed, healing visualizations required detailed knowledge of a growing vocabulary of mantras. These syllables were considered to have great cosmic or spiritual significance and are often contrasted to the more utilitarian *dhāraṇīs* of ordinary Mahāyāna. However, the distinction between the two kinds of incantation is slippery in practice, and both continued to be popular.

Whatever larger spiritual or religious potencies were promised of mantras, they nearly always could also be used to provide relief from illness. Tantric practitioners thus chanted, wore, and displayed mantras associated with Bhaiṣajyaguru, Tārā, Avalokiteśvara, and a wide range of other buddhas, bodhisattvas, gods, and goddesses to protect themselves from ailments and a range of other mundane forms of suffering or discomfort {1: 26, 28, 30, 35, 45}. Mantras could likewise be virtually "installed" in the body of the practitioner—particularly in the hands or fingers, which could then be used to neutralize ailments or poisons with merely a touch (see a related practice in {1: 47}).[20]

Mantras were frequently combined with visualizations to create complicated practices necessitating great concentration skill. For example, the *Tantra of the Great Vairocana* (Skt. *Mahāvairocana tantra*), composed in mid-seventh century India and becoming centrally important in the Japanese Shingon sect, promised that all illnesses caused by negative karma accumulated in previous lives could be eradicated.[21] It advises practitioners to visualize a *vajra* sitting upon a "wondrous lotus" floating above the eight peaks of the sacred Mount Meru. Above this *vajra*, one visualizes the syllable A with "awesomely blazing light."[22] All of this is to be visualized while the practitioner ingests mantra-empowered medicines.

Another key aspect of the Tantric repertoire that continued and extended Mahāyāna rituals was the use of mandalas (Skt. *maṇḍala*, literally "circle"). Consecrated circular ritual spaces demarcated by cow dung, mustard seeds, string, or other blessed objects were a regular feature of Mahāyāna ritual practice. The *sūtras* associated with Bhaiṣajyaguru incorporated the construction of a mandala into the core ritual for that deity, and manuals from medieval China specify how such rituals should be carried out {1: 28§8}. Taken up by Tantric Buddhism, such practices developed over time into far more complex mandalas representing sacred geometries or cosmic maps.[23]

Constructed, drawn, or visualized mandalic cosmograms became integrated into Tantric healing practice. For example, one of the principal Supreme Yoga texts, *Binding of the Wheels Tantra* (*Cakrasaṃvara tantra*), composed in India in the late eighth or early ninth century, introduced a practice known as the "body mandala" (*kāyāmaṇḍala*). Here, the practitioner visualizes the principal mandala of the text pervading the entire body, purifying it, and transforming it from an ordinary physical body into a "divine abode."[24] The abovementioned *Fundamental Spell Book of Mañjuśrī* also gives instructions for constructing healing mandalas.

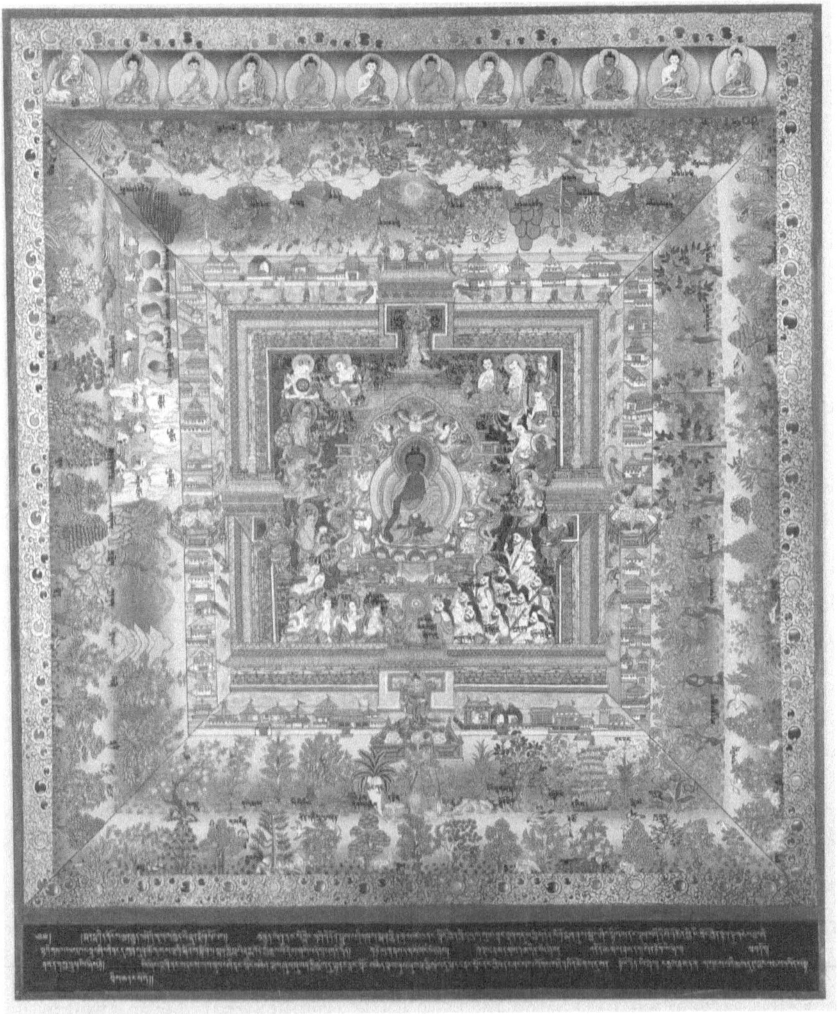

**3.2** Mandala depicting the lineage of Tibetan medicine, centering on Bhaiṣajyaguru and including Jīvaka Kumārabhṛta, Yutok Yönten Gonpo, and other figures discussed throughout this book. Modern copy of a *thangka* painting commissioned by Sangyé Gyatso (1653–1705). Image courtesy of Wikimedia Commons, public domain.

In addition to these developments that extended Mahāyāna ritual practice in new directions, Tantra, like other forms of Buddhism, continued to draw extensively from conventional Indian medicine.[25] Despite their reputation for transcendent and otherworldly ritual practices, even some of the most mature Supreme Yoga *tantras* continued to recommend a range of remedies for illness not at all dissimilar to what one would find in conventional Āyurvedic texts. A particularly significant source is the *Wheel of Time Tantra* (*Kālacakra tantra*), which was the last of the major *tantras* to be composed in India in the eleventh century. This text contains an encyclopedic synthesis of various sciences or realms of knowledge, including copious information on medicine.[26] These sections discuss a wide range of therapies, including herbal medicines, fumigation, dietary regimens, medicinal baths, and topical ointments. The *Wheel of Time Tantra* is replete with concepts borrowed from medical contexts when it discusses diagnosis, prognosis, and the signs of imminent death.[27] It also contains knowledge about embryology, gynecology, obstetrics, and healing childhood illnesses similar to the information found in the classic Indian medical literature.[28]

## UNIQUE FEATURES OF TANTRIC HEALING

Tantric healing rites exhibit many continuities with Mahāyāna Buddhism, which were amplified, enhanced, or expanded in new directions. However, the Tantric movement also introduced several new techniques and doctrines that represented more radical breaks with Buddhist precedents. Like the visualization techniques discussed in the previous section, many of these new developments emerged in dialogue with non-Buddhist Tantric and yogic systems that were developing in India in the medieval period.[29]

One of the most important features distinguishing Tantric Buddhism from previous forms of Mahāyāna is the practice of "deity yoga" (*devatāyoga*). As discussed in the previous chapter, the purpose of deity invocation, visualization, mantras, mandalas, and other ritual elements in conventional Mahāyāna practice was to make the transformative powers of the buddhas and bodhisattvas present in the here and now. The practitioner used rituals to invoke the presence of the deities and to transfer their blessings to particular objects, spaces, or bodies. In Tantric deity yoga practice, on the other hand, these ritual elements (as well as others, such as hand gestures called *mudrās* and the *homa* fire sacrifice) could be used to merge the identity of the practitioner with that of the deity.

This type of practice often began with practitioners placing themselves inside a visualized or physically constructed mandala. They then used rituals to invoke a tutelary deity (*iṣṭadevatā*) and merge their bodies and minds with it. This presented a departure from the Mahāyāna logic of calling on deities for assistance. The presumption of deity yoga was that, through merging with the deity, practitioners could not just gain blessings but also take on a range of divine powers for themselves. These included the ability to conquer disease, within both their own bodies and those of others {1: 40}.

Another notable departure from previous forms of Buddhism was Tantra's antinomianism. Like the Mahāyāna aspirant who practiced worldly pursuits as skillful means in their quest to liberate the suffering of all beings across the cosmos, Tantric practitioners were encouraged to acquire techniques from a broad range of sources. However, unlike their conventional Mahāyāna counterparts, *tāntrikas* were not limited to socially acceptable bodies of knowledge. Deviant practices previously considered beyond the pale for practitioners—such as sorcery, necromancy, transgressive sex, and other taboos—were now considered legitimate sources to be mined for efficacious techniques.[30]

Tantra authorized a range of occult knowledge that could be downright dangerous if one were not properly prepared, trained, and supervised. Buddhists had long considered demonic possession a cause of serious illness, but now possession could also be the means of cure.[31] Tantric practitioners could transfer disease-causing spirits from the bodies of the sick to the body of a spirit medium to interrogate, chastise, punish, or defeat them. While the specialists officiating over such exorcisms were usually male monastics, the use of virginal women or young children as mediums became common in many Buddhist cultures.[32] In China and Japan, such practices were widespread in the medieval period, providing opportunities for female specialists to play a central role in Buddhist ritual healing {1: 21§10}.

Tantric practice could also result in the acquisition of abilities that could easily be used for evil or selfish goals. Rituals for killing or neutralizing one's enemies, invoking and harnessing the powers of dangerous spiritual beings, and other black magical arts all were legitimate parts of the Tantric repertoire.[33] Out of concern that such powers might fall into the wrong hands, *tāntrikas* typically were required to be initiated into practice lineages to gain access to the most well-guarded secret teachings and had to study under the supervision of a perfected teacher or guru.

Other antinomian practices contravened traditional concepts of pollution or physical feelings of disgust or repulsion. The *Wheel of Time Tantra*, for example, touts the healing effects of tabooed substances. One passage calls for ingesting menstrual blood through the nose to increase one's vitality and reverse the effects of old age.[34] Another passage prescribes eating a combination of semen and menstrual blood for the elimination of ailments.[35] (This combination, especially if removed from the female vagina after sexual intercourse, was often considered highly potent and was used for various ritual purposes in many Tantric traditions.) Another passage from the same text calls for ingesting feces, urine, semen, blood, and human flesh mixed with honey to prolong one's life.[36]

Its willingness to engage in this range of antinomian practices is one way that Tantric Buddhist healing can be distinguished from previous forms of Buddhism. In the hands of a well-trained practitioner who had the best intentions for all beings in their heart, such rites were considered beneficial, legitimately part of the Dharmic practice of skillful means. Tantric Buddhism also stands apart from previous forms of Buddhism in its acceptance of all aspects of human experience—including desire, sexuality, and negative mental-emotional states, which conventional Buddhists had shunned as detrimental and misguided.

Underlying the Tantric approach to unwholesome or distasteful aspects of human life was a new and pervasive alchemical metaphor.[37] Through the alchemy of Tantric practice, so the argument goes, any poison can be transmuted into a blessing, converted from a hindrance into something conducive to one's spiritual progress. References to alchemical healing practice in Tantric texts are not always merely metaphorical, however. Alchemical remedies (Skt. *rasāyana*), particularly those involving mercury, played a major role in Tantric practice in Tibet, as well as in Tibetan medicine.[38] The *Wheel of Time Tantra* discusses the preparation of gold, lead, copper, and other metals for making elixirs to rejuvenate the physical body and eradicate the signs of old age.[39]

In Tantric Buddhism, alchemy also commonly refers to a process of distillation and refinement that takes place within the mind and body of the adept Tantric practitioner. This internal practice of alchemy enables the practitioner to transform anger, sexual arousal, and other internal poisons into positive states. Internal alchemy also allows the practitioner to extract the spiritual power or the "vital essence" (*rasa*) of certain objects in the physical world. Through the power of Tantric practice, the essences of medicines, minerals, the wind, or the Elements could be extracted and transmuted into a subtle nectar or elixir (*amṛta*). This elixir, in turn, could be used to confer spiritual powers or magical attainments on the participants in a ritual to nourish body and mind, heal disease, or increase longevity {1: 42}.

This practice of "essence extraction" (Tib. *chülen*) became a routine part of the Tantric repertoire, incorporated into healing rites alongside visualization, mantras, mandalas, deity yoga, and the rest. For example, during one ceremony dedicated to White Tārā, the officiating master calls upon participants to visualize the "distillation" of the Five Elements into yellow-, white-, vermillion-, emerald-, and indigo-colored light and nectar.[40] Next, they visualize all five essences emanating from a flask held by the Buddha of Infinite Life (Amitāyus) and dissolving into Tārā's body. From there, this "nectar of deathless life" is visualized being poured through the top of each person's head, filling up their body. This nectar is said to wash away all karmic faults and diseases, heal the bodily Elements, and clear any impediments that would prevent one from living a full life of one hundred years.

Later in the same rite, the master distributes small pills to the participants. These "precious pills" (Tib. *rinchen rilbu*)—when empowered through ritual practice also referred to as "Dharma medicine" (Tib. *chömen*), "nectar pills" (Tib. *dütsi rilbu*), "accomplished medicines" (Tib. *mendrup*), and other similar names—are frequently found playing a role in Tantric rituals.[41] According to Tibetan texts, they represent concrete manifestations of "all the distillations of this world and Nirvana," the "essence of the 404 sorts of medicine," and the "quintessence of glorious foods that make firm your good fortune and life" {1: 60}.[42] When consuming the pills, the devotees are guided to visualize the destruction of all diseases. This is followed by various mantras to prolong longevity.

## THE SUBTLE BODY

Later Tantric developments—particularly those associated with the Supreme Yoga texts—were influenced by the notion of a deeper dimension of the human body that can be affected by forces on an unseen plane of reality. A vision of this subtle body (in Buddhist sources also known as the "*vajra* body") coalesced in Indian Buddhist literature in the eighth to tenth centuries.[43] This represented a novel notion of embodiment not present in earlier Nikāya and Mahāyāna Buddhism.

The Buddhist subtle body did have deep historical precedents, however. Similar models of the body were recorded in India as early as the first millennium BCE, in the *Upaniṣads*, and likely had been circulating since that time. Scholars have long thought that at least some part of this system derives from Chinese forms of self-cultivation practiced in Daoist circles, which would easily have been able to be transported along the Silk Road or the maritime routes from China to India.[44] Central Asia is also a possible origin point of this system, where, in the mid-fifth century, the aforementioned *Secret Essential Methods for Curing Meditation Sickness* records a surprisingly early description of the Tantric Buddhist subtle body system and how to manipulate it using visualization meditation.[45] The Buddhist subtle body is also clearly the result of pervasive competition and dialogue between Buddhism and other Tantric traditions in India itself which were developing their own similar systems contemporaneously.[46] While the jury is still out on the exact steps by which these various ingredients led to the development of the Buddhist subtle body, it is clear that this model did not develop in a vacuum but rather in constant contact and exchange with a wide range of non-Buddhist traditions from around Asia.

As a complete system of theory and practice, the Buddhist subtle body never became as significant in other parts of Asia as it was in Indian and Tibetan cultural regions. In East Asia, Tantric Buddhist theorization and practice concerning the subtle body more often used the East Asian model of the body and concepts such as *qi* (such practices of localization will be discussed in greater detail in chapter 7). However, parts of the Indian subtle body system can be found in East Asia and in various parts of Southeast Asia.[47]

One of the most important features of the Tantric subtle body was that it represented a new understanding of how the individual human body was interconnected with the mind, the environment, and the cosmos at large. These connections hinged on an elaboration of the concept of Wind. As discussed in chapter 1, the classical Buddhist model held that the corporeal body was constructed out of the Great Elements. According to the Elemental doctrine, all of the body's movements represented manifestations of Wind (*vāyu*). Some Buddhist texts additionally specify that there are five principal manifestations of the Wind Element within the body, an idea also found in the foundational texts of the Āyurvedic medical system, as well as in some of the *Upaniṣads* and other Indian religious materials.[48] Each of the Five Winds was located in a different part of the body and controlled distinct bodily, sensorial, and even psychological functions. Buddhist texts often mention additional types of Wind representing karma, the force behind conception and fetal development, the force sustaining life, and other cosmic influences (see, e.g., {1: 5}).

Texts on the subtle body tend to accept the doctrine of the Elements, including the notion of multiple Winds, as an accurate description of the "outer" (i.e., the corporeal or physical) body. They also continue to recognize *vāta*, the Wind *doṣa* or pathogenic corruption of the Wind Element, as one of the chief factors of illness.[49] Wind thus continued to be understood both as a normal dynamic feature of the physiology of the body and one of the principal causes or symptoms of disease. However, Tantric texts added to *vāyu* and *vāta* a third type of Wind. Usually called *prāṇa* in Sanskrit, this Wind referred to very fine influences operating at a much subtler level than the corporeal Elements and *tridoṣa*.[50] Representing mind and body simultaneously, these subtle Winds intricately connected one's physical embodiment with one's mental and emotional fluctuations. These Winds also represented vital energies that ensured the optimal functioning of the human organism {1: 41–43}.[51]

The subtle Winds moved through the body along an intricate network of pathways or channels (Sk. *nāḍīs*). Literally meaning "pipe," "tube," or "vein," this generic term could also refer to any number of physical anatomical structures (such as blood vessels, for example). The subtle channels were sometimes said to be separate structures that existed at a deeper level than the corporeal flesh, although exactly how (or whether) these corresponded to physical anatomy was a point of contention among Buddhist theorists and medical specialists alike.[52] Texts also differ on the number of subtle channels they recognize (72,000 and 350,000 are commonly cited). They likewise differ on exactly where these subtle channels are located in the body, with each tradition providing a map considered valid within the context of the particular practices of that group. The *Tantra of the Secret Community* (*Guhyasamāja tantra*), the *Hevajra Tantra*, the *Binding of the Wheels Tantra* (*Cakrasaṃvara tantra*), and the *Wheel of Time Tantra*, each representing major Tantric traditions, describe the subtle body in different ways.[53]

Given these divergent interpretations, it is impossible to precisely describe the anatomy of the Tantric subtle body in any detail here. Speaking in general terms, most Buddhist Tantric systems recognized three central channels: *avadhūtī*, *lalanā*, and *rasanā*.[54] (In Hindu traditions, these channels are usually called *suṣumna, iḍā*, and *piṅgala*.) *Avadhūtī* runs along the midline of the body (sometimes simply called "the middle," *madhyamā*), with *lalanā* on the left side and *rasanā* on the right. Broadly speaking, the central channels begin in the lower abdomen near the navel or at the genitals and run upward along the spine to the head. Sometimes, these three channels run parallel to one another, whereas some traditions describe them intersecting at regular intervals. *Avadhūtī* often ends at the crown or between the eyebrows, while *lalanā* and *rasanā* often end at or near the nostrils. Typically, *lalanā* is associated with the moon, masculinity, semen, action, and skillful means, whereas *rasanā* is associated with the sun, femininity, blood, passivity, and wisdom.[55]

Located along the three central channels are a series of spinning chakras (Skt. *cakra*, literally "wheel"). Usually numbering between four and six in Buddhist traditions (but potentially numbering seven or more), these are *prāṇa* centers, nexus points where different types of energy can be cultivated and stored. At each chakra, subsidiary channels branch off from the central lines to connect with the rest of the body. Knots and blockages (*granthi*) can form at nodes where channels meet, potentially hindering the flow of *prāṇa* through the system, leading to spiritual stagnation and poor health. One of the principal goals of subtle body practice is therefore to untangle these knots and smooth out the flow of *prāṇa* through the subtle body.

Channels emanating from the heart chakra are considered especially important, as they represent various types of consciousness. (In some texts, these channels appear in the head rather than the heart.)[56] Some of these branches are responsible for the senses.[57] Subtle influences thus constantly enter into the subtle body system via the heart depending on the things one sees, hears, smells, tastes, and thinks. Negative mental or emotional states or disturbances in one's surroundings can easily impact the *prāṇa* throughout one's entire body and thereby influence one's overall mental and physical well-being.

It is not only sensory inputs that affect the subtle body. Whereas the gross bodily Winds are influenced by the seasons, the food one eats, the medicines one takes, and other factors in the immediate environment, the subtle body is an open system that responds to myriad subtle energy flows throughout the cosmos. Through such influences, one's channels are inextricably intertwined with the vast universe and everything in it. One of the major themes in the *Wheel of Time Tantra* is the complex connections between the cyclical rhythms of the movements of subtle energies in the individual body and the cosmic cycles of the planets, stars, and other celestial objects.[58] A whole system of medical astrology is deduced based on understanding these connections.

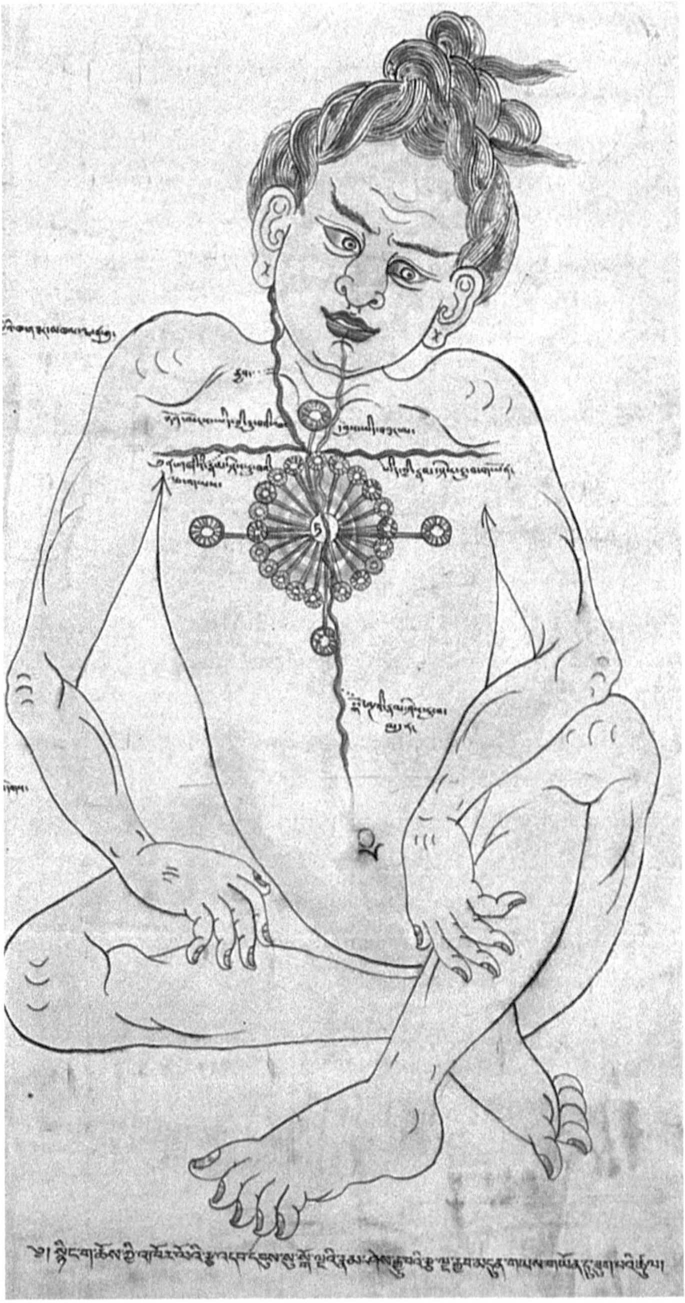

**3.3** Depiction of the heart chakra with branching energy channels (Skt. *nāḍīs*). *Thangka* painting commissioned by Sangyé Gyatso (1653–1705).

Tantric practices to maintain the health of the subtle body and cure its disorders vary widely. At the most basic level, any practice that promotes positive mental states or surrounds the practitioner with beneficial sensory stimuli can contribute to good health by soothing the subtle body. Any number of powerful objects—such as mandalas, empowered ritual implements, gemstones and other auspicious material—can be used to infuse the subtle body with healing or strength. One reason that Tantric Buddhism calls for the practitioner to use visualization, mantras, mandalas, essence extraction, and other such practices is to cultivate or store specific positive influences in different parts of the body.

Tantric Buddhist approaches to subtle body cultivation also can call for a range of physical postures (*āsana*) and breathing exercises (*prāṇāyāma*) designed to regulate, move, or enhance specific vital essences within the channels and chakras. As is the case in systems of *haṭhayoga* associated with Hinduism, such exercises are often connected with specific health benefits. The *Wheel of Time Tantra*, for example, prescribes certain breathing patterns for a range of illnesses, longevity, and rejuvenation of the body.[59] It also recommends headstands for the alleviation of phlegm and the "*vajra* posture" for the elimination of backache.[60]

Such exercises, while mentioned only sporadically in the root *tantras*, came to be organized into sophisticated systems of practice in Tibet, where various lineages of "magical movements" for the subtle body channels and Winds (Tib. *tsalung trulkhor*) emerged.[61] These practices call for combinations of physical postures, movement, and breath control to cultivate health and longevity, as well as to prepare the body for higher spiritual attainments. Such practices circulated widely within secretive lineages of Tantric practitioners around Asia. *Trulkhor*, *tummo*, and *yantra* yoga are still practiced for spiritual advancement and health maintenance within Tibetan contexts.[62] A related contemporary Thai system called "stretching of the sages" (Th. *ruesi dat ton*) even more explicitly emphasizes therapeutic applications.

Aside from physical postures and breathing exercises, some subtle body practices called for advanced practitioners to work with a substance called *bodhicitta* (literally "thought of awakening"). In Mahāyāna Buddhism, *bodhicitta* referred to the compassionate determination to become enlightened for the sake of all sentient beings. In some Tantric subtle body practices, however, *bodhicitta* was conceived of as a physical manifestation of the essence of the mind.[63] *Bodhicitta*, in this interpretation, was understood to be a vital energy or generative force that could be collected and cultivated within the body. Meditations focusing on storing and moving *bodhicitta* through the subtle body system could be used to

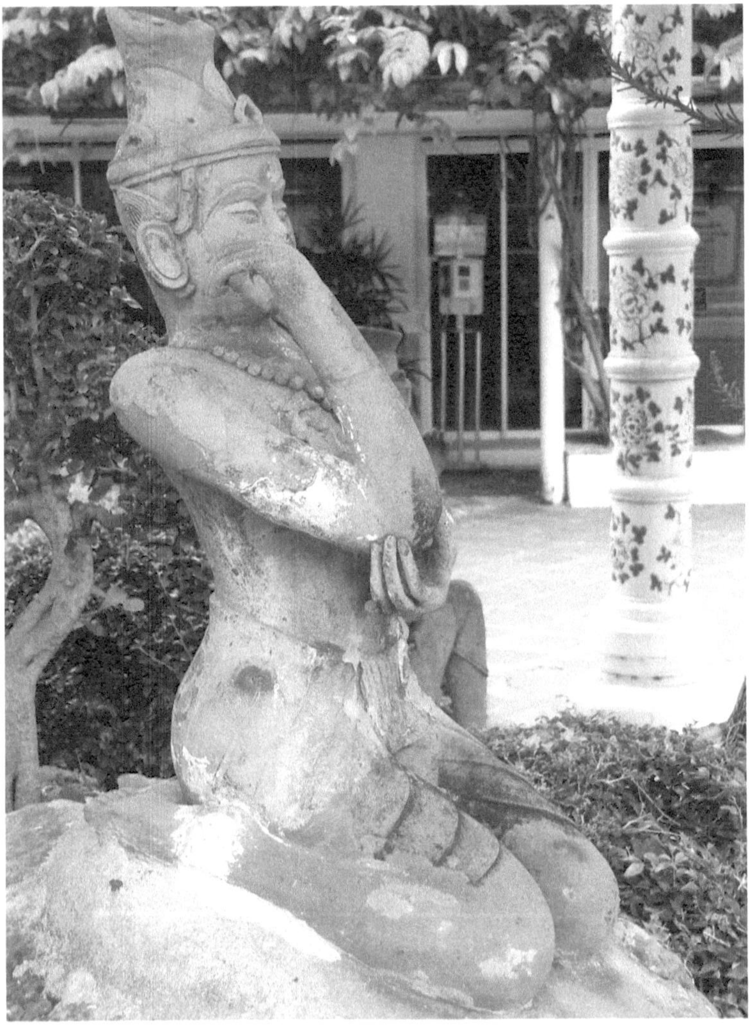

3.4 Nineteenth-century sculpture depicting a Buddhist yogi (Th. *ruesi*) named Vyādhipralaya practicing "stretching of the sages" (Th. *ruesi dat ton*), a Tantric influenced tradition of bodily cultivation similar to *haṭha* and *yantra* yoga. An accompanying manuscript describes this posture as a therapy for stiff feet and hands. From the Wat Phra Chetuphon temple in Bangkok, Thailand.
Photo by the author.

empower skillful means, promote one's health, and increase one's vitality and longevity.

*Bodhicitta* was also sometimes described as the subtle essence or distillation of the sexual fluids. This correlation was relevant in a variety of visualizations focused on manipulating sexual essences within the subtle body system {1: 40§1}.[64] In one common version of this meditation, the practitioner visualizes white and red "drops" (*bindu*), representing the subtle essences of male and female *bodhicitta*, respectively, within the central channel. In some texts, the fiery red essence in the lower chakras is personified as the goddess Caṇḍālī, who (like her Hindu counterpart, Kuṇḍalinī) ascends the central channel into the crown.[65] In other meditations, the heat of the red essence rises and melts the white essence, which descends. Meeting in the middle, their union symbolizes the unification of sun and moon, female and male, wisdom and skillful means.

The unification of red and white could also be achieved through visualized sexual intercourse or actual intercourse enacted in a ritualized manner and accompanied by meditations or visualizations. For males, the retention of semen during any such sexual encounters, real or virtual, was of utmost concern. Loss of semen meant a loss of vital essence, leading to both mental and physical illness. As the thirteenth-century Tibetan *Hidden Description of the Vajra Body* (*Dorjé lükyi beshé*) explains, loss of semen leads to the dissipation of the body's Fire, the Life-Sustaining Wind being compromised, the body becoming cold and weak, and the mind becoming discontent.[66]

While these practices are invariably enveloped within a program of self-transformation aimed at nothing less than full buddhahood, the *tantras* often specifically enumerate the health benefits of sexual cultivation. These benefits are mentioned, for example, in the *Wheel of Time Tantra*, which considers semen retention and sexual cultivation an effective treatment for "white leprosy," as well as halting the effects of aging.[67] The use of visualized sexual intercourse for health purposes is also mentioned in two commentaries attributed to the semi-legendary eighth-century Padmasambhava (also known as "Guru Rinpoche," the most revered Tantric master in Tibet). These short texts are included in a fourteenth-century Tibetan collection called the *Seminal Heart Essence in Four Parts* (*Nyingthig yazhi*). To treat illness, the texts call for the practitioner to visualize female spirits (*ḍākinī*) in sexual embrace at various chakras.[68] The meditator visualizes a vital essence or energy arising from "the point of sexual contact" of each spirit. This essence or energy then moves throughout the subtle body, restoring the digestive fires or counteracting the *tridoṣa*. The text also states that "composite illnesses" (i.e., those caused by more than one *doṣa*) are to be treated over the course of three days by practicing a *prāṇāyāma* exercise that involves holding the breath while "applying holds from below and above." Meanwhile, the practitioner visualizes spirits in sexual embrace throughout the entire network of channels in the body and a nectar flowing from their point of contact, filling "the whole body like milk." This visualization is said to expel disease from the body.

Such sexual cultivation practices may seem inconsistent with the Buddhist monastic culture of celibacy. (Although, we have already seen that monastic involvement with childbirth was commonplace, and practices to increase fertility and sexual virility were not unknown either; see {1: 49§2.}) But it is important to realize that this was not a case of a few libertine practitioners engaging in transgressive practices from non-Buddhist traditions. A whole range of Buddhist Tantric sexual techniques appears to have developed in close dialogue with the larger constellation of subtle body practices sweeping through Indian religious circles, and significant innovations were contributed to that centuries-long conversation by Buddhists.[69] While it certainly did not constitute the sole or even main focus of Tantric Buddhism, sexual cultivation is by no means marginal and was discussed in detail in some of the most historically significant Tantric texts.

* * *

This chapter has outlined Tantric Buddhist approaches to health and healing in a general and thematic way rather than strictly chronologically. Although many historical details and sectarian interpretations have not been covered here, the purpose was to broadly outline how Tantric healing built upon and differed from what came before. Stepping back to look at the entire range of ideas and practices discussed in this chapter, we can conclude that Tantra continued the process of integrating healing with the Dharma that had begun with the Mahāyāna. Not only were *tāntrikas* expected to master healing skills as expedient means of advancing their bodhisattva path but Tantra also provided a range of more diverse, more potent therapies.

As this book has progressed, healing has moved into a more and more prominent position within the Dharma. In fact, according to the nondual philosophy that undergirded Tantric movements both inside and outside Buddhist circles, the worldly and the otherworldly were two sides of the same coin. Thus, in Tantric discourses, physical healing and spiritual enlightenment were always different facets of the same thing. For *tāntrikas*, to possess the power of healing, or to accomplish the perfection of the physical body, was synonymous with expressing the enlightenment of the universe. Tantric practices such as those described in this chapter were considered means of progressing toward the realization of enlightenment, but they also are consistently described as being useful for acquiring this-worldly benefits, such as maintaining good health and curing illness.

## FURTHER READING

Garrett, Frances. 2008. *Religion, Medicine and the Human Embryo in Tibet*. London: Routledge. An analysis of Tibetan Buddhist discourses on conception, gestation, and childbirth, integrating perspectives from both Buddhist and medical history.

Orzech, Charles D., Henrik H. Sørensen, and Richard K. Payne, eds. 2011. *Esoteric Buddhism and the Tantras in East Asia*. Leiden and Boston: Brill. A large compendium of essays on various aspects of East Asian Tantra. Includes chapters on *dhāraṇīs* and other healing rituals, as well as background on numerous relevant deities.

Samuel, Geoffrey. 2008. *The Origins of Yoga and Tantra: Indic Religions to the Thirteenth Century*. Cambridge: Cambridge University Press. A general introduction to early Indian Tantra, placing Buddhist developments within a larger historical framework.

Strickmann, Michel. 2002. *Chinese Magical Medicine*, edited by Bernard Faure. Stanford, Calif.: Stanford University Press. A readable overview of Tantric Buddhist healing based on Chinese sources, with an emphasis on cross-fertilization between Buddhism and Daoism.

Wallace, Vesna, trans. 2001. *The Inner Kālacakratantra: A Buddhist Tantric View of the Individual*. New York: Oxford University Press. A general introduction to the *Wheel of Time Tantra*, with a chapter on its medical and scientific contents.

CHAPTER 4

# *Common Questions*

Thus far, this book has concentrated on the teachings about illness and health that emerged within Nikāya, Mahāyāna, and Tantric Buddhism in India. We have also been exploring these traditions' divergent approaches to therapeutics. In part 2, I will trace how these core features underwent enormous change as Buddhist medicine was transmitted over time and across geographic regions over two millennia. At the same time that it has been constantly transforming throughout this long global history, it is also true that certain themes have appeared again and again across divergent times and places. This chapter surveys some of these commonalities. It does so by outlining certain areas of doctrinal inquiry that have been perennial topics of debate and discussion. Buddhists have rarely agreed on the answers to these questions; however, they represent common concerns and problematics that have shaped, informed, and guided Buddhist engagement with medicine across many contexts throughout history and that remain salient today.

## ILLNESS AND SUFFERING

Buddhists consider illness to be one of the principal forms of suffering encountered within a human lifetime. Along with birth, old age, and death, it is one of the so-called fourfold afflictions (Skt. *catasro-duḥkhatāḥ*) that Buddhism is principally concerned with alleviating. Buddhist traditions have tended to agree that, for the unenlightened person, the impermanent nature of the physical body is a profound source of suffering. We wish to enjoy eternal pleasure, ease, and health, but it cannot be so. The body is prone to imbalance and disease. A period of relatively good health offers only a temporary respite from the essentially dissatisfactory and unpredictable nature of human embodiment.

In response to this situation, Buddhist discourses often speak of illness as something that must be borne with patience and equanimity.[1] Many forms of meditation practice from across the Buddhist world involve contemplating the impermanence of the Elements, physical structures, and bodily sensations as a way of realizing that the material body is empty (Skt. *śūnyatā*) or devoid of self (Skt. *anātman*). Through this insight, one lets go of the unrealistic expectation that we can control our health.

Contemplating illness thus provides a particularly good opportunity to cultivate detachment from the body, and Buddhists past and present have often expressed appreciation for bouts of illness as poignant and illuminating experiences {1: 7; 2: 34§3}.[2] This perspective is found not only in didactic texts that teach contemplative practices but also in narratives that illustrate how the realization of emptiness or non-self can deeply transform a person's response to illness. Medieval East Asian collections of stories about eminent monks and nuns, for example, frequently emphasize the awareness and equanimity with which adept practitioners of the Dharma die {1: 21§5}. Recent reporting on the stroke and end-of-life care of the Vietnamese Buddhist leader Thích Nhất Hạnh (b. 1926) have taken a similar tone toward this beloved contemporary figure.[3] In all of these accounts, the stoicism of the patient in the face of illness and death is taken as proof of the individual's spiritual attainment. Such stories of detachment have helped to model the proper "sick role" for Buddhists and provided ideal depictions against which devotees have habitually judged themselves and one another.

The notion that human embodiment is indelibly marked by suffering was a feature that Buddhism shared with other renunciate traditions that emerged in ancient India. (For example, Jainism held that forbearance was the only sensible response to illness, and Jain monastics were supposed to accept illness without seeking healing.)[4] While many Buddhists have expressed a detached perspective, Buddhism nevertheless has always supplemented its stoic stance with concrete health-seeking techniques. As discussed earlier in this book, Nikāya Buddhism authorized medical care for monastics; held lay doctors in high esteem; and taught *parittas*, contemplations, and other remedies to combat or alleviate the suffering of illness. Later forms of Mahāyāna and Tantric Buddhism seem to take for granted that it is possible to eradicate illnesses through their expanded repertoires of Buddhist practices. Seeking to do so was considered advisable, even a required part of the process of enlightenment.

Modern secularized and medicalized Buddhists continue to make claims about Buddhism's medical efficacy today, promising a litany of health benefits from the practice of mindfulness and other Buddhist-inspired practices. Of course, Buddhist traditions past and present have differed in their recommendations, each offering its own opinions concerning the best therapeutic treatments for various diseases. However, two positions have persisted across sectarian divides and across time. On one hand, the sick body has always been for Buddhists something of a heuristic device: an object of contemplation used to develop insights into deeper truths about the impermanence of human life and to cultivate acceptance in the face of the inevitability of suffering. On the other hand, the sick body has always also been a site of inquiry and experimentation for the development of a range of contemplative, ritual, and material therapeutics. These two seemingly contradictory sides of the Buddhist response to illness have produced a certain level of ongoing tension, which can be observed informing Buddhists' reflections upon and experiences of illness across cultures throughout history.

## BUDDHIST BODIES

In Nikāya and Mahāyāna texts, the ordinary unenlightened human body is a source of much dissatisfaction and suffering.[5] In Nikāya Buddhism, the body is thought of as a prison to be escaped. In Mahāyāna, the body is seen as a vehicle that allows bodhisattvas to use skillful means to benefit others. In both cases, however, the body is often described as unrefined and unclean, or even defiled.[6]

Some authors call particular attention to the repulsive nature of the body's various excretions, fluids, and organs, characterizing the body as riddled with illness and filth {1: 6§4}. Various texts prescribe visualizations that heighten practitioners' awareness of these putrid bodily defilements. For example, they often encourage contemplation of a host of parasites or worms (Skt. *kṛmi*) infesting every nook and cranny of the body, sapping its strength and causing disease.[7] Such "meditations on impurities" (Skt. *aśubhabhāvanā*) are said to evoke a distaste for the sensual pleasures of the body and detachment from the allures of the physical form.

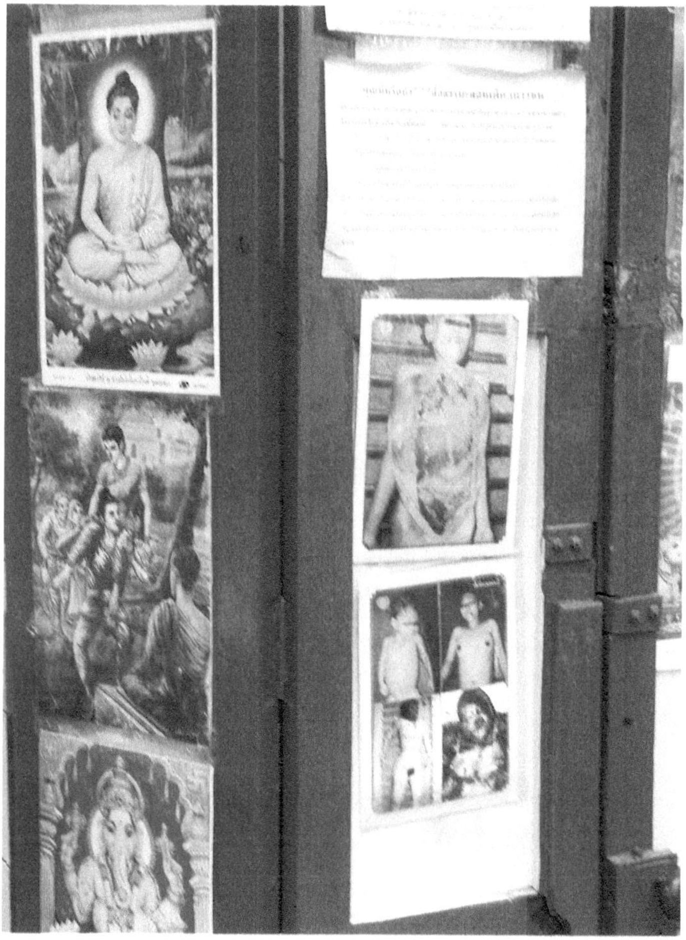

**4.1** Along with the devotional images and meditation aids in a Bangkok poster shop, gruesome scenes of accident victims are sold as reminders of the impermanence and loathsomeness of the human body.
Photo by the author.

There is an obvious gendered dimension to traditional Buddhist discourses on disgust. If all unenlightened bodies are repellent, female bodies are often considered especially so. Intensely negative portrayals of female anatomy and physiology are rampant in historical texts, appearing virtually any time topics such as sexuality, menstruation, conception, gestation, or childbirth are mentioned.[8] For example, Buddhist *sūtras* describing the week-by-week development of the fetus in Sanskrit, Chinese, and Tibetan characterize the womb as a place of filth and stench {1: 5}.[9] Other *sūtras* refer to the female sexual organs as "a dead pig's uterus," "a bag of excrement," or "horse intestines."[10] Modern texts often continue to connect female bodily processes with defilement; for example, when trying to dissuade practitioners from smoking, Buddhist teachers have described tobacco as the defiling product of a demoness's spilled menstrual blood {2: 8}. Such attitudes fit with and contribute to the generally misogynistic treatment of women across the Buddhist tradition, particularly by predominantly male monastic authorities.[11] Despite a few notable moments of inclusion, this type of sexist rhetoric has been a common feature of most forms of Buddhism throughout history.

At the same time that ordinary bodies are characterized in such negative ways, the bodies of enlightened beings are often viewed as clean and pure. The Buddha himself is often said to have had a special body adorned with a number of unusual features (webbed digits, golden-hued skin, and a protuberance on his crown, among other things) that visibly marked him as a "great man" (Skt. *mahāpuruṣa*).[12] Adept members of the sangha are also often said to have developed special bodies that mark them as particularly wise or enlightened. For example, one popular medieval Chinese story tells of the Central Asian monk Fotucheng, whose intestines could be removed through a hole in his abdomen and washed in water. Once cleansed, they shone light by which the monk could read scripture at night.[13] Such details closely connect spiritual advancement with bodily purification.

Tantric texts differ from Nikāya and Mahāyāna texts in that they often reverse the usual rhetoric of repulsion and disgust by expressing an appreciation for the beauty, sensuality, and even sexuality of the ordinary human body. Some of the very aspects of the body that were for other Buddhists emblematic of pollution—for example, menstrual blood, sexual fluids, and excrement—became parts of the sacred rites and antinomian symbolic imagery of Tantra.

Regardless of how they see the body, miraculous physical transformation and spontaneous healing are featured across virtually all Buddhist traditions. These are not just things of the past but continue to play a role in modern Buddhism. Many contemporary Buddhists consider it possible for certain monks to transform their bodies through ardent asceticism and deep meditation to the point of preventing decomposition upon death.[14] Claims of miraculous signs also accompany the death of Buddhist masters, in tribute to their spiritual attainments.[15] The bodies of *tāntrikas* at the highest levels of cultivation are said to be so pure that they are transformed into light. This so-called rainbow body (Tib. *jalü*) is a visible confirmation of the adept's achievement of ultimate wisdom, representing the highest level of refinement by altogether transcending the corporeal body.

As discussed in chapter 3, bodily transformation in Tantric Buddhism is normally done through complex visualizations, deity identification, internal alchemy, sexual yoga, and other subtle body practices. However, it is also a common expression of the nondual philosophy of emptiness to say that the normal body is perfect just the way it is, defilements and all. The notion that every human body is sacred is thus one of the basic concepts of Tantra.[16]

In fact, many contemporary Buddhist groups say that bodily perfection is not about actual physical transmutation but rather shifting one's attitude or perception toward one's body. The body's cellular or genetic structure, for example, may be perceived as an expression of Buddha Nature that is perfect in and of itself {2: 11}. Likewise, in some of the most common contemporary therapeutic meditation protocols, participants are taught to develop an accepting and loving stance toward their physical imperfections as part of psychological healing.

Generally speaking, it is a truism in Buddhism that the more virtuous and wise one is, the more perfect one's body becomes or the more perfect one's body is perceived as being.[17] This juxtaposition of the shortcomings of the ordinary body with the possibility of its perfection through Buddhist practice has provided a productive ground for the development of many healing rituals and ideas throughout Buddhist history. It continues to offer devotees "tools to think with" today.

## THE HEALING POWERS OF ENLIGHTENMENT

Across Buddhist traditions, the possibility of bodily transformation has not always meant that all enlightened people are impervious to disease. Nikāya Buddhist texts speak frankly about the illnesses that afflicted the Buddha at various points during his lifetime. Although the Pāli Canon states that he was generally healthy, it also mentions that he experienced headaches, backaches, injuries, a case of the *doṣas*, and other complaints.[18]

As recounted in the *Sūtra on the Great Liberation* (Pāli *Mahāparinibbāṇa sutta*), the Buddha was able to foretell the time and place of his death and to forestall it for several months. Nevertheless, in the end, he became ill and died after eating a kind of food called "pig's delight" (*sūkaramaddava*, generally considered to have been either a toxic mushroom or spoiled pork flesh).[19] For the devout, the moment of the Buddha's *parinirvāṇa* (literally "full cessation") signifies his complete and final liberation from the long chain of rebirths and his ultimate victory over karmic ensnarement. However, the narrative of the Buddha's death also has provided something of a script for the ideal way for the sick to die, with clarity and peace of mind. Rising above bodily pain, and without succumbing to despair, the Buddha spent his last moments on Earth quietly teaching the Dharma and meditating.

In contrast to this Nikāya Buddhist vision, Mahāyāna traditions have tended to see the Buddha and other enlightened beings as altogether different from ordinary humans. With superhuman bodies whose physical form can be changed at will, they are impervious to disease and able to vanquish the illnesses of others with the wave of a hand or a single-syllable mantra. The story of the Buddha's death, as reimagined in the Mahāyāna version of the *Sūtra on the Great Emancipation* (Skt. *Mahāparinirvāṇa sūtra*), speaks of the Buddha's true body as being made of indestructible adamant that is immortal and unsullied by disease.[20] While it appears that the Buddha is sick and dying, he is in fact simply "manifesting" the illness as an expedient charade to teach a higher truth. The deeper teaching in this case is the Buddha's transcendence of the limitations of physical embodiment.

This depiction is in harmony with the Mahāyāna doctrine that buddhas and bodhisattvas have multiple bodies. The ordinary fleshly body that appears on Earth represents a mere manifestation, while the deity's perfect and eternal "truth body" (Skt. *dharmakāya*) exists beyond ordinary space and time.[21] Enlightened beings frequently are depicted as being able to transform their manifestations at will, appearing in any form they wish. They sometimes mask their divine status behind decrepit or sick bodies only to reveal their true identities at a dramatic moment {1: 22}. The plotline of one of the most popular Mahāyāna *sūtras*, the *Vimalakīrti Sūtra* (Skt. *Vimalakīrti-nirdeśa sūtra*), revolves around the enlightened character Vimalakīrti, who feigns an illness to teach an assembly of bodhisattvas, gods, and monastics about the ultimate truth of the Emptiness of all illnesses.[22]

Whether enlightened beings and deities have the ability to heal themselves, Buddhist devotees across the globe have continually reached out to them for help in times of need. Mahāyāna bodhisattvas such as Avalokiteśvara routinely show up in narratives to conquer disease with a minimum of effort. Adept monks and nuns have also frequently been credited with awe-inspiring healing powers. Powerful Tantric practitioners such as the Tibetan hero Padmasambhava are said to be able to exert control over the phenomenal world and effortlessly overcome illness and even death through ritual manipulation. The spirit of Jīvaka, the Buddha's doctor, is regularly invoked in Thailand to heal illness or empower healing practice {2: 16}.[23] In Myanmar, Buddhist "wizards" (Br. *weikza*) representing deified individuals, historical and legendary, are called upon by the faithful for divine intervention {2: 19, 31}. Objects associated with such individuals are thought to exude healing powers by virtue of having been in contact with them {2: 34}.

Of course, some contemporary practitioners would object to these beliefs as superstitious "hocus-pocus."[24] But, even self-described secular Buddhists often value a blessing from the Dalai Lama or other Buddhist figures and may express the feeling that a set of *mālā* beads from a particular temple is "lucky" or "healing." With such a rich well of Buddhist doctrine and lore to draw upon, ongoing conversation about the relationship between enlightenment and illness is to be expected. Like the other dilemmas or open questions mentioned throughout this chapter, this has been over the centuries a fruitful area for much philosophical exploration, doctrinal innovation, and hearty disagreement.

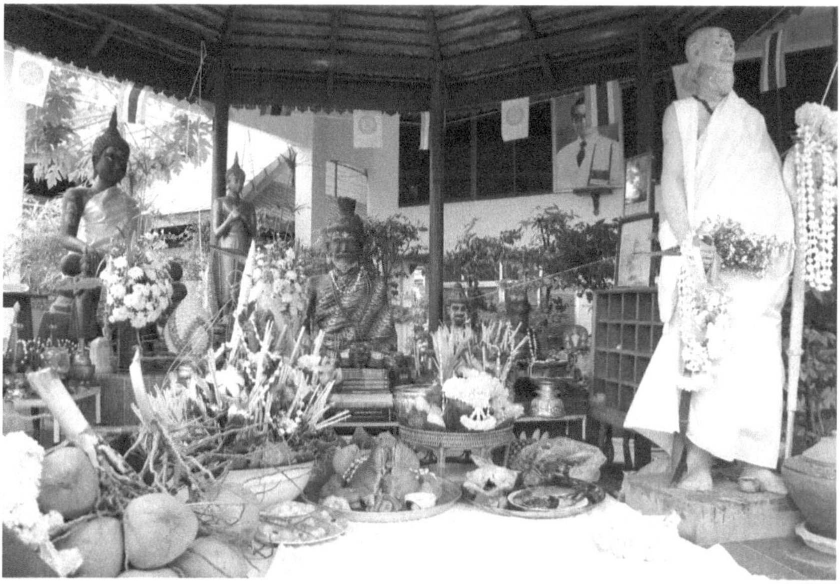

**4.2** An elaborate altar at a traditional medicine hospital and school in Chiang Mai, Thailand, where patients and practitioners pray for Jīvaka to empower medical procedures. The altar is festooned with offerings before an "honoring the teacher" (*wai khru*) ritual.
Photo by the author.

## KARMA'S ROLE IN HEALTH AND ILLNESS

Karma is a controversial doctrine for secular modern Buddhists, whose scientific understanding of the world does not allow for the acceptance of rebirth as literally true. For most Buddhists throughout history and around the world, however, karma has been and continues to be one of the most important areas of inquiry related to health and illness. Why is it that people get sick? Buddhists have routinely turned to the concept of karma to answer this question. Predictably, they have understood this doctrine in different ways.[25]

At the most abstract level, most Buddhists throughout history would have acknowledged karma as the ultimate cause of all of the physical conditions one experiences in a lifetime. As unenlightened beings, we do not have a buddha body or enjoy complete command over the physical realm. As we continue to be trapped in *saṃsāra*, the seemingly endless karmic cycles of birth and death, we repeatedly are born into material bodies inevitably plagued by myriad problems and insufferable ailments. Many Buddhist texts more explicitly connect the strength, shape, and resilience of our bodies in a particular lifetime to the karma we generated in previous lives. Negative karmic accumulations result in various disfigurements or disabilities, physical or mental illnesses, bodily weakness, and vulnerability to premature death {1: 18§2}.[26] Positive karmic merits, on the other hand, result in physical beauty, robust health, and long, relatively pain-free lives {1: 8}.

In addition to these more general ways that karma influences one's health, it can also be more directly involved in causing specific instances of illness. However, not all illnesses are directly caused by karma in this way. In one passage from the Pāli Canon, the Buddha is challenged by an ascetic espousing precisely that view. The Buddha acknowledges that some ailments are indeed directly caused by karma. But he insists that others are caused by Bile, Phlegm, Wind, the combination of the three, the seasons, "uneven care of the body," and harsh treatment {1: 1§1}.[27] Many narratives from across the Buddhist world likewise depict the illnesses of the Buddha, eminent monks, and other adepts and heroes as having no direct connection with karma.[28]

At the same time, Buddhist doctrine also postulates that the effects of one's faulty actions can directly manifest in one's body, exhibiting the same qualities as the initial fault. For example, early narratives of the Buddha's physical ailments often characterize them as directly resulting from karmic misdeeds in past lives or from rivalries, feuds, or antagonisms between the Buddha and other people that recurred over many lifetimes.[29] In one passage, for example, the Buddha is said to have suffered from diarrhea as a result of having in a previous life as a doctor wrongly prescribed a laxative to a patient out of greed for payment.[30]

This so-called boomerang karma can also be a force leading to positive outcomes. Certain *sūtras* say that good health and a strong, attractive body can be achieved by means of medically oriented merit-making. The *Bathhouse Sūtra* (Ch. *Wenshi jing*), for example, promises concrete health rewards for those who donate bathhouses for the promotion of the sangha's health and hygiene {1: 8}. As mentioned in chapter 1, the Buddha's good digestion is said to have resulted from his

4.3 A wooden plaque inscribed with a passage from the *Bathhouse Sūtra* adorns a wall in a modern bathhouse in downtown Seoul. This treatise on the karmic and health benefits of donating bathing supplies to the sangha was translated into Chinese in the early medieval period {2: 8}.

Photo by the author.

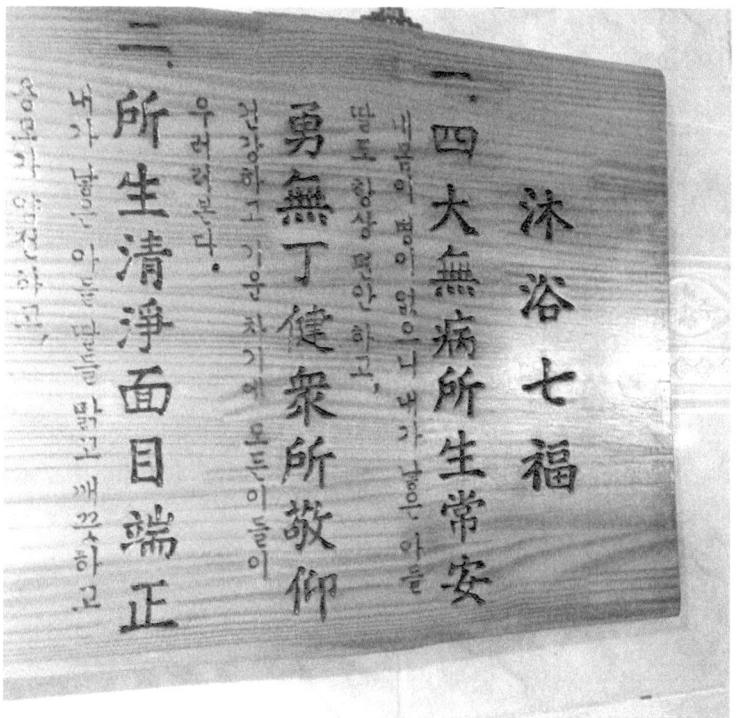

reincarnating as a medicinal fish and feeding himself to the public in a previous life. Such connections between karma and health continue to be drawn today by many Buddhists the world over, who continue to argue that good health is directly tied to the intentional cultivation of ethical and generous behavior {2: 14}.

Another consequence of this belief is that, because of the ever-present dangers of karmic retribution, Buddhists often feel that maintaining good health means being constantly vigilant against incurring karmic faults. General morality—especially adhering to the five precepts (*pañcaśīlāni*; i.e., abstaining from killing, stealing, sexual misconduct, lying, and intoxication)—is seen as crucial for one's health {1: 44}. In some, but by no means all, Buddhist societies, moral expectations also have included vegetarianism {2: 14}.[31] However, even in the strictest traditions, frequent exceptions to prohibitions against meat or alcohol have been made for the sick insofar as were medically necessary.

Buddhists in various cultures have often interpreted illnesses impossible to treat with current medical technologies as being karmic in origin {1: 56}. Since these illnesses lie beyond the reach of conventional medicine, they are impossible to cure without direct intervention by higher powers. In different historical settings, different disease categories have been especially associated with karmic retribution. Historical *sūtras* most often mention a disease called *kuṣṭha*. Commonly translated as "leprosy," but involving a complex cluster of ailments that do not correspond to any one biomedical condition, these incurable, disfiguring skin conditions were often understood to be the direct result of slandering the Dharma or committing other egregious offenses.[32] Today, many Buddhists likewise feel that incurable cancers are karmic diseases {2: 14}.

Nikāya Buddhist texts usually stress that, once negative karma is accumulated, individuals—even the Buddha himself—must live out its effects. However, narratives from across the Buddhist world often suggest that the abrogation of past karma and the spontaneous curing of illness are indeed possible. In Nikāya Buddhism, this normally happens through the intervention of some kind of spirit or god (Skt. *deva*), though occasionally the Buddha himself plays a role.[33] For Mahāyānists, who much more readily accept the omnipotence of enlightened beings' powers over the phenomenal world, divine intervention is much more frequent and accessible. While a host of deities are thought to be waiting to assist the faithful when called upon, Bhaiṣajyaguru is particularly propitiated for karmic illness because he is seen as the remover of karmic obstacles of last resort {1: 20}. Finally, for *tāntrikas*, who work to acquire the powers of the deities for themselves, the ability to cleanse karmic stains is said to be one of the benefits of advanced Buddhist practice. Tales of the celebrated hero Nāgārjuna, famous for his healing powers, say that he once healed a farmer of a goiter on his neck.[34] Although the goiter had been caused by past karma, Nāgārjuna taught the farmer to use the mandala of the *Tantra of the Secret Community* (*Guhyasamāja tantra*) to gain control over his karmic fate and thus eradicate the illness.

Both the general role of karma in health and its specific role in boomerang karma and karmic illnesses continue to be widely accepted across the Buddhist world. If we wish to make a generalization, we might safely say that in Buddhist thought karma tends to provide the preconditions for illness—that is, it is the reason one is reborn into a physical body with particular weaknesses and propensities for certain ailments. Although it is thus the ultimate reason we must suffer from illness, karma is only the proximal cause of some ailments. Working out the details of the role of karma in particular instances of illness, establishing what those karmic faults might be, and determining how to remedy the situation are thus open questions that have been, and continue to be, important areas for discussion and analysis for Buddhists.

## MENTAL VERSUS PHYSICAL HEALTH

The relationship between mind and body is a complex area of Buddhist doctrine that has been the subject of centuries of sustained investigation, explication, and debate. With a few prominent exceptions, most schools of thought have understood the mind (*nāma*) and the body (*rūpa*) as separate, though interrelated, things {1: 6}.[35] Once we move past that basic starting point, however, we find that the mind, the body, and the connection between them has been understood quite differently. There is no way to do the entire subject justice in this short section. However, for our present purposes, it is important to mention that a prominent commonality between virtually all forms of Buddhism is that they find the cause of physical disease to lie at least partially in the mind.

Buddhists have generally identified unwholesome or agitated mental states as causes of ailments both mental and physical. Conversely, they have tended to hold that positive mental states positively affect one's overall health and vitality. Even when these connections are not elaborately explained, the assumption that mind and body are interrelated in this way is often at work in the background.

This is the logic behind narratives of the Buddha and his disciples being cured of illnesses through contemplating the Awakening Factors {1: 2}, for example, and of sick people being cured through the happiness they experience upon hearing the confidence in a skilled doctor's voice {1: 4}.

Monastic authors and other writers in various Buddhist cultures across historical epochs have worked to understand and elaborate these mind-body connections more precisely {1: 6§1, 7; 2: 2, 5, 32}. As discussed in chapter 1, a connection commonly made in earlier texts is a parallelism between the *tridoṣa* and the three "mental poisons." In the standard version of this formulation, the mental poison of greed or craving (Skt. *rāga*) aggravates defects of the mind and body related to Wind, anger or hatred (Skt. *dveṣa*) aggravates Bile, and ignorance or delusion (Skt. *moha*) aggravates Phlegm.

A different theory, common in Mahāyānic and Tantric Buddhist writings, relates the mind and body via the Wind Element. Because Winds of various types are agents linking the physical and mental, they are healing if properly harnessed but can cause madness, physical disease, and even spontaneous death if not. A countless variety of therapies for managing the Winds and preventing Wind illnesses have consequently been developed within diverse Buddhist circles {1: 41–43}. In modern contexts, theories of the Winds are often connected with, compared with, or translated into modern psychological language, and their management is sometimes even called "Buddhist psychiatry" {2: 32}.[36]

The basic premise of all of these correlations is that too much of a negative mental state will cause imbalances in both mental and physical health. Conversely, Buddhist practices designed to overcome undesirable habits of mind can lead to long-term mental and physical health. This is one major reason meditation is so often seen by Buddhists as benefitting health and well-being. Texts from across traditions have for centuries attributed concrete therapeutic effects to all manner of contemplative practices (e.g., {1: 36–43, 2: 20–24, 27, 35}). Many of these texts prescribe specific visualizations, words, or other objects of meditation that target particular ailments. The proliferation of healing meditations notwithstanding, "meditation illness" (Ch. *chanbing*) has also been a widely recognized phenomenon. This category includes mental instabilities and physical disorders that can result from improper or excessive meditation practice {1: 36–38}. Given these dangers, Buddhist traditions often have considered the serious practice of meditation to be safe only for renunciants living in controlled environments practicing under direct supervision.

As I will discuss in chapter 8, lay involvement in meditation has become much more significant in the modern era. Today, scientific research affirms that certain types of Buddhist-inspired meditation practice can play a beneficial role in mental health and well-being. This proposition has become mainstream enough that even some Western governments have begun adopting meditation into national health-care policies {2: 22}. As will be discussed in chapter 9, however, some meditation researchers are beginning to point out potentially harmful side effects, indicating that "meditation illness" is an empirically verifiable phenomenon.[37]

Although there is certainly much that is new about the incorporation of scientific research into these debates, the question of the health benefits and risks of meditation—which has become so salient today thanks to the "mindful revolution"—is not necessarily a novel dilemma of the twenty-first century. Rather, this is the latest manifestation of a millennia-long investigation that continues to unfold. Today, as in previous eras, there is no single position that all Buddhists accept defining the relationship between mind and body or how one might influence the other. However, it is safe to say that learning to use these interrelationships for healing purposes has been one of the most prominent features of Buddhist medicine in all times and places.

## MEDICAL ETHICS

Medical ethics is another area of perennial concern and discussion for Buddhists. As mentioned in previous chapters, Buddhist literature has introduced various idealized physicians who have served as role models for the ethical behavior of lay and monastic healers. In the Nikāya tradition, Jīvaka has played this role {1: 1§4, 20}.[38]

Jīvaka is a complex character. While he is adopted into the king's family and treated like a son, the various versions of his biography say that he was either the son of a courtesan or the product of an illicit affair. In classical times, this would have meant that both his lineage and caste status were suspect. On top of his dubious origin, all of the extant versions of Jīvaka's biography depict him using trickery and lies in the process of curing patients. He deceives powerful kings, and in the Sanskrit version of the tale, even his own teacher. In one story separate from his biography, Jīvaka makes a moving automaton in the form of a beautiful woman out of medicinal substances.[39] He then allows patients to have sex with his creation to cure them of certain conditions. The intentions behind all of these narrative elements seem to be to make clear that a lay doctor is not held to the same standards of conduct as a monastic. He can freely break even some of Buddhism's most fundamental moral precepts when he knows that his actions will achieve the higher purpose of healing.[40]

However, even if the ideal physician is not required to be rigorously honest, he is expected to be exceedingly generous. In the Pāli version of the narrative, Jīvaka starts his career as a rather selfish character concerned only with earning his fee.[41] By the end of the story, he has accumulated great wealth from his medical practice, which he uses to heap lavish gifts upon his adoptive family. He becomes famed in Buddhist literature as a great lay donor, giving clothes and even donating his mango grove as a place for the sangha to live during the rainy season. Jīvaka is particularly noted for giving gifts that promote the health of the monastic community, and he is repeatedly applauded for the enormous karmic merit he has thereby accumulated {1: 8}. All of these acts are important precedents that set forth the parameters for the moral behavior of physicians in Buddhist societies.

In contrast to Jīvaka, whose goals are largely limited to earning a living and earning merit by serving the monastic community, idealized Mahāyānic doctors are called to the medical profession by their desire to promote the health of all sentient beings. Perhaps the most iconic doctor in Mahāyāna literature is the young bodhisattva Jalavāhana, from the *Sūtra of Golden Light*, who takes over his father's practice when he witnesses intense suffering during a severe epidemic {1: 4}. Another model healer, the sagacious Samantanetra from the *Sūtra of the Entry Into the Realm of Reality* (*Gaṇḍavyūha sūtra*), is a compounder of aromatics in the marketplace {1: 9}. The operation of his stall, immersed in the hustle and bustle of commerce and society, is the ideal setting for him to reach the masses with the compassion and skillful means of a bodhisattva.

When writing down their thoughts on medical ethics, physicians across Asia have often been inspired by the Mahāyāna value of compassion for all beings. The celebrated late seventh-century Chinese physician Sun Simiao, for example, while not avowedly Buddhist himself, was obviously inspired by Buddhist notions of compassion, universality, and nonviolence in his advice to aspiring physicians {1: 53}. His declaration on medical ethics is commonly referred to among Western practitioners of Chinese medicine today as the "Chinese Hippocratic Oath." This same ethos can be seen in action today when, for example, the fourteenth Dalai

Lama's physician called for more compassion in the modern medical system in an interview with PBS,[42] or when Buddhists draw upon Buddhist values to call for universal health care and more enlightened models of medicine.[43]

Closely related to the ethos of compassion, Buddhists have historically valued the free distribution of medical knowledge, care, and resources to the population at large. The Mauryan king Aśoka (304–232 BCE) is much celebrated in Buddhist narratives as a model of royal generosity, and care for the sick is an important theme in stories about him.[44] In another vein, Buddhist donors in medieval China inscribed one of the grottoes at Longmen (modern-day Henan Province) with dozens of common medicinal recipes, so that they would be preserved for general use in an accessible format {1: 46}. In coming chapters, we will explore the activities of many other historical rulers, foundations, and private individuals.

One of the most trenchant critiques of the contemporary mindfulness movement has been that, in being extracted from the Buddhist ethical system and instead being offered through expensive private training, it has been separated from the central Buddhist values of compassion and non-commercialism in which the meditation practice developed. Many secular contemporary meditators are becoming increasingly cognizant of the importance of integrating ethics into the practice of therapeutic meditation {2: 24}.

Another area of ethical concern that has been important in Buddhism is the relationship between humans and the environment. Because most forms of Buddhism see the body as a microcosm, most Buddhists understand one's health to be constantly affected by the wider world. While the notion of "the environment" is a modern idea, Buddhists have traditionally thought it necessary to regulate oneself in accordance with many environmental factors to maintain optimal health. These have included the Elements, the weather, the seasons, one's immediate surroundings, the seen and unseen beings in one's vicinity, planetary configurations, cosmic energies, and other forces, depending on the tradition. Many forms of Buddhism have advised making changes to one's diet and daily regimen according to the logic of the Great Elements. In East Asian cultures, on the other hand, owing to the processes of localization that will be discussed in chapter 7, such changes would normally be interpreted according to the Chinese logics of *qi*, *yin-yang*, and the Five Phases (*wuxing*) instead. In certain forms of contemporary Buddhism, this understanding of interconnectivity has translated into environmental activism.[45] Modern Buddhists have seen matters of individual health to be intimately tied not only to environmental

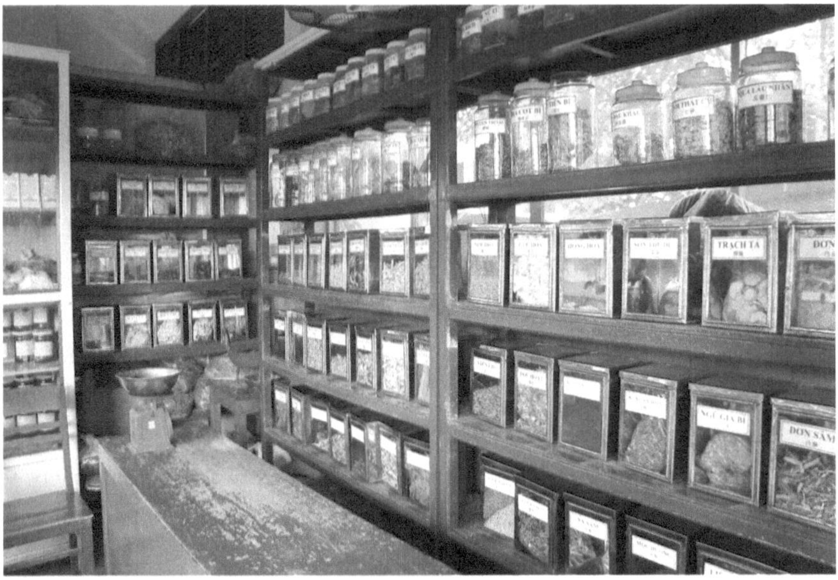

**4.4** Herbal dispensary at the Tuệ Tĩnh đường Hải Đức charitable medical clinic in Hue, Vietnam. Staffed largely by monastics, this facility provides free medical care for the sangha and the surrounding community.
Photo by the author, courtesy of the Jivaka Project (http://jivaka.net), Creative Commons license.

sustainability but also to other contemporary moral issues such as income inequality and social justice.

For many Buddhists, both historically and today, ethics and health concerns have come together around the issue of vegetarianism. Historically, Buddhism's position has been mixed. Abstention from eating meat has been a basic feature of East Asian Mahāyāna since the medieval period, mostly a nonissue for Nikāya Buddhists, and hotly debated throughout Tibetan history.[46] Contemporary authors have connected vegetarianism with health benefits, using both modern nutritional arguments and karmic arguments for why eating animals leads to ill health {2: 14}.[47]

Throughout history, Buddhists have expressed opinions and formulated responses to questions of medical ethics by drawing from the full range of Buddhist teachings and practices.[48] They have continued to weigh in on contemporary health-care debates—including the most fraught issues in bioethics today, such as abortion, euthanasia, cloning, and organ donation.[49] They have connected individual human health with larger ethical concerns in many ways but have not always agreed on the specifics of what ethical health-care practice should look like. Because of this diversity of opinions, the Buddhist tradition offers a rich trove of resources for thinking about the ethics of health care in a variety of cultural and historical settings.

* * *

This chapter has introduced several areas of doctrinal inquiry that have been focal points for discussion, debate, and development across centuries and spanning significant cultural divides. These questions have not only been key in shaping Buddhist discourses and texts throughout history but also have affected Buddhist social realities. How different Buddhist communities have answered these questions has in no small part influenced their health-care practices, organizations, and social movements. They have influenced the formation of government health-care services and institutions in Buddhist societies, and they have informed Buddhists' understandings of their bodies in sickness and health. While the more recent trends of modernization and globalization (discussed in chapters 8 and 9) have introduced a gamut of new issues, the six themes discussed here have continued to drive Buddhist engagement with medicine in the modern and contemporary periods. All of these topics remain relevant open questions today for Buddhists across the world, who would undoubtedly agree that they are extremely important to discuss and debate, even if they may answer them in markedly different ways.

## FURTHER READING

Bronkhorst, Johannes. 2011. *Karma*. Honolulu: University of Hawai'i Press. A short book providing a detailed history of the concept of karma in Indian religions, comparing Buddhist uses of the notion with those of Jainism and Brahmanism.

Keown, Damien. 1995. *Buddhism and Bioethics*. New York: Palgrave Macmillan. An application of Buddhist ethics to contentious contemporary bioethical issues concerning the beginning and end of life (e.g., birth control, abortion, death, euthanasia).

Langenberg, Amy Paris. 2017. *Birth in Buddhism: The Suffering Fetus and Female Freedom*. Abingdon-on-Thames: Routledge. An analysis of gender discourses in Indian Buddhism based on the study of Buddhist accounts of gestation and birth.

Mrozik, Susanne. 2007. *Virtuous Bodies: The Physical Dimensions of Morality in Buddhist Ethics*. New York: Oxford University Press. An exploration of the Buddhist doctrine that karma affects the health, beauty, and longevity of the physical body.

Siderits, Mark. 2015. *Buddhism as Philosophy: An Introduction*. Aldershot, Hampshire, UK: Ashgate. A readable general introduction to Buddhist philosophy.

# PART II

# *Historical Currents and Transformations*

## CHAPTER 5

# *Circulations*

The first part of this book introduced the basic medical orientations, doctrines, practices, and questions that developed in the context of the three main forms of Buddhism. The second part now turns to tracing their circulation, development, and transformation over the last two millennia. Since Buddhism spread throughout Asia, and eventually globally, it is impossible to cover every detail of the history here. Rather, each of the following chapters will present a specific lens that will illuminate macro-level processes. Throughout, I will use examples or case studies drawn from current scholarship to illustrate how these larger processes played out in specific times and places.

We begin our investigation with an overview of the circulation of Buddhist medicine in Asia in the premodern period. Buddhism was one of the most important catalysts for the cross-cultural exchange of medical knowledge in that period. Despite the fact that medicine rarely receives much attention in general accounts of the history of Buddhism—and despite the even greater dearth of Buddhism in general histories of medicine—the spread of Buddhism played a fundamental role in the circulation of medical ideas and practices across a huge swathe of territory, from Persia to Japan and from Mongolia to Java.

## NETWORKS AND NODES

If the traditional accounts are to be believed, the transmission of Buddhism within the Indian subcontinent had already begun during the lifetime of the Buddha.[1] The Buddha is said to have instructed his followers to fan out and spread the Dharma across the land. In the centuries following, Buddhism's expansion was supposedly assisted by King Aśoka, who ruled over a large territory in northern India in the third century BCE.[2] Legend says that Aśoka both adopted Buddhism personally and dispatched the first missionaries to take the religion beyond India to neighboring lands. While these details may or may not be accurate, we know that Buddhism did come to be established in Sri Lanka as early as the third century BCE. Archaeological evidence from modern-day Afghanistan, Pakistan, Tajikistan, and Uzbekistan also attests to vibrant Buddhist cultures in those parts of the world in the last centuries BCE and the first few centuries CE.

The relative isolation of the western and eastern halves of Eurasia came to an end at around this time, as well, with the emergence of the Silk Road and Indian Ocean maritime routes as arteries of cross-continental trade. From this point onward, kingdoms across the Eurasian landmass came to be increasingly interconnected. As people, goods, and institutions began to move more freely between India, Southeast Asia, and East Asia, Buddhism began to spread along those trade routes as well.[3] The first records of Buddhism arriving in China date from as early as the first century CE. It was flourishing among Iranian peoples in Central Asia, along the Silk Road, and in the Tarim Basin by the second century.[4] It had also arrived in Vietnam by the second century.[5] It was introduced to Korea in the fourth century, to mainland Southeast Asia around 500 CE, to Japan in the sixth century, and to Tibet in the seventh.

Different forms of Buddhism flourished within these diverse cultural, linguistic, and political spheres, and these differences related to both local and regional factors. Nikāya Buddhism developed mainly in Sri Lanka and mainland Southeast Asia, although also in certain city oases along the northern route of the Silk Road. Mahāyāna was predominant elsewhere along the Silk Road and in East Asia, including in Vietnam. Tantra flourished in the Himalayas and Japan, as well in kingdoms located in modern-day Cambodia and Indonesia.

Ironically, the new interconnections across Eurasia also contributed to the spread of epidemics, plagues, and other diseases, as a result of the increased mobility of people and goods.[6] Disease was thus both the product of, and stimulus for, cross-cultural exchanges of medical ideas and practices. In other words, Buddhism, disease, healing, and cross-cultural exchange came to be entangled in a self-reinforcing feedback loop.

Many of the aspects of Buddhist medicine discussed in the first part of this book were well ensconced within Buddhist texts, practices, and institutions by the time these began to spread outside India. Wherever Buddhism went, Indian medical ideas and practices went along for the ride. Over time, Buddhist notions of health, disease, and the body were translated into many new languages, introduced to many new cultures, and incorporated into many new social contexts and political regimes. However, as we will explore in more detail in the next chapter, the reception and development of Buddhist medicine abroad, like Buddhism itself, were shaped by local processes of adaptation, localization, and translation.

When discussing the patterns of cross-cultural exchange, certain ways of modeling the process may be more helpful than others. Speaking in terms of "flow" encourages us to think of Buddhism as a liquid that moved freely across the land, indiscriminately swallowing up or inundating whatever stood in its path. "Transmission," on the other hand, might evoke an image of India broadcasting messages, as though by telegraph or email, that traveled in direct lines and were straightforwardly received in other parts of Asia. In fact, the cross-cultural circulation of Buddhist knowledge cannot be characterized as either amorphous free-flows or direct point-to-point communications. A better metaphor might be that the crosscultural movements of Buddhism constituted a network with distinct nodes, between which specific packets of information circulated. Given the fragmentary nature of the sources available to us, we must accept that we do not have a crystal-clear picture of the totality of this network. But historians know enough that we can begin to describe its contours.

Some nodes in the network of the exchange of Buddhist medical knowledge were major centers of Buddhist learning and pilgrimage across India and the rest of Asia. While medicine was never the sole focus of learning at these nodes, many were renowned for this. One important early example is the city of Taxila (also known as Takṣaśilā), one of the major cities in the region of Gandhāra that flourished from the third century BCE until the fifth century CE. Conquered by Alexander the Great between 327 and 325 BCE, this far northwestern corner of the Indian subcontinent was, in the early Common Era, still ruled by kings with Greek heritage and heavily influenced by Hellenistic culture. This so-called Indo-Greek region, with Gandhāra as its hub, was a major funnel for Mediterranean thought—including ideas of medicine, astronomy, and other sciences—into India.[7]

Taxila looms large in early Buddhist accounts of medicine. It was here that the renowned Buddhist physician Jīvaka, the heroic doctor featured in the *vinayas* and early *sūtras*, was said to have learned the craft of medicine from a "world-famed doctor."[8] While not all versions of the Jīvaka biography name his teacher, some imply that he was Ātreya, the supposed author of *Caraka's Compendium*, the foundational Āyurvedic medical text {1: 20}.[9] We need not take this story literally to understand that Gandhāra in general, and Taxila specifically, were renowned in the ancient period as a confluence point for surgical, medical, and Buddhist learning. Archaeological evidence from Taxila and other sites in the area, including copper surgical instruments and a number of pharmaceutical tools, has underscored the advanced state of medical knowledge in the region.[10]

The nearby sites of Gilgit and Bamiyan were significant too. Multiple copies of the *Bhaiṣajyaguru Sūtra* dating from the sixth or seventh century suggest that these places were important for the development of the Medicine Buddha's cult {1: 25}.[11] Other relevant Gilgit manuscripts include a set of *dhāraṇī* texts that pertain to neutralizing snakebite, healing childhood ailments, protecting pregnancies, and seeking sons, among other benefits.[12]

On the far eastern side of India, perhaps the most important node of Buddhist learning in the world in the first millennium was the "Great Monastery" (*mahāvihāra*) of Nālandā, which flourished from the fifth to twelfth centuries CE in modern-day Bihar.[13] Often referred to as a monastic university, this institution's lecture halls, libraries, and dormitories attracted around three thousand students from across Asia. The curriculum of learning centered on Buddhism but also included the Vedas, Sāṁkhya philosophy, and the so-called Five Sciences, including medicine.

It was at Nālandā that the great scholar Vāgbhaṭa supposedly composed the *Compendium of the Essence of the Eight Branches [of Medicine]* (*Aṣṭāṅgahṛdaya saṃhitā*), below abbreviated as *Essence of the Eight Branches*. This text, which synthesized the major streams of Indian medicine, became widely revered in both Āyurvedic and Buddhist medical traditions. Vāgbhaṭa is also credited with the authorship of a second text, *Treatise on the Eight Branches* (*Aṣṭāṅga saṃgraha*), a longer tome whose content overlaps with and expands upon the *Essence of the Eight Branches*. Both works contain passages that appear to give homage to the Buddha.[14] While these may hint at Vāgbhaṭa's own religious commitments, scholars have long debated the authorship of these texts and caution that very little is known about Vāgbhaṭa as a historical person.[15]

Historians are fortunate that the Chinese Buddhist pilgrim Yijing (635–713 CE) left a detailed account of his experiences while studying at Nālandā. He observed many medical and health-promoting practices undertaken by the monastic residents {1: 16} and seems to have noticed the popularity of the *Essence of the Eight Branches*.[16] Accounts of another nearby monastic center, Vikramaśilā, are also abundant. Flourishing from the first half of the ninth century to the end of the twelfth, this was a renowned location of Tantric learning and a major source of inspiration for the Tibetan tradition.[17]

Beyond the Indian subcontinent, other important nodes emerged along the Tarim Basin, in China, Korea, Japan, Tibet, Sri Lanka, Southeast Asia, and other locations. Such nodes were not constant or permanent features of the network. They came in and out of prominence over the centuries, and their rise and fall shaped and reshaped the network through which Buddhist ideas and practices moved across Asia. I will discuss these locations and developments in more detail throughout this and the next two chapters. For reference, the major sites discussed throughout the book dating from the first millennium are included on the map in figure 5.1.

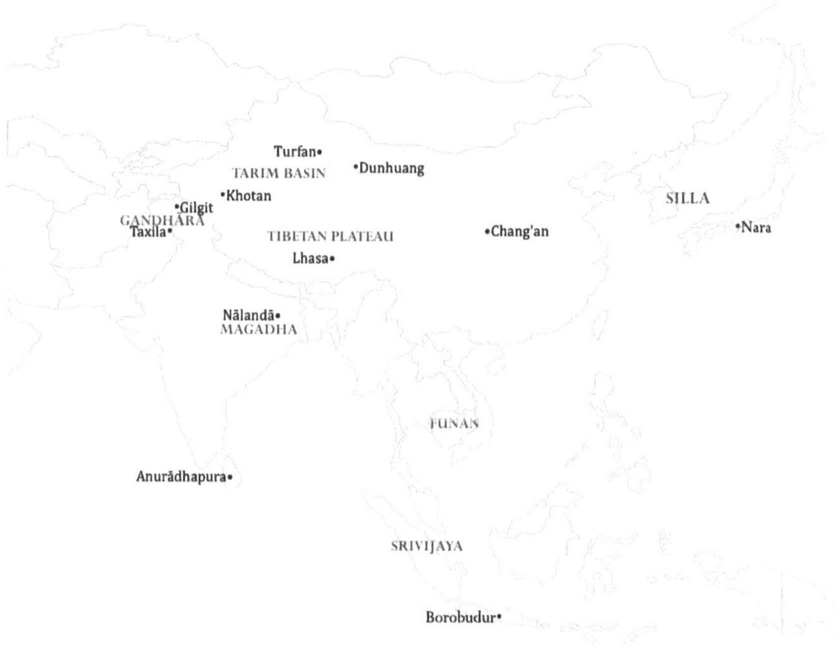


**5.1** Map of important nodes in the network of Buddhist exchanges from the first millennium CE mentioned in this book.

Image by the author.

## OBJECTS OF EXCHANGE

Many details about the circulation of Buddhist medical knowledge through the network cannot be reconstructed from our vantage point in the present, so many mysteries remain. Why does the first mention of the Buddhist subtle body system appear in a mid-fifth century Chinese translation of a text composed in Khotan? Was Tantric healing in part inspired by preexisting Daoist models? What connections did the physical movements of Tibetan yoga have with Thai practices that look quite similar? In the absence of concrete historical evidence, the answers to such questions remain obscure. However, despite the fact that there are a lot of places where our knowledge is incomplete, historians do have a number of concrete data points we can examine. Although scattershot, these records provide hints at the overall patterns of circulation within the network as a whole.

One type of object of exchange is texts, whose circulation will be discussed in detail in the next chapter. From looking at the movement of texts, we can understand certain nodes in the network as "centers of calculation" for medical knowledge.[18] All manner of Buddhist writings were brought from around Asia to the major monasteries in China, Tibet, Japan, and so forth, and a significant percentage of these dealt with health, illness, and the body. At these same nodes, commentators and exegetes labored to systematize, explain, promulgate, put into practice, and otherwise use this new health-related material. Both new translations and new explanations were subsequently compiled and disseminated onward from these locations. These not only circulated domestically but also were exported abroad, where they became objects of further study and veneration in entirely new cultural contexts.

In addition to *sūtras* and other texts that were patently Buddhist, it is also clear that certain medical treatises were circulating widely in Buddhist hands. For example, Vāgbhaṭa's *Essence of the Eight Branches* appears to have been known across the Buddhist world. It was highly influential in India, Sri Lanka, mainland Southeast Asia, Tibet, and parts of Central Asia, where it contributed to the formation of local traditions of Buddhist medicine (see chapter 7). Another notably mobile treatise is the *Tantra of Rāvaṇakumāra*, a text on obstetric and pediatric illnesses of demonic origin, which is available today in Sanskrit, Tamil, Tibetan, Chinese, Khmer, and Arabic.[19]

Medicinal substances were other notable objects circulating throughout the network.[20] Many of the most widely traded medicines and aromatics in Eurasia originated in Buddhist territories. Musk from Tibet was prized in the Middle East and Europe, which played a major role in incorporating the Himalayan region into the transcontinental trade networks.[21] Aromatic medicinals native to Southeast Asia, such as cardamom, nutmeg, turmeric, and zedoary, were also widely sought after.

The movement of these medicinal substances was closely tied to patterns of trade and commerce. Detailed historical records from the capital of Tang dynasty China (618–907), for example, bear witness to the importation of medicinals from Buddhist kingdoms as both imperial tribute and commodities for sale in the city's bustling multiethnic marketplaces.[22] The materia media texts produced in China during this period are replete with foreign substances imported from across the Buddhist world.[23] The Tang emperor, Taizong (r. 626–649 CE), who developed a keen interest in Indian medicine, even sent a group of emissaries to India to the court of King Harṣavardhana (ca. 590–ca. 647 CE) to acquire medicines and seek out a doctor skilled in their use.[24]

While not all of this pharmaceutical trade was associated specifically with Buddhism, Buddhism played a significant role in generating demand for all kinds of spices, aromatics, animal parts, minerals, and magically potent substances considered medicinal. Prominent Buddhist texts called for the ingestion of exotic South Asian plants such as black pepper, cassia, saffron, chinaberry, *gulgulu* (Commiphora wightii), and the three myrobalans: *harītakī*, *āmalaka*, and *vibhītakī* or *bibhātakā* (Terminalia chebula, Phyllanthus emblica, and Terminalia bellirica).[25] The three myrobalans, either taken individually or combined in a famous Indian recipe called the "three fruits" (*triphalā*), were particularly celebrated across the Buddhist world as panaceas for many common ailments {1: 4, 26}. Other texts advocated the use of foodstuffs such as ghee, yoghurt, and sugar common in India but unknown in many parts of Asia before the spread of Buddhism.[26] Exotic substances such as bezoar, sandalwood, coral, and various gemstones were thought to have potent magical properties and were called for in many Buddhist healing rituals {1: 26, 32, 33, 45}.[27]

Demand was further stoked by Buddhist stories that extolled the medicinal power of such items. For example, the biography of the idealized King Aśoka tells of a time that the king lost his wealth and became so poor that all he had left to donate to the sangha was half of a medicinal *āmalaka* fruit.[28] Because of the healing power of this fruit, the merit he earned from this simple gift was enough to propel him back to his former glory. Indian medicinals also frequently appeared in Buddhist iconography; for example, many Tibetan images of Bhaiṣajyaguru depict the all-powerful healer holding a *harītakī* fruit in a bowl, symbolizing its potency and identifying Bhaiṣajyaguru as the lord of medicines.[29]

Buddhists invariably incorporated locally available pharmaceuticals into their rituals and regimens as well. In China, for example, realgar, orpiment, and cinnabar—all of which were celebrated as potent numinous substances by Daoist ritualists and alchemists—became prized ingredients in Buddhist healing {1: 45}. Tea, a plant native to East Asia, became widely used as a stimulant and medicine in Buddhist institutions in that region.[30] In Tibet and Central Asia, butter played a starring role in many healing rituals and visualizations {1: 36}. Native plants and domestic products were convenient substitutes for, or supplements to, the medicinals called for in Indian Buddhist texts. While a rising Buddhist population in any given place stimulated interest in foreign medicines, it also led to an intensification in the cultivation and distribution of prized local products.

Aside from texts and medicines, another critically important object circulating between the nodes of the Buddhist world was people. I have already mentioned the legend of Jīvaka, the physician said to have traveled from his home in Rājagṛha (in the modern-day Indian state of Bihar) across all of northern India to Taxila to study medicine. Stories told about the founding figure of Sowa Rigpa, the doctor Yutok Yönten Gonpo, who will be discussed more in chapter 7, tell of his crossing the Himalayas into India to gain the healing knowledge that contributed so materially to the Tibetan medical tradition.

Narratives and tales from the premodern period depict individuals of Indian, Tibetan, Central Asian, East Asian, and Southeast Asian extraction actively propagating Buddhist medicine around the network {1: 21}.[31] Buddhist monks are frequently said to have attracted fame, fortune, and followers in new lands because of their healing activities. These narratives are characteristically tinged with legendary elements, and we cannot take literally their accounts of wondrous healings. For example, the most famous Korean protagonist, Hyetong, a monk from the Silla kingdom, is said to have heroically cured a princess from an affliction by defeating a dragon {1: 21§9}. Such fantastical details notwithstanding, the fact that such stories circulated widely suggests that itinerant Buddhists were closely associated with healing in the minds of many. The fact that the narratives show healer monks treating commoners, the elite, and members of the royal or imperial family also attests to their wide appeal across the social spectrum.

While narratives are inadmissible as solid evidence of the activities of historical people, the evidence for long-distance travelers is in some cases quite reliable. Over the course of the first millennium, a string of Buddhist pilgrims left travelogues and other records of their journeys around the Buddhist network. These travelers undertook voyages with the intention, they tell us in their own words, of acquiring Buddhist education and texts. By no means did all—or even most—of this transcontinental travel involve medicine. However, extant records suggest that the long-distance movements of the most famous of these monastics and missionaries often contributed materially to the transcontinental circulation of medical ideas, objects, and practices.

The aforementioned Chinese pilgrim Yijing is a prominent example, as his account of his time in India includes a number of chapters detailing Indian monastic practices concerning health, medication, and personal hygiene {1: 16}.[32] Two of Yijing's predecessors, Faxian (337–422 CE) and Xuanzang (602–664 CE), also reported on medical practices and ideas they had encountered during their travels in India.[33] Another celebrated example is the Tibetan monk Rinchen Zangpo (958–1056), who traveled to India as an adolescent to learn Buddhism.[34] He is also credited with making an early translation of Vāgbhaṭa's *Essence of the Eight Branches*.[35]

Such intercontinental travel was multidirectional and did not necessarily always privilege India. Puṇyodaya (fl. mid-seventh century), for example, was a Tantric master from Central India who traveled to study in Sri Lanka, teach in China, and gather texts and medicines in Funan (modern-day Cambodia).[36] The Japanese monk Kūkai (774–835 CE) spent two years in China studying Esoteric Buddhism and brought home the *kaji* empowerment rituals that would become a mainstay of healing ritual practice in Japan into modern times {1: 23}.[37] His contemporary Saichō (767–822 CE), after a similar trip, played a major role in reshaping the Japanese cult of Bhaiṣajyaguru.[38] Several centuries later, in 1385, the Vietnamese Buddhist monk and physician Tuệ Tĩnh (ca. 1330–ca. 1389) was sent by the Vietnamese Trần dynasty, along with nineteen other monks, on a tribute mission to Ming China (1368–1644). When the mission concluded, Tuệ stayed behind, living the rest of his life in China. While far from his homeland, he wrote a guide on Vietnamese medicinals, *Miraculous Drugs of the South* (*Nam dược thần hiệu*), which explained to the Chinese the traditions of "Southern medicine" {1: 57}.[39]

Long-distance travel by members of the sangha appears to have been a strongly gendered phenomenon. From the insistence of the *vinayas* on regulating female healers more stringently than males (as mentioned in chapter 1), one supposes that monastic women may originally have been more involved than men in healing and nursing activities. In later Buddhist history, women continue to appear in medical narratives, being valued as loyal and skilled healers, nurses, caretakers, attendants, or fundraisers {1: 21§5}. However, they tend not to be depicted as magic-wielding workers of healing miracles in their own right, and they are never shown engaged in transcontinental travel.

Aside from monastics, there also were countless numbers of other travelers: merchants, caravan workers, soldiers, itinerant lay healers, and many others. Because these individuals were not attached to durable and politically powerful institutions, their voices were not well preserved in the historical record. However, regardless of whether they left records of their missions, the movements of all of these "go-betweens" throughout the network played a crucial role in translating Buddhist medical knowledge across languages and intemediating between different parts of the Buddhist world.

The concentration of polyglot and multicultural people, both lay and monastic, at nodes such as Taxila, Nālandā, Chang'an, Nara, Lhasa, Dunhuang, and Khotan naturally led to these locations becoming what scholars call "contact zones" or "trading zones." These were places where practitioners of different systems of knowledge and practice met, allowing for much cross-fertilization of ideas.[40] Buddhist monastic complexes at these nodes often included special accommodations in which sick members of the sangha received medical, nursing, and hospice care.[41] As international travel increased, the stunningly diverse backgrounds of the residents no doubt contributed to the cosmopolitanism of the medicine practiced in such spaces.

Of course, there were always more conservative monastic disciplinarians who criticized hybridity, arguing that the sangha should follow closely the "pure" or "original" teachings.[42] However, such appeals are likely to have fallen largely on deaf ears. With the opportunity to combine imported and local therapies, nodes throughout the network became places for experimentation with new medicinals, medical procedures, healing rituals, and other therapeutic approaches.[43] It was Buddhism that provided the institutional spaces in which to experiment and innovate, as well as the motivation to accumulate knowledge of what was efficacious and worthy of being passed on to future generations. Thus, Buddhism was a major reason that this period of Asian history was marked by such medical cosmopolitanism, syncretism, hybridity, and exchange.

## BUDDHIST MEDICAL NETWORKS AND LOCAL POLITICS

The go-betweens discussed in the previous section comprised something of a pan-Asian intelligentsia.[44] Given their willingness to take up positions in foreign lands, many of these mobile individuals likely would have felt stronger allegiance to the Dharma writ large than to any particular local ruler or regime. Nevertheless, the shape and success of the network as a whole inevitably depended on local and regional politics and was subject to the whims and policies of individual rulers. Buddhist medical practitioners and institutions, wherever they were located, were therefore intrinsically motivated to pursue funding and patronage from local rulers, officials, and elites.

Supportive rulers often played a pivotal role in the expansion of the Buddhist network and the birth of new nodes. Legends of King Aśoka, which were known throughout the Buddhist world, had long held him up as a shining example of how a devout Buddhist ruler should take care of his population's needs.[45] The model of "benevolent" or "humane" Dharma kings presented in numerous Mahāyāna and Tantric Buddhist texts also inspired generations of rulers to support Buddhist charitable medical institutions.[46] Historical rulers often strove to live up to these expectations, and Buddhist medical charities often provided attractive opportunities to prove their generosity to their populations. The reputation of a ruler's generosity could spread internationally. The Indian king Harṣavardhana, for example, was described in Chinese reports as a good Buddhist ruler who supported charitable institutions such as dispensaries and "merit halls" (Skt. *puṇyaśālā*) that provided medical care for the poor.[47]

In no small part because of such models, Buddhist medicine enjoyed increasing official support in China throughout the first millennium. The first permanent public hospitals, hospices, and dispensaries for which there is historical record were established in the late fifth and early sixth centuries by Buddhist rulers.[48] Emperor Wen (r. 559–66 CE) of the Chen dynasty (557–589 CE) organized elaborate rituals and vegetarian banquets dedicated to Bhaiṣajyaguru to protect his state from epidemics and other disasters.[49] By the first decade of the eighth century, an empire-wide network of monastic charities—including not only hospitals but also leprosaria, orphanages, hostels for travelers, and care for the elderly and the poor—came under the centralized administrative control of the government bureaucracy.[50] It is not coincidental that the ruler at this time was Empress Wu Zetian (r. 690–705 CE), who mobilized Buddhist ideology—including presenting herself as a reincarnation of the bodhisattva Maitreya—in an effort to legitimize the rule of the empire by a woman.

In the late twelfth century, similar efforts by the Khmer king Jayavarman VII (ca. 1122–1218) involved building a network of 102 "health houses" (*ārogyaśālā*) across his kingdom {1: 24}.[51] Dedicated to Bhaiṣajyaguru, these institutions featured altars with statues of that healing deity flanked by bodhisattvas and adorned with inscriptions and mandalas. The grounds of the health houses included medicinal baths for patients, storehouses for medications and equipment for medical alchemy. Aside from building these institutions, Jayavarman patronized monastic universities where the training of physicians could be undertaken.[52] Jayavarman's efforts to promote medicine in his empire have been interpreted as an integral part of an effort to win over the population, particularly in newly acquired territories in the western part of the kingdom. For Jayavarman, like Empress Wu and many other rulers in medieval Asia, it was essential to his political career that he portray himself as a generous and devout ruler through his support for Buddhist medicine.

Not only did rulers build Buddhist medical institutions but they also hired Buddhist specialists to conduct protection or healing rites for the royal family, organize empowerment rites for armies, and protect their realms from epidemics. Jayavarman, for example, supported cults dedicated to Bhaiṣajyaguru and Avalokiteśvara in an effort to ritually prevent epidemics from harming his newly expanded realm. In eighth-century Japan, the emperor retained the Tantric specialist Kūkai to cure his intractable illnesses {1: 23}. Buddhist ritual specialists also presided over the birth of the Japanese imperial heir in the twelfth century {1: 32}. Opportunities for employment by ruling families meant that something like an international job market existed for especially qualified healer monks. Specialists were often "headhunted" by rulers, enticed to move across the continent with lavish gifts and opportunities for power.

Tantric Buddhist healing methods also received official support among Khitans and Tanguts in Central Asia in the Liao (916–1125) and Xixia (1038–1227) dynasties. In the thirteenth century, these territories were absorbed by the Mongols, who went on to establish the largest land empire in world history

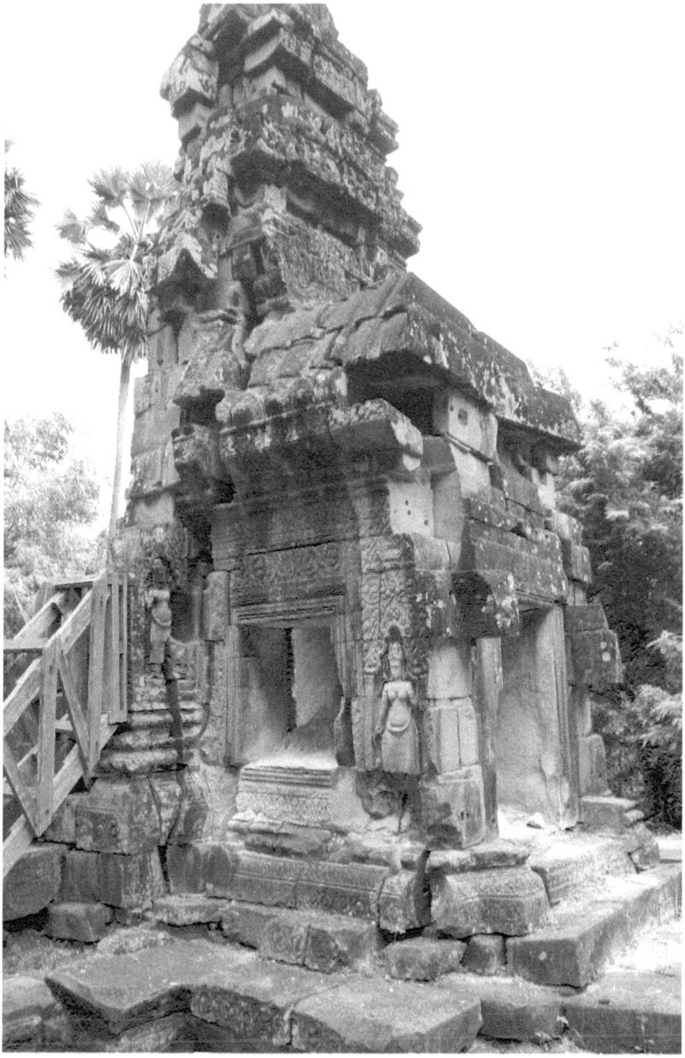

**5.2** One of the few *ārogyaśālās*, or "health houses," built by Jayavarman VII across the Khmer empire in the late twelfth century still standing today. Ta Phrom Kel is part of the Angkor archaeological complex in Siem Reap, Cambodia.
Photo by the author.

(1206–1368). Stretching from Eastern Europe to Korea, the Mongol empire caused many ruptures in the global order but also created new opportunities for Buddhist medicine to proliferate. Tradition holds that the Mongols first converted to Buddhism in 1247 when the Tibetan monk Sakya Paṇḍita (1182–1251) cured the khan's leprosy while on a diplomatic mission to the Mongol court.[53] Whether or not that is true, the Mongol rulers became great patrons of Tibetan medicine. Once Tibet had been absorbed into the empire, Tibetan clerics from the Sakya order were given positions of power at the Mongol court, and their tradition of Buddhist medicine, Sowa Rigpa (literally "knowledge of healing"; see chapter 7), became a significant influence throughout the region.[54]

Centuries after the fall of the Mongol empire, official support for Sowa Rigpa again rose markedly during the rule of the fifth Dalai Lama (1617–1682), who sponsored the authorship and editing of a number of medical texts, created an examination system for physicians, and established monastic schools of medicine and astrology.[55] He also personally designed new rituals for the *Bhaiṣajyaguru Sūtra* and other Tantric healing rites, which were adopted throughout the medical establishment he was building.[56] Many of these innovations were centered at the monastic medical college at Chagpori ("Iron Mountain"), established in 1694.

Shortly thereafter, both Tibet and Mongolia were absorbed into the Qing dynasty (1636–1911), which controlled a massive territory including Taiwan, Manchuria, and the rest of modern-day China. Many Qing rulers, who were of the Manchu ethnicity and committed Buddhists, patronized Tibetan Vajrayāna ritual specialists and became personally invested in Tibetan religious politics. While Sowa Rigpa was by no means the only form of medicine supported by the state, Qing rulers established a network of Tibetan monastic medical institutions across Inner Asia {2: 4}.[57] These served as important sites for the promulgation of Sowa Rigpa to far-flung corners of the multiethnic empire. Similar to other examples mentioned throughout this section, these institutions gave the Manchu court the opportunity to demonstrate their largesse and generosity. They also ensured the continuity of the practice of Sowa Rigpa throughout large parts of Inner Asia into the modern period.

* * *

During the premodern period, devotees around Asia employed Buddhist solutions for the suffering of illness. Across a vast territory, people used common

Buddhist medical metaphors, told similar stories about heroic Buddhist healers and deities, employed therapies and interventions prescribed in Buddhist texts, and engaged in debates about health and disease that centered on widely shared Buddhist concepts. This diffusion of Buddhist medicine from India to the rest of Asia was not the result of indiscriminate spread nor direct transmission. Rather, a multilingual, multicultural, and multidirectional network of monastics and missionaries contributed to the creation of a transcontinental conversation about medicine within Buddhist contexts.

Rulers across the region facilitated this circulation by funding Buddhist medical institutions, adopting Buddhist ritual healing methods, and employing Buddhist medical specialists. The relationship with secular power was not always so rosy, however. In many parts of Asia, Buddhist institutions came into conflict with secular authorities. The sangha's power was periodically checked by political rivals, which sometimes resulted in disruptions in the networks of exchange or even the disappearance of certain nodes of Buddhist learning. Some of the resulting reconfigurations had temporarily stultifying effects, such as when Hinduism became preeminent over Buddhism in Chenla in the sixth century or when Buddhism began to lose prestige and official support in China in the mid-eighth century after a significant rise in antiforeign sentiment.[58] Buddhism also receded in importance in Tibet during the so-called Dark Age, from the mid-ninth century through the end of the tenth, as a series of rulers persecuted Buddhist institutions.

While Buddhism eventually recovered in Cambodia, China, and Tibet, other geopolitical disruptions were more permanent. Particularly devastating were the abandonment and destruction of many Buddhist centers of learning that took place during the gradual Islamization of Western Asia, which will be discussed in more detail in chapter 7.

## FURTHER READING

Lo, Vivienne, and Christopher Cullen, eds. 2005. *Medieval Chinese Medicine: The Dunhuang Medical Manuscripts.* London and New York: RoutledgeCurzon. An illustrated introduction to the medical manuscripts, including Buddhist materials, discovered at the important node of Dunhuang.

Naqvi, Nasim H. 2011. *A Study of Buddhist Medicine and Surgery in Gandhara.* Delhi: Motilal Banarsidass. A discussion of archaeological and textual materials related to Buddhist medicine found at Gandhāra.

Neelis, Jason. 2011. *Early Buddhist Transmission and Trade Networks: Mobility and Exchange Within and Beyond the Northwestern Borderlands of South Asia*. Leiden: Brill. An analysis of the Buddhist networks, with a focus on the Indian subcontinent.

Sen, Tansen, ed. 2014. *Buddhism Across Asia: Networks of Material, Intellectual, and Cultural Exchange*. Singapore: Institute of Southeast Asian Studies. An analysis of the Buddhist networks, with a focus on long-distance exchange beyond India.

Yoeli-Tlalim, Ronit. 2021. *ReOrienting Histories of Medicine: Encounters Along the Silk Roads*. London: Bloomsbury. An overview of the history of premodern Silk Road medical exchanges between Chinese, Tibetan, and Muslim cultures.

# CHAPTER 6

## *Translations*

This chapter briefly introduces textual sources for the premodern history of Buddhist medicine and some of the larger historical questions and concerns raised by their cross-cultural circulation and translation. A note of caution is necessary at the outset: although texts constitute the historian's most valuable source for reconstructing the past, we must always remember that they are in many ways a false record of what was actually practiced on the ground. While certain texts might contain authoritative statements about doctrine and practice, they always reflect the opinions, ideals, agendas, and expectations of authors and audiences rather than the actual everyday practice of healing most people experienced in any given time or place.

One of the main arguments of the previous chapter is that Buddhist medicine is the product of thousands upon thousands of discrete moments of exchange of written, oral, and tacit knowledge among individuals across many multicultural social contexts. If we imagine those countless interactions as a deep ocean of swirling currents, then much of the specifics of the innovation and experimentation that went on lie in the invisible depths. Indeed, the voices of entire categories of participants who did not author texts (e.g., women, nonliterate practitioners) are almost completely missing.

The historian's viewpoint is always limited, as it can be based only on whatever small amount of information floats up from the depth of the ocean of practice into the textual record. As such, the historian's process can be likened to inspecting the seafoam on the surface of the ocean to try to understand what is going on below. Therefore, we must ensure that our mindset in approaching historical texts remains humble and always be cognizant of our own ignorance.

At best, texts can give us just a hint about the churning currents that lie beneath the surface; we can never take them to be the full picture.

## GENRES

Tradition holds that when the Buddha died, his followers convened an assembly to collect and codify his teachings. At this so-called First Council, the Buddha's foremost students are said to have recited what they had heard the master say over his lifetime, and the assembly committed that to memory. While legendary, this story is indicative of the fact that, for centuries, the transmission of the Buddhist canon—usually referred to as the *Tripiṭaka* (literally "three baskets")—took place via memorization and oral recitation.[1] Over time, different factions or sects evolved that interpreted these teachings differently or developed different "memories" of what the Buddha had spoken. Although scholars and practitioners have their own theories, at present, there is no definitive way to tell if any extant tradition accurately represents the original teachings. Most historians of Buddhism doubt that any of the texts we have in our possession represent faithful renditions of the words of a historical Buddha. Rather than approaching Buddhist texts as a univocal whole, or trying to determine which of the many competing Buddhisms is the true original, historians are generally interested in focusing on the different voices and divergent perspectives within the corpus and learning what these can tell us about changes in the religion and its social context over time.

The main scriptural genres available to us for the historical study of Buddhist medicine are the *vinayas*, *sūtras*, and *tantras*. As discussed in chapter 1, the six *vinayas* that remain today each contain a section that sets forth monastic regulations on the storage and use of medicines and other therapeutics developed by different sects of Indian Buddhism. Many *sūtras* from across the Buddhist world contain descriptions of the origins and makeup of the body and mind, the physical and mental causes of disease, various methods of cure, and the healing powers of particular Buddhist divinities and heroes. The *tantras* teach adept practitioners to marshal the subtle energies of the universe to cultivate healing powers. Across all genres, there are many colorful stories about Buddhist healers and their patients, and healing is routinely mentioned as a benefit of practicing Buddhist ethics, devotion, rituals, and meditation.

While the scriptures are critical for understanding Buddhist medicine, it is in the commentaries and treatises (*śāstras*) that ideas about disease, healing, and the body are often most clearly and most extensively elaborated. These genres were not understood to have the status of "Buddha-word" (*buddhavācana*) but rather were acknowledged to have been composed by scholars and exegetes. (Making such distinctions was of crucial importance to Buddhists, although these decisions were often controversial; see {1: 62}). The various Buddhist collections differ in terms of the proportion of Buddha-word versus commentary, but the latter frequently outweighs the former. The Tibetan canon, for example, is divided into the *Kangyur* ("translated words") and *Tengyur* ("translated treatises"), the former containing about 108 titles (the exact number varies by edition) and the latter more than 3,600.

Descriptions of medicine in these voluminous texts vary across time and space, bearing witness to the continual transformation and development of the tradition over time. While *vinayas*, *sūtras*, and *tantras* are often anonymous composite texts difficult to pin down to a specific author, commentaries and treatises more often can be traced to historical writers. Such texts can therefore tell us about the doctrines, narratives, and ideas people were interested in at particular times and in particular places. They also can reveal processes of authorship, translation, and intercultural adaptation. They tell us about the local dynamics of reception in places to which Buddhism spread. They can reveal, for example, what doctrinal, sectarian, ideological, political, economic, and social concerns influenced how a particular healing practice was interpreted or implemented in particular settings. Or what influence the personal biography, aspirations, and commitments of the author or authors had on a text's popularization. They also tell us how Buddhist medicine was adapted to or integrated with local medical and cultural traditions.

## PROVENANCE

Generally speaking, historical texts of the genres described here are available today in either "excavated" or "received" form. "Excavated" refers to manuscripts or other writings that have been discovered at historical or archaeological sites. Although they are not without their problems, these texts are valued by historians because they were not edited or altered when passed down through generations. As material objects, such texts can also tell us something about the text-making technology and material culture of the past and are therefore interesting for those reasons as well.

The earliest Buddhist writings in Sanskrit to have been excavated in this way date from the first century CE in the Gandhāra region. These birch-bark manuscripts, written in the Gāndhārī language (related to Sanskrit) and in the Kharoṣṭhī script, represent the oldest known pieces of Buddhist writing. In fact, they are thought to represent the earliest texts extant from the Indian subcontinent on any subject.[2] However, they contain only small fragments concerning medicine, so on the whole they do not concern us.

A more important archaeological discovery for our purposes is the Gilgit manuscripts, a collection found in Pakistan, written in Sanskrit, that contains a number of editions of the *Bhaiṣajyaguru Sūtra* {1: 25} dating from the sixth to seventh centuries. Even more significantly, further up the Silk Road in the town of Dunhuang and the surrounding area, a cache of tens of thousands of documents was preserved by the desert climate.[3] These include texts in Chinese, Sanskrit, Sogdian, Syriac, Tocharian, Tibetan, Uighur, and other languages dating from the fourth to tenth centuries. These predominantly concern Buddhism but also relate to a wide range of other religious and cultural traditions from around Eurasia, such as Eastern (Nestorian) Christianity, Manichaeism, Zoroastrianism, and Judaism from farther west and Confucianism and Daoism from farther east.

Buddhist manuals describing rituals, pharmacology, and other kinds of therapies are extant as part of this collection {1: 29, 31}. Medicine was apparently quite cosmopolitan at Dunhuang, and Buddhist institutions played a major role. Historians have been able to ascertain that a charitable hospital was operational in the mid-eighth century and that monastic medical personnel circulated among the large monasteries providing healing services.[4]

Some excavated texts were not lost but had simply lain forgotten and uncatalogued for many centuries in monastic libraries or private collections. Texts related to Buddhist medicine previously unknown to historians have been discovered in archives all over the Buddhist world.[5] Such excavated texts have revolutionized the study of the history of Buddhism, allowing scholars to gain a sense of what premodern Buddhism was like in specific historical locations. These collections also sometimes contain valuable information relevant to the history of the intersection of Buddhism and medicine in those locations.

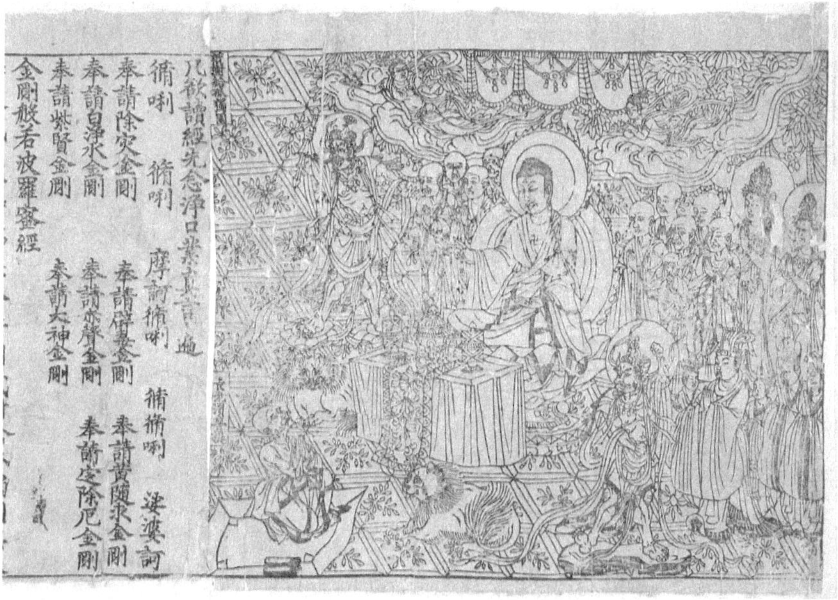


**6.1** A copy of the *Diamond Sūtra* dated 868 CE, discovered at Dunhuang, represents the earliest printed book in the world. The *Diamond Sūtra* is frequently chanted by Mahāyāna Buddhists for relief from illness and is among the most popular texts in East Asian Buddhism. From the British Library. Image courtesy of Wikimedia Commons, public domain.

Although excavated texts reveal much information about the time and place of their composition, historians also value texts that remained in circulation, continually being handed down through the generations via oral transmission, copying, and eventually printing. These "received" texts are far more numerous than the excavated texts and thus represent the largest body of sources for the study of Buddhist medicine. Scholars use received texts with caution because of the significant changes they often underwent through the process of transmission across the centuries, but these texts are considered the most authoritative by various contemporary Buddhist traditions.

One important collection of early Buddhist texts preserved and passed down in this way is the Pāli Canon, a collection first written down in Sri Lanka in the first century BCE in the Pāli language, a close relation of Sanskrit. This canon is an invaluable source for understanding early Buddhism and also early Buddhist medicine. The Pāli Canon is most likely the earliest collection of texts that mentions the Elements and *tridoṣa* in Indian history, as it appears to predate the writing down of the principal Āyurvedic texts by a few centuries. Now serving as the foundation of the Theravāda tradition in Southeast Asia, this collection is also relevant to the study of contemporary Buddhism in Sri Lanka, Myanmar, Thailand, Laos, and Cambodia.

Over the course of the first millennium CE, both the Chinese and Tibetans imported, translated, and preserved texts associated with many Buddhist sects active in India and other parts of Asia. Thus, the received canons in Chinese and Tibetan languages contain a much wider range of ideas and doctrines than the Pāli Canon. Other major collections of received Buddhist writings available today include *Tripiṭakas*, or parts thereof, written in Manchu, Mongol, Tangut, and other languages. Received collections such as these contain many individual texts related to health, medicine, and therapeutics—many more than in the excavated texts.[6] The frequency with which medical topics are taken up in these received sources is a strong indication that medicine was thought to be an important part of the Buddhist tradition across cultures, important enough to translate, preserve, and recopy over time.

## MEDIA

All of the texts discussed here—whether excavated or received, written in whichever language or script—are important records of ideas but also material objects in their own right. Scholars interested in the history of writing practices call our attention to how messy and contingent much of this historical record is. While modern readers might be accustomed to encountering well-prepared translations of historical texts, the premodern source base is filled with scribal errors, scratched-out characters, comments in the margin, and other anomalies common to handwritten manuscript texts. (One such multilayered document is translated in {1: 51}.) In the premodern period, writing out a text meant copying it by hand onto a piece of birch bark, palm leaf, paper, or other perishable item. Often, these texts are damaged, missing pieces, or survive only in fragments.

At the other end of the spectrum lie the texts written on more durable media like stone. At many times in history, rulers, elites, or groups of donors pooled resources to carve texts into stela or onto the walls of caves. An example of the latter pertinent to our investigation is the inscription of medical recipes onto the walls of the Longmen grottoes at a Buddhist site in central China {1: 46}.

Beginning in the late first millennium, Buddhist texts also began to be printed. The earliest extant printed document in the world, in fact, is a copy of the *Diamond Sūtra* from Dunhuang—a text that was and is still today frequently recopied or chanted to protect devotees against illness.[7] The earliest complete printed *Tripiṭaka* extant is a thirteenth-century set of woodblocks housed today in the Haeinsa temple in South Korea. This collection contains dozens of texts related to Buddhist medicine derived from medieval China.[8] Producing an entire printed *Tripiṭaka* was a complex and expensive undertaking; thus, these documents were useful as official gifts or tribute among rulers in the premodern period. In many Buddhist countries, *Tripiṭakas* were produced on a regular basis by governments to patronize, control, or promulgate Buddhism.[9]

The explosion of printing and the emergence of the worldwide book trade in the early modern period meant that printed editions of Buddhist texts

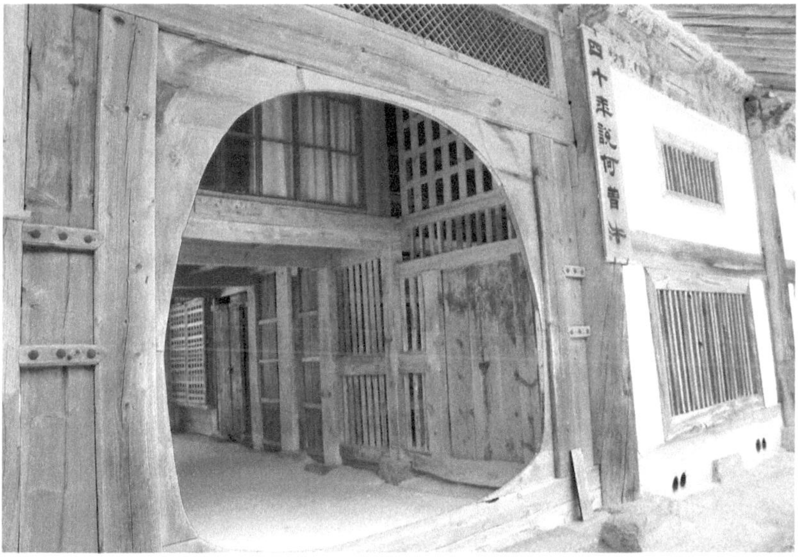


**6.2** The Haeinsa temple complex houses 81,350 woodblocks from the thirteenth century that were used for printing the Korean *Tripiṭaka*. Located in South Gyeongsang Province, South Korea.
Photo by the author.

could be produced cheaply and disseminated widely (for discussion of Buddhist medicine and modern print culture, see {1: 58; 2: 9}). One consequence of this fact is that, today, both excavated and received Buddhist medical writings from virtually all traditions and in virtually all languages can be readily accessed by scholars and practitioners around the world. In the last two decades, these sources have increasingly been digitized. This means that the most important texts suitable for the study of Buddhist medicine can now easily be found online and can be searched, shared, and downloaded onto a computer or mobile device. For researchers or practitioners with adequate skills in Asian languages, a huge number of Buddhist sources on medicine are now literally available in one's pocket.

At present, the most important collections of texts for research of Buddhist medicine include the portions of the Pāli Canon made available online by the Vipassana Research Institute and Sutta Central,[10] the Pāli and Sanskrit materials in the Göttingen Register of Electronic Texts in Indian Languages,[11] the comprehensive collections of East Asian sources available through the Chinese Buddhist Electronic Texts Association and the SAT Daizōkyō Text Database,[12] and the Tibetan canons from the Buddhist Digital Resource Centre and Columbia University's American Institute of Buddhist Studies.[13] A comparative display of texts translated into Sanskrit, Chinese, Tibetan, English, and other languages is available on the Thesaurus Literaturae Buddhicae website.[14] Texts excavated from Silk Road archaeological sites are available through high-resolution photographic scans on the International Dunhuang Project's website.[15] In addition, a one-hundred-volume compilation of texts focused on Buddhist medicine was recently made available in print by the Shaolin Temple, which claims to be a complete collection of sources on that topic in Chinese.[16]

Today, Buddhist writings about health, medicine, and therapeutics from all eras and geographical locations are more readily available, accessible, and portable than ever before. It is now possible that, with the right combination of language skills, an individual scholar can rapidly compare medical ideas across a number of Buddhist traditions from around the world and across time. Such comparative projects are becoming possible even for nonspecialists, assisted by the growing number of modern languages into which Buddhist texts from many traditions are being translated. (Of course, the two anthology volumes that accompany this book are intended to facilitate such comparisons.) While we will never be able to recover the totality of the ocean of practice, the ability to readily compare many editions of Buddhist texts across various collections in different languages allows us to begin to understand some of the ocean's currents. Tracing the movement of texts—and hence of certain ideas and practices—across time and space allows us to discover more about how people read, understood, and practiced Buddhist medicine.

## TRANSLATION AND ADAPTATION

Devotees across the world typically have considered Buddhist *sūtras* to be infallible transmissions of the Buddha's words. Historical research, on the other hand, paints a more complicated picture. In fact, the vast majority of the extant Buddhist literature has been shown to have been edited, compiled, or composed outside of India. As they were transported and translated across linguistic and cultural boundaries, Buddhist texts were continually adapted and transformed. The medical materials contained in extant Buddhist texts, like other types of Buddhist knowledge, were regularly modified, elaborated, reinterpreted, and adapted while in transit across time and space.[17]

Some of the changes introduced through these processes of cross-cultural exchange and translation were unintentional. As they were encoded and re-encoded in new languages and new scripts, translators occasionally made errors.[18] Even when every effort is made to ensure accuracy, the act of translation invariably introduces a number of inconsistencies, adaptations, and transformations into a text.

It was also frequently the case that translators and editors intentionally tweaked the contents of texts to adapt Buddhist ideas for local audiences. On the one hand, authors could insert their own comments and interpretations into existing texts because they were interested in clarifying, elaborating, or developing upon certain aspects of doctrine. On the other hand, such modifications also included edits to suit the current political, cultural, or intellectual climate. Often, Buddhist authors even fabricated "apocrypha" or "pseudo-translations," entirely new texts made to look like authentic translations, which could be passed off as part of the received tradition (for an example related to Buddhist medicine, see {1: 44}).[19] Tibetan "treasure texts" (Tib. *terma*), said to have been hidden by the Buddha or other sages centuries before and only now revealed or rediscovered by people with special powers, are one recurring example of this phenomenon.

Questions of provenance, authorship, and authenticity were frequently debated by Buddhist exegetes and physicians {1: 62}.

While some cross-cultural translators had few compunctions about taking editorial liberties, others were more concerned about departing from original Indian source texts. A range of translation strategies and tactics were employed depending on the translators' goals. Some translators tried to minimize the adaptation or customization of Buddhist teachings by using transliterated Sanskrit terminology (sometimes even writing out Sanskrit words in the Indian *siddhaṃ* script). Others translated the terms into the target language using the closest equivalents for Sanskrit terminology in the local language. Because of their high degree of fidelity, texts produced with these more conservative tactics tend to preserve a fairly accurate representation of Indian medicine, even though they were produced thousands of miles away from India. Over time, Indian medical terms expressed in transliterated Sanskrit or in closely equivalent translation terms also began to appear abundantly outside of Buddhist texts. Ideas and practices introduced into new cultures via Buddhist texts came to be separated from their original Buddhist contexts and disseminated through indigenous medical writings as well.

However, the process of translation almost always resulted in transformations in the opposite direction as well: indigenous terms, frameworks, and ideas infiltrated Buddhist writings during the act of translation. Such introjections could be subtle: in some cases, it may simply have been a translator's choice to gloss a Sanskrit medical term with an indigenous term that had a slightly different meaning or connotation. On the far end of this "domesticating" spectrum of translation practice, the presentation of Indian medicine could be expressed entirely with indigenous vocabularies and doctrinal adaptations that make the ideas difficult, or even impossible, to trace back to India.[20]

Usually, the details of why such adaptations did or did not happen lie below the surface of the ocean of practice. Nevertheless, sometimes a hint about the translators' motivations can be gleaned. For example, the biography of Jīvaka is extant in a number of versions in the Pāli, Sanskrit, Chinese, and Tibetan languages {1: 1, 20}. From our vantage point in the present, it is impossible to tell whether all of the extant versions derive from a common source, when exactly they developed, or who changed them and why. However, what is clear is that the extant versions of the story show signs of having been adapted to appeal to different audiences.[21] In the Chinese version of the story, for example, Jīvaka is said to have been born with acupuncture needles in his hands (acupuncture is a paradigmatically Chinese medical procedure) and to have been versed in various Chinese medical arts. In the other versions, different details are introduced, presumably because these spoke more strongly to local audiences.

While the Jīvaka biography was rewritten for different cultural contexts, other texts were modified by a gradual process of accretion instead. An example of this process is the *Sūtra of the Great Compassion Dhāraṇī of Avalokiteśvara* {1: 26}. Different versions of this *sūtra* are extant in the Chinese, Tibetan, and Mongolian Buddhist canons, as well as in a manuscript fragment written in Tibetan from Turfan.[22] Some of these editions include lists of rituals and recipes for the treatment of specific ailments appended to the core text. These sections invariably reveal what kinds of illnesses people were concerned about in specific times and places and include localized content relating to specific materia medica and ritual therapeutics.

Aside from translation and adaptation, another transformation that some texts underwent when being introduced into new cultural contexts was anthologization. Anthologies are collections of passages of Buddhist literature removed from their original contexts and placed into a new relationship within a new composition. One example of anthologization is a Chinese encyclopedia by the seventh-century Daoshi (?–683 CE), which organized Buddhist knowledge about medicine, nursing care, and hospice from across the *Tripiṭaka* under the heading of "The Suffering of Illness" {1: 3}.[23] A different example, a text from twelfth- to thirteenth-century Japan, contains a range of materials about the demonic "corpse-vector" disease {1: 51}. Although they originated in different contexts—some Buddhist, some Daoist, some Chinese, some Japanese—the pieces in this composite text, along with the compiler's annotations, were brought together into one document. The multilayered text provided a guide for monks in the practice of moxibustion against the dreaded disease, but, like all anthologies, it also gives modern historians a peek into the interests and reading practices of the person or people who created it at a specific time in a specific place.

Finally, our discussion of the cross-cultural translation and adaptation of texts cannot be complete without acknowledging the large number of treatises, commentaries, reference works, travelogues, lectures, and other historical sources that do not represent translations or anthologies per se but were equally involved in introducing Buddhist medicine to new cultural contexts. Though they often worked in only one language, the authors of these works were no less involved in cross-cultural transmission and reception. The Chinese monks Zhiyi (538–597 CE) and Daoxuan (596–667 CE), for example, each composed works that systematized Buddhist approaches to healing for their contemporaries in the form of a meditation manual {1: 37} and a guide to monastic discipline {1: 14}, respectively.[24] In the twelfth century, the Tibetan physician Yutok Yönten Gonpo composed a major medical treatise that combined influences from India and elsewhere in Asia (discussed in detail in the next chapter). Just over a century later, in Japan, the contemporaries Kokan Shiren (1278–1346) and Kajiwara Shōzen (1265–1337) each wrote treatises that tried to reconcile Buddhist perspectives with their own experiences as patients and physicians {1: 7, 56}. Despite their monolingual nature, all of these compositions can tell us something about how individual teachers or practitioners were putting into practice in local contexts the information they were receiving from across the broader Buddhist networks. A close reading of these texts also can reveal the complexity of the choices, preferences, strategies, and idiosyncrasies of individual authors.

## MAJOR TEXTS ON BUDDHIST MEDICINE TRANSLATED INTO WESTERN LANGUAGES

What follows is a brief overview of the most important texts related to Buddhist medicine with scholarly translations in Western languages. Many of these texts are discussed in more detail in other chapters but are here brought together into a systematic list, grouped by genre.

### *Monastic Disciplinary Texts*

Developed by the early Indian Buddhist schools and translated into various languages across Asia, the six extant *vinayas*, or monastic disciplinary codes, each contain a section of rules about the collection, storage, and provisioning of medicines that pertained to a particular monastic community or sect in ancient India. These sections often give a sense of the treatments in use at the time for common disorders. Complete English translations are available of the medical sections of the Pāli *vinaya* and the *vinaya* of the Mahīśāsaka school, while partial translations are available of medical content from the *vinaya* of the Lokottaravādin nuns

{1: 1, 10, 11, 13}.[25] In these *vinayas*, certain points of discipline are often illustrated with founding stories that present medical practices in narrative form {1: 12}.

This category of literature also includes disciplinary treatises and commentaries on the *vinayas* that were composed in various parts of the Buddhist world. Either synthesizing the monastic codes for local audiences or representing independent efforts to establish a set of rules, such texts often contain much information on the understanding, implementation, and adaptation of Buddhist medical knowledge locally. The *Samantapāsādikā*, a commentary on the Pāli *vinaya* translated into Chinese in the fifth century, contains much material on both elemental and demonological medicine scattered throughout the text.[26] Other examples that are particularly rich in medical content that have been partially translated into English include an influential synthesis of *vinaya* texts by the Chinese master Daoxuan (596–667 CE) {1: 14} and various "Rules of Purity" (*qinggui*) manuals that guided East Asian monastic conduct {1: 15}.[27]

## *Foundational Scriptures*

Major *sūtras* and *tantras* served as focal points for devotion, exegesis, and commentary in Buddhist circles across Asia. Because of their importance and wide circulation, they are extant in many editions and languages. One key text, the *Bhaiṣajyaguru Sūtra* (Skt. *Bhaiṣajyaguru-vaiḍūrya-prabhā-rāja sūtra*), details the previous lives and vows of the buddha Bhaiṣajyaguru. This text is extant today in Chinese (in four versions), Khotanese, Sanskrit, Sogdian, Tibetan, and Old Uighur, and several of these have been translated into English {1: 25}.[28]

Some of the most important Mahāyāna scriptures were vehicles for the wide circulation of medical information. A chapter of the seminal *Lotus Sūtra* (Skt. *Saddharmapuṇḍarīka sūtra*), for example, introduced the bodhisattva Bhaiṣajyarāja ("Medicine King") as an object of worship and contemplation.[29] The *Sūtra of Golden Light* (Skt. *Suvarṇaprabhāsa sūtra*) contains a chapter that outlines the basic doctrine of *tridoṣa*, including the correlations among the arising of illnesses, the seasons of the year, and the medicinal flavors {1: 4}.[30] A chapter of the *Vimalakīrti Sūtra* (Skt. *Vimalakīrti-nirdeśa sūtra*) introduces the basic Mahāyāna philosophical position on the ultimate emptiness of illness.[31] The Mahāyāna version of the *Sūtra on the Great Liberation* (Skt. *Mahāparinirvāṇa sūtra*) contains several sections that deal with medicine in a metaphorical way or as a heuristic device for understanding Buddhist teachings. The most important section in that regard is the chapter of the *sūtra* called "Manifesting Disease."[32]

Important scriptures of the *tantra* class include the *Binding of the Wheels Tantra* (*Cakrasaṃvara tantra*), the *Hevajra Tantra*, and the *Wheel of Time Tantra* (*Kālacakra tantra*), all of which discuss the anatomy and physiology of the subtle body.[33] The latter text presents something of a compendium of conventional and Tantric healing practices, discussed in more detail in chapter 3.

## *Ritual Manuals*

Ritual manuals give instruction on how to invoke divine or spiritual assistance for conquering diseases or maintaining health, as well as how to perform exorcistic rites and incantations to dispel demons or treat particular ailments {1: 25–35}. The rituals usually involve interactions with buddhas, bodhisattvas, protector deities, nature spirits, or demonic entities that have been incorporated into the Buddhist pantheon. Ritual healing texts might be exoteric or esoteric and may be classified as *sūtras*, *tantras*, or otherwise.

The *Bhaiṣajyaguru Sūtra* details the rites that can be carried out to save oneself from disease and untimely death. Some Chinese ritual manuals that elaborate on the *sūtra*'s procedures have been translated into English {1: 28§8}. A chapter of the *Sūtra of Golden Light* prescribes a ritual for invoking the protection and healing of the goddess Sarasvatī by bathing with thirty-two aromatic medicines, making offerings, and chanting *dhāraṇī*.[34] Another key ritual manual is the *Great Compassion Dhāraṇī of Avalokiteśvara*, a text that contains a number of ritual and medicinal therapies appended to the main text {1: 26}.[35] The *Fundamental Spell Book of Mañjuśrī* (*Mañjuśrī[ya]mūlakalpa*) is a Tantric compendium composed in the late sixth or early seventh century in India.[36] From Tibet, several short ritual manuals on the Six Teachings of Naropa provide a range of Tantric practices related to health and vitality.[37] Additionally, Gyalwa Yangönpa Gyaltsen Palzang's (1213–1258) *Hidden Description of the Vajra Body* contains a rich description of the subtle body and the practices most relevant for its cultivation.[38] Other examples of short healing ritual manuals are available from India {1: 27}, China {1: 28–31, 45}, Japan {1: 33, 51}, and Mongolia {1: 35, 2: 4}.[39] Not included in this section are manuals focused on healing meditations, which are discussed next.

### *Manuals on Meditation and Other Contemplative Practices*

Many Buddhist texts provide advice on how to use meditation to come to terms with the suffering of illness while not necessarily curing it.[40] However, texts from across Buddhist traditions do often give explicit instructions on how to treat ailments with some kind of contemplative practice. As mentioned in chapter 1, a number of early Nikāya texts describe the immediate healing effects of contemplating the Factors of Enlightenment {1: 2}. The *Girimānanda sutta*, for example, mentions ten contemplations that cure a sick disciple.[41]

Mahāyāna and Tantric texts have much more to say on meditation proper. A Mahāyāna perspective on the healing power of visualization is presented in two texts dedicated to the bodhisattva brothers Medicine King and Supreme Medicine.[42] A number of Tantric meditation techniques for health and longevity have also been translated into English from the Tibetan {1: 40–42}. A much later sixteenth- or seventeenth-century Pāli text called *The Yogāvacara's Manual* (a *yogāvacara* is a practitioner of meditation) describes mantra recitation, visualization, and the movement of a point of light through the body.[43] Such techniques also were collected in various Southeast Asian meditation texts in the early twentieth century {1: 43}.[44]

Also included in this category are texts with instructions on how to counter the negative effects of meditation itself, which was often acknowledged as potentially dangerous for one's health if done incorrectly. Perhaps most notable in this area is a fifth-century text from Khotan that teaches a range of visualization exercises that can be done to counter "meditation illness" {1: 36}.[45] Compositions by the sixth-century Chinese meditation master Zhiyi include both short and long treatises on ailments that can arise in meditation and a wide range of interventions to treat them {1: 37} and texts from Korea and Japan also tackle this subject {1:38}.[46]

### *Narratives*

As illness and healing are frequent tropes, many canonical Buddhist narratives are relevant to the study of the history of medicine. The *vinayas* are full of narratives, many with medical content {e.g., 1: 1, 12}. One of the most important *vinaya* narratives is the biography of Jīvaka, the model Buddhist doctor

{1: 1§4, 20}.[47] Other notable stories depicting the Buddha, deities, and members of the sangha as healers are found in collections of *avadānas* and *jatakas*, as well as in biographies of monks, *mahasiddhas*, and other Buddhist heroes from across Asia {1: 18–21}.[48]

## *Philosophical Treatises*

Buddhist philosophical treatises often purport to explain the nature of illness and health and how healing is related to various doctrines such as karma, dependent origination (*pratītyasamutpāda*), and emptiness. Important examples of texts in this category include *Questions of Milinda* (*Milindapañhā*), which introduces perspectives on the body and health within a philosophical discourse.[49] The Elements and *tridoṣa* are introduced in the context of Buddhist philosophical teachings in the *Great Elephant Footprint Simile* (*Mahāhatthipadopama sutta*) and the *Great Exhortation to Rāhula* (*Mahārāhulovāda sutta*).[50] A series of texts, including the *Vimuttimagga*, *Visuddhimagga*, and other related compositions detailing the "path" or "stages" of spiritual development often broach medical matters in the course of explaining how the body and mind are interrelated.[51] A later exemplar of this genre, the *Yogācārabhūmi* {1: 6}, describes the origin and makeup of the body, as well as its relationship to the mind, making frequent reference to Indian medical doctrines.[52]

## *Medical Treatises*

This category includes medical texts that, despite their origin outside Buddhism, came to be adopted or incorporated into canonical collections. For example, twenty-two Indian medical texts are included in the Tibetan *Tengyur*, the division of the Tibetan Buddhist canon dedicated to commentaries.[53] Of these, the texts that have been translated into English include the *Essence of the Eight Branches* (*Aṣṭāṅgahṛdaya saṃhitā*), the seminal text written by Vāgbhaṭa in the early seventh century.[54] Disseminated widely and translated into multiple languages, this compendium became a foundational text for Āyurveda and Buddhist medicine alike and unquestionably represents the most influential Indian medical treatise in history. The *Tengyur* includes the root text, as well as four commentaries on it, including an auto-commentary attributed to Vāgbhaṭa not extant in Sanskrit. Another Indian medical text from the *Tengyur* that has been translated into English is the *Siddhasāra*, a seventh-century treatise also partially available in

Arabic, Khotanese, and Uighur translations.[55] Another is the *Yogaśataka*, a practical manual traditionally attributed to the Buddhist philosopher Nāgārjuna but which also likely dates to the seventh century.[56]

Other important examples of medical treatises adopted into Buddhist canonical collections include *Kāśyapa's Compendium* and *Tantra of Rāvaṇakumāra*, two Indian medical texts on demonological ailments of pregnancy and early childhood that were incorporated into the Chinese Buddhist canon and also circulated widely in other languages.[57] Finally, the *Sūtra of the Descent of the Embryo* (*Garbhāvakrānti sūtra*), preserved in a number of Chinese and Tibetan editions, describes the processes of conception, gestation, and birth in ways that closely parallel Indian medical treatises {1: 5}.[58]

### *Extracanonical Texts*

Last are a number of miscellaneous texts that have remained unintegrated into the Buddhist canons but that attribute themselves to, quote extensively from, or otherwise bear witness to the circulation of medical knowledge in Buddhist contexts. These include, for example, medical manuals excavated from Buddhist sites on the Silk Road. The *Bower Manuscript* is an untitled sixth-century birch-bark compilation made in a Kuchean Buddhist monastery that includes texts on divination, incantation, and medicine.[59] The *Weber Manuscript* is a collection of Kuchean translations of medical and magical therapies dating from no later than the seventh century.[60] The *Book of Jīvaka* (Skt. *Jīvakapustaka*) is a text dating from between the seventh and eleventh centuries attributed to Jīvaka, written in alternating Sanskrit and Khotanese.[61]

A number of Tibetan works on medicine relate closely to Buddhism but are not part of the official Buddhist canon. Most notable is the *Secret Essence of Ambrosia in Eight Branches: An Instructional Tantra* (commonly known as the *Four Tantras*, Tib. *Gyushi*), a twelfth-century Tibetan composition that forms the basis of Tibetan medicine to this day {1: 60–61}.[62] Two important works produced by the regent of Tibet at the turn of the eighteenth century include the *Blue Beryl* (*Baidurya ngönpo*), which is a commentary on the *Four Tantras* accompanied by a series of seventy-nine paintings,[63] as well as a history of Tibetan medicine called *Beryl Mirror* (Tib. *Vaidurya melong*).[64]

We also must mention here the *Casket of Medicine* (Pāli *Bhesajjamañjūsā*) from thirteenth-century Sri Lanka, the only extant medical treatise written in Pāli.[65]

Additionally, several of the most important East Asian medical treatises make explicit or implicit reference to Indian teachings on ethics, massage, recipes, and surgery, including *Prescriptions Worth a Thousand in Gold* (Ch. *Qinjin yaofang*), *Prescriptions at the Heart of Medicine* (Jp. *Ishinpō*), the *Classified Collection of Medical Prescriptions* (Kr. *Ŭibangyuch'wi*), and others {1: 52–55}.[66] Also to be mentioned here are the huge number of historical records, popular narratives, poetry, and other miscellaneous writings from across Asia that talk about Buddhist healers or therapies, whether approvingly or disapprovingly, in detail or in passing.

* * *

While the ocean of practice is deep and its currents mostly unfathomable, historians are nevertheless interested in examining the extant textual evidence for what information it can reveal. Historians agree that no Buddhist text anywhere unproblematically reflects a pristine, original form of Buddhism. Instead, texts from across Asia are the products of centuries of translation, adaptation, synthesis, and cross-cultural influence. Comparing extant versions of translated, adapted, rewritten, and recompiled texts from around Asia can help us to gain a sense of how transmitted Buddhist knowledge was reconfigured to suit particular local medical cultures, social dynamics, and political and economic realities. It can help to reveal the unique and locally specific factors that governed the reception and recirculation of Buddhist medical knowledge.

To understand the motivations that drove the work of individual authors and translators, however, it is critical to investigate them on a case-by-case basis. With this in mind, I highly recommended readers to explore in depth the major textual sources of Buddhist medicine currently available in translation in Western languages listed above. In addition, the local, microhistorical, and biographical materials presented in the anthologies that accompany this volume and mentioned in the citations in the endnotes throughout this book will greatly enrich the general discussion presented in this chapter.

## FURTHER READING

Mizuno, Kogen. 1995. *Buddhist Sutras: Origin, Development, Transmission*. Tokyo: Kosei. A readable introduction to the history of Buddhist literature that addresses many of the central questions in this chapter.

Salguero, C. Pierce. 2014. *Translating Buddhist Medicine in Medieval China*. Philadelphia: University of Pennsylvania Press. Focuses on the strategies and tactics used in the translation, adaptation, and assimilation of Indian medicine in medieval China.

Silk, Jonathan A. 2015. *Brill's Encyclopedia of Buddhism*, vol. 1, *Literature and Languages*. Leiden: Brill. A detailed, up-to-date reference work on historical Buddhist literature in a number of languages.

Web-based English translations of Buddhist scriptures:

- From Pāli: Access to Insight (http://www.accesstoinsight.org)
- From Chinese and Japanese: BDK English Tripiṭaka Project (http://www.bdkamerica.org)
- From Tibetan: Translating the Words of the Buddha (http://84000.co)

# CHAPTER 7
## *Localizations*

The previous two chapters talked about processes of circulation and translation in the broadest terms. Here, we will dive into some specifics about how Buddhist medicine was localized in various parts of Asia during the premodern period. This chapter identifies three long-term historical trajectories that predominated in different regions. The first, which I will for convenience call "displacement," pertains to those places in Central, South, and Southeast Asia where Islam or Hinduism replaced Buddhism as the major religious and cultural influence. The second, "domestication," unfolded in East Asia, where Buddhist approaches to health and medicine were in the long run largely absorbed into indigenous cultural and intellectual frameworks. The third trajectory, "translocation," characterizes those parts of Central and Southeast Asia where ideas received from India formed the basis for long-lasting local or regional traditions of Buddhist medicine that grew and thrived independently.

Let us not get hung up on this particular terminology. Of course, each of these words are problematic in their own way. Future historians will come along and argue that these metaphors bias our understanding of certain important processes and obscure our view of others. That our generalizations are not able to do justice to all of the complexities of the historical events. That is as it should be. As was the case in previous chapters, we are interested in identifying macro-level patterns—while periodically zooming in to examine particular examples—to provide the scaffolding for future scholars to do precisely this work of refinement.

## DISPLACEMENT

As mentioned in previous chapters, archaeological discoveries in northwestern India, Pakistan, and Afghanistan and along the Silk Road have given us some of the earliest evidence for the practice of Buddhist medicine. Buddhism was transmitted even further west early in the Common Era, reaching as far as modern-day Iran. While records of Buddhist medicine are nonexistent in that region, the first recorded translator of Buddhist texts to arrive in China, An Shigao (fl. ca. 148–180 CE), is said to have hailed from the Parthian empire (247 BCE–224 CE). The explanations of the Elements, *tridoṣa*, flavors, and other Indian medical doctrines in texts translated and composed by him thus likely preserve unique evidence of how those ideas were understood in Iranian areas.[1] Incidentally, these same texts also represent the earliest appearances of Indian medical concepts in the Chinese language.

Despite being an early Buddhist outpost, An Shigao's homeland underwent a process of Islamization.[2] Originating in the Arabian Peninsula in the early seventh century, Islam spread rapidly to Iran and Afghanistan during that century. Much of the Silk Road territories and present-day Xinjiang (western China) were Islamized by the end of the tenth century, with Khotan following in the beginning of the eleventh. Small pockets of Buddhist adherents remained across this area. However, prestige and official support for exchanges with non-Muslim regions markedly diminished in the second millennium. Buddhism no longer played the dominant role it once had in providing the context for economic, artistic, intellectual, and cultural exchange.

Meanwhile, Buddhism in India was being severely threatened by a resurgent Hinduism, and soon would all but disappear. The last major Buddhist state in India proper was the Pāla dynasty in the eighth to twelfth centuries. At their height, the Pālas controlled a territory that stretched from eastern Pakistan to Bangladesh. Buddhism flourished under the dynasty, the monastic university at Nālandā increased in stature, and learned Indian Buddhist scholars were in high demand around the Buddhist world. However, the Pāla rulers were eventually defeated by Hindu rivals, marking the end of major official patronage for Buddhism in the subcontinent.

Muslim armies had been staging incursions into northern India since the seventh century, in large part to exert their dominance over the trade routes running through the area. Between the twelfth and sixteenth centuries, these invaders pressed increasingly eastward across India. Around the year 1200, they razed the monastic center at Nālandā, leaving India without a major node of Buddhist learning. By the end of this period, the majority of northern India had been Islamized, and Buddhist culture was mostly eradicated in the land where the Buddha had lived and taught.

Indonesia went through its own process of Islamization a few centuries later. Although little scholarship has been done on Buddhist medicine in this area, archaeological evidence from the region speaks to the circulation of *dhāraṇī* rituals for protection and healing.[3] Borobudur, built in the eighth to ninth centuries, was a major pilgrimage site. Certain areas of the archipelago had been closely tied to Buddhist networks in the first millennium CE. The Chinese pilgrim Yijing spent some time in the kingdom of Srivijaya (modern-day Sumatra), studying Sanskrit on his way to India. Despite this long history, the area was Islamized in the fourteenth and fifteenth centuries.

Anxieties in the face of this drastic geopolitical reorientation are palpable in the Buddhist textual record. For example, the *Wheel of Time Tantra*, the eleventh-century treatise mentioned in chapters 3 and 6, espoused a millenarian prophesy about Islam conquering the world. The text promised that a Buddhist savior would appear to definitively defeat the foreign religion and usher in a golden age of the Dharma and a kingdom of peace called Shambhala.[4] Despite this apocalyptic vision pitting the two religions against each other in all-or-nothing terms, the historical reality was more nuanced, and many fruitful interreligious and intercultural exchanges took place between Buddhism and Islam.[5]

The primary medical tradition of the Islamic world, *yūnānī tibb* (literally "Greek medicine"), was closely related to Greco-Roman medicine and thus had certain theoretical similarities with both Āyurveda and Buddhist medicine (an emphasis on the same Great Elements, for example). Given the large amount of pharmaceutical and technological exchange that had been taking place across Eurasia for centuries by this point, these traditions also had come to share many specific therapies or procedures. Thus, although explicit references to Buddhist texts, legends, and institutions were discouraged in Islamized areas, it is plausible that, in practice, the rupture may have been largely unnoticeable to many patients—and maybe even to some practitioners as well.

Connections between Buddhist and Islamic medicine abound. In the heart of the Islamic world, the famous Bīmāristān hospital built in eighth-century Baghdad—one of the most significant institutions in the history of medicine—was built according to a model described in the Āyurvedic classics. Those texts, in turn, seem to have been introduced to the area by Buddhists from the kingdom of Bactria.[6] Farther east, potent substances from the Middle East such as theriac and snakestone circulated widely in Buddhist Asia.[7] Initially translated into Chinese during the Tang dynasty, Islamic medicine eventually became highly influential during the Mongol-ruled Yuan dynasty (1279–1368) and was known as far away as Kamakura Japan (1185–1333).[8]

While Tibetans often identified with the myth of Shambhala and thought of themselves as the prophesied defenders of the Buddhist faith, they also interacted and exchanged with their Islamic neighbors. I have already mentioned the brisk trade of Tibetan musk in western Central Asia, the Middle East, and Europe. Going in the opposite direction, concrete evidence of Islamic influence in Tibet includes the incorporation of Middle Eastern medicines into the local pharmacopoeia, the introduction of the diagnostic practice of urinoscopy (which originated in Greek medicine but came east via the Islamic world), certain aspects of alchemy, and other ideas and practices.[9]

The significant contribution of Islamic medical culture in Tibet was later acknowledged by Tibetan physicians in one of the founding myths of the origin of their medical system.[10] Written in the sixteenth century, this legend speaks of a time nearly a thousand years earlier when the ruler of Tibet fell ill. Physicians were recruited from far and wide, including Bharadhaja, the reputed founder of Āyurveda; the Yellow Emperor, the mythological founder of Chinese medicine; and Galenos from "Tazig or Phrom" (i.e., Persia or Byzantium). The latter figure, bearing the name of the famous Roman physician Galen, is without a doubt here meant to stand for the Greco-Roman-Islamic tradition. Meeting in the Tibetan king's service, the story tells us, these seminal figures together composed a medical text that gave birth to Tibetan medicine, which was a combination of the best aspects of Indian, Chinese, and Western practices.

In addition to these explicit exchanges and influences, the similarities between medical systems also made it possible for certain originally Buddhist ideas or practices to go underground, so to speak, continuing to be employed by healers, although now beneath a Hindu or Muslim veneer.[11] One example of this phenomenon is a series of block-printed amulets written in Arabic but apparently modeled after Buddhist talismans.[12] Traces of Buddhist healing still circulated among some Muslim and Hindu practitioners even in the twentieth century. An Indian folklorist working in Bengal in the late 1970s found lay healers in that region chanting incantations that could be traced directly to Buddhist matrans or *dhāraṇīs*, although their Buddhist origins had been long forgotten {2: 25}.[13]

Despite the prevalence of such cross-pollinations, as the process of Islamization intensified, the Buddhist and Islamic worlds became increasingly separated. Huge areas of previously Buddhist territory—a great swathe from Iran to Xinjiang, from Pakistan to Bangladesh, and southeastward all the way to Indonesia—did not permanently exit the stage of the history being described here. However, the significance of Buddhist medicine in those regions receded dramatically as it was increasingly displaced by Islamic alternatives.

## DOMESTICATION

While Buddhist medicine disappeared in much of Western Asia, India, and Indonesia, a second, quite different historical trajectory played out in East Asia. Here, Buddhist medical ideas and practices received from India persisted and remain important features of the medical landscape today. Their long-term viability resulted in large part from the fact that foreign aspects of Buddhist medicine were translated and adapted in ways that facilitated their absorption into native cultural and intellectual frameworks, a process I refer to as "domestication."

From the time of the arrival of Buddhism in East Asia, proponents of Indian methods of healing had to contend with the codified, literate, and prestigious medical system native to East Asia, which scholars usually call "classical Chinese medicine." This tradition had been closely aligned with Chinese imperial ideology as far back as the Han dynasty (206 BCE–220 CE).[14] Buddhist institutions and practitioners began to compete successfully with classical medicine during the so-called Period of Division (220–589 CE) that followed the collapse of the Han dynasty. They were able to do so because this period was for the most part marked by the absence of a centralized state and a sense that classical political models were no longer working.

The so-called medieval period between the collapse of the Han and the beginning of the Song dynasty in the tenth century was a high point in the history of Chinese Buddhism. The Chinese capitals of Chang'an, Luoyang, and Jiankang, emerged as major nodes in the Buddhist world at this time. All manner of Buddhist texts were brought from around Asia to the major monasteries and translated into Chinese by multiparty and multicultural translation assemblies who themselves had come from all over the Buddhist world.[15] Various forms of Indian knowledge were introduced to China through this massive translation project, including many Buddhist approaches to health and well-being.

The significance of Indian medicine in China peaked in the first half of the Tang dynasty (618–907 CE).[16] In this period, exotic items from around the world were considered desirable by the cosmopolitan elite, and major Chinese cities were filled with foreign people, ideas, and fashions. The capital's markets, closely intertwined economically with the rest of Asia, brimmed with foreign spices, aromatics, and other pharmaceuticals.[17] Indian medical concepts such as the Four Elements, *tridoṣa*, and other doctrines—introduced through Chinese translations of the *Sūtra of Golden Light* {1: 4}, the *Sūtra of the Entry Into the Realm of Reality* (*Gaṇḍavyūha sūtra*) {1: 9}, and other texts discussed previously—influenced the medical authorities of the period, whether or not they identified as Buddhist.[18] Travelogues written by the monastic pilgrims Faxian (ca. 320–420 CE), Xuanzang (602–664 CE), and Yijing (635–713 CE) introduced Chinese readers to Indian hospitals, public dispensaries, and monastic medical education.[19] Narratives about foreign healer monks treating commoners, the elite, and members of the royal or imperial family generated interest in Buddhist medicine across the social spectrum {1: 21}.

Translations of important Buddhist medical texts continued to be made in China as late as the eleventh century.[20] However, a backlash of xenophobia, nativism, and neoclassicism had begun in the second half of the eighth century that soured elite Chinese attitudes toward explicitly foreign knowledge. Between the years 842 and 845 CE, a severe repression of Buddhist institutions in the "Huichang Persecution," left the Buddhist order decimated and its power base hobbled. When the Song dynasty (960–1279) took over, it ushered in a period of neo-Confucian and neoclassicist reforms. Moving to standardize imperial medical training in the mid-eleventh century, the Song government chose to emphasize texts from the pre-Buddhist era.[21] Although a handful of Buddhist ideas were represented in the authorized books—most notably in the writings of Sun Simiao {1: 52, 53}—this decision effectively wrote Buddhist therapies out of the official Chinese medical canon.

Many aspects of Buddhist tradition were reformulated during this time to better align with domestic frameworks of thought and practice and not appear so foreign.[22] Schools of Buddhism such as Chan (Jp. Zen) that prioritized indigenous Chinese philosophical, religious, and aesthetic traditions emerged. Likewise, classical Chinese medical models came to be preferred over their Indian counterparts in most Buddhist discourses.[23] Buddhist medicine did not disappear; however, from this period onward, Buddhists came to be more interested in native forms of therapy, such as acupuncture, moxibustion, self-cultivation (*yangsheng*), martial arts, Chinese herbal medicine, and Chinese divination than in Indian concepts or practices. Buddhist exegetes and lay physicians alike still occasionally wrote about Indian medicine, but when they did, they most often expressed those ideas in the indigenous terminology of Chinese medicine (e.g., *qi*, *yin-yang*, *wuxing*) rather than Sanskrit {1: 39, 48}. When justifying their involvement in such activities, they were more likely to appeal to ancient Chinese medical authorities than foreign Buddhist physicians {2: 3}.

This is not a narrative of displacement, however. The core Mahāyāna teachings on healing continued to be prominent throughout the remainder of Chinese history. Engaging in Buddhist healing rites, propitiating Buddhist healing deities, and calling on Buddhist monastics to perform healings or empower medicines continued to be popular across all segments of Chinese society.[24] Buddhist values, such as selflessness, universal compassion, and vegetarianism, continued to inform the ethical foundation and personal ideologies of physicians {2: 3, 9}.[25] Patients continued to patronize Buddhist institutions in search of healing, and Buddhist temples continued to be famed for their involvement in medicine (notable examples include the famous Shaolin Temple in Henan Province,[26] as well as several lesser-known locations that specialized in female medicine).[27] The influence of Buddhism can also be seen in the popular literature of the premodern period.[28] In short, Buddhist medicine was everywhere. The difference was that, with few exceptions, the benefits of these health-seeking activities were spoken of using native Chinese medical terms rather than Indian medical concepts such as the Elements or *tridoṣa*.[29]

The domesticated form of Buddhist medicine created in China was also adopted throughout East Asia, where Buddhism for the most part arrived via China, not directly from India. East Asian cultures were introduced to Chinese Buddhism and classical Chinese medicine simultaneously as part of a "package" that included literature and the arts, systems of governance and social organization, material culture and architecture, and other aspects of continental Chinese civilization. (Unfortunately, owing to a lack of sources, not much is known about the indigenous medical cultures of Korea and Japan before the introduction of the writing system from China.)

In Korea, where Buddhism was introduced in the late fourth century, the textual records from the Silla (57 BCE–935 CE) and Koryŏ (918–1392) dynasties suggest that Buddhism contributed significantly to health care.[30] Temples served as important locations for healing, and monks were famed for their medical knowledge {1: 21§9, 49}. Devotees chanted, recopied *sūtras*, used *dhāraṇī*, and made talismans for health.[31] The worship of Bhaiṣajyaguru (Kr. Yaksabul) was especially popular, particularly at Tonghwasa Temple, which became a major cultic site.[32]

Although these aspects of Buddhist medicine became extremely popular throughout Korean society, Indian medical doctrines never became a major influence for physicians. Lip service was occasionally paid to the Great Elements—even in key medical compilations produced by neo-Confucian physicians in the fifteenth and seventeenth centuries {1: 55}. However, these references are few and far between and of a superficial nature, suggesting that much of the theoretical substance of Indian medicine was not in circulation.

Meanwhile, in Japan, the Buddhist and classical Chinese therapies introduced simultaneously in the sixth century were understood to be largely compatible.[33] In many other parts of Asia, physicians and monastics belonged to separate social categories, but Japan was home to many monastic physicians (*sōi*), practitioners who specialized in combining Buddhist and Chinese medicine {1: 56}.[34] Because of this integration, passages from Buddhist texts frequently appear in some of the most important Japanese medical treatises. The earliest surviving medical encyclopedia, the *Prescriptions at the Heart of Medicine* (*Ishinpō*), published in 984 CE by Tanba no Yasuyori (912–995 CE), for example, includes quotes attributed to the bodhisattva Nāgārjuna explaining classical Indian ophthalmology {1: 54}.[35]

In Japan, temples had a particularly important role to play in protecting the populace from disease and epidemics. The Shōsōin, an eighth-century monastic storehouse located at the Tōdaiji temple in Nara, is a valuable time capsule providing a snapshot of these kinds of activities.[36] The collection includes imported medicinals such as the "five-color dragon's tooth" (a fossilized elephant tooth used as a sedative), realgar, and plant medicines deriving from China, India, and Silk Road territories. Records show that sixty medicinal substances were offered to the temple by Queen Consort Kōmyō in 756 CE. Consecrated by Vairocana Buddha, these medicines were to be dispensed to the public to prevent diseases.

**7.1** Votive plaques (*ema*) placed by the faithful seeking healing at Tanukidanisan Fudōin temple in Kyoto. Devotees have circled "recover from illness" or "suppress cancer" and have indicated the afflicted parts of their bodies.
Photo by Justin Stein.

Japanese monastics were also important as cross-cultural brokers facilitating medical exchanges with the wider world. One area that seems to have been particularly ripe for cross-pollination was women's reproductive health. Indian fertility formulas and other interventions for women's health care were introduced from

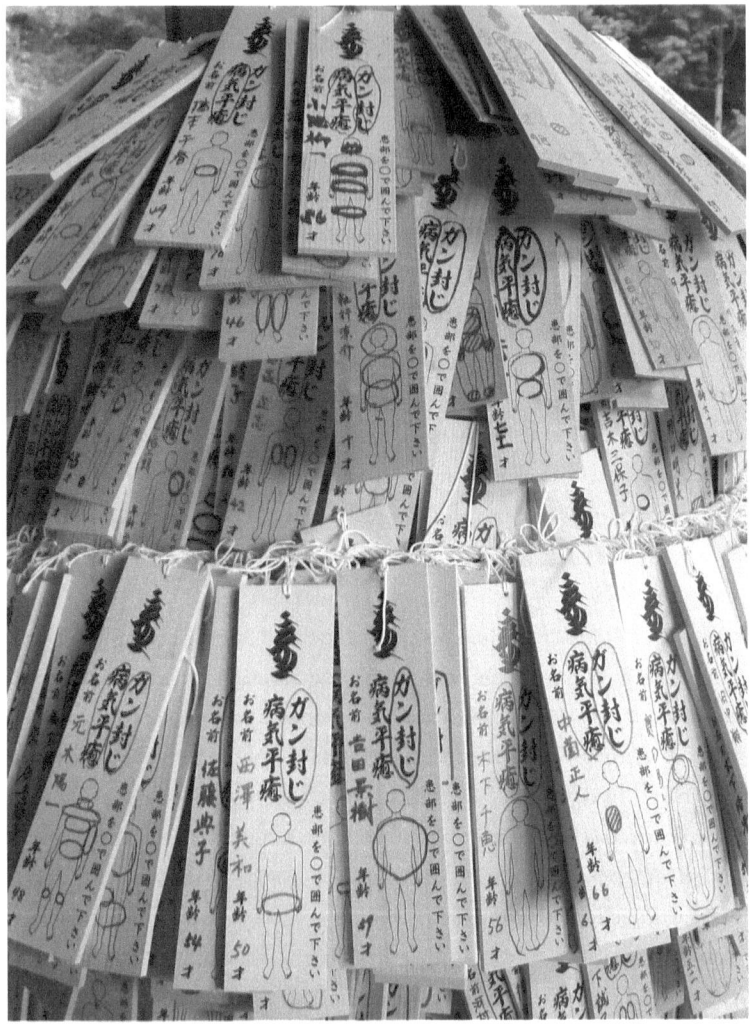

China possibly as early as the ninth century, and records from medieval Japan indicate that Buddhist monastics were active in obstetrics and pediatrics {1: 32}.[37] Over a century later, the monk physician Kajiwara Shōzen (1265–1337), a member of a Buddhist order dedicated to medical charity, continued to blend and innovate {1: 56}. He authored a comprehensive Japanese medical treatise and the first Japanese medical work written for a popular audience, both of which introduced readers to medical theories, pharmaceutical formulas, and diagnostic techniques from China, the Middle East, and Buddhist treatises.[38]

As in China and Korea, however, it was ritual healing that seems to have been the Buddhist health intervention with the most currency among the general public. Japanese Buddhist groups frequently invented healing rituals to enhance their popularity and vie for patronage {1: 51}.[39] *Dhāraṇī* healing and esoteric rituals were prevalent, and rituals propitiating Bhaiṣajyaguru, Avalokiteśvara, Kṣitigarbha, and Mañjuśri were also particularly well received {1: 21§11, 23, 32, 33}.[40] The same ritual repertoire was also used in veterinary medicine.[41] Japanese monks frequently traveled to the mainland to keep abreast of the newest developments in Chinese Buddhism, since access to specialized knowledge could translate into official support. The monk Kūkai (774–835 CE), for example, spent two years in China studying Esoteric Buddhism and brought back the *kaji* empowerment rituals that he would employ to preserve the ruler's personal health {1: 23}.[42]

Japanese Buddhist rituals often emphasized or accentuated exotic aspects of Indic culture, such as the sounds of Sanskrit syllables or the use of the *siddhaṃ* alphabet {1: 51}. However, the overall impact of Indian doctrines on the Japanese medical landscape was still much less significant than that of classical Chinese medical concepts. The benefits of Buddhist medicine were usually explained in terms of Chinese vocabularies rather than Sanskrit. Authors most often discussed the efficacy of Buddhist interventions in terms of cultivating *qi* (Jp. *ki*), balancing *yin-yang* (Jp. *onmyō*), regulating the *wuxing* (Jp. *gogyō*), or nourishing the viscera (Jp. *gozō*) {1: 38}.[43] Detailed discussions of Sanskrit medical concepts such as the Elements or *tridoṣa* are extremely rare. Buddhist healing rites also heavily incorporated ideas derived from Daoism and Chinese self-cultivation traditions, as well as spirit-manipulating and purification practices associated with the native traditions of Shintō {1: 32, 51}. For example, hot springs were locations long associated with healing in indigenous Japanese culture that became especially important focal points of Buddhist healing activities {1: 22}.[44]

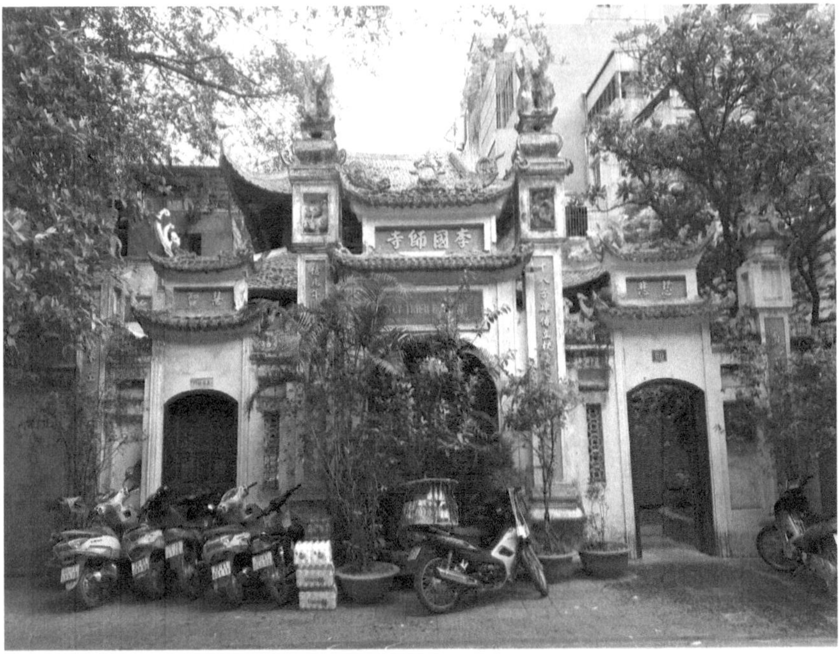


**7.2** The Lý Quốc Sư Pagoda in Hanoi, Vietnam, is dedicated to a monk living in the eleventh and twelfth centuries noted for his healing activities. He is reputed to have healed the king of an illness that doctors could not relieve.
Image courtesy of the Jivaka Project (http://jivaka.net), Creative Commons license.

As we round out our tour of East Asia, it must be noted that very little scholarship has been done on the history of Buddhist medicine in premodern Vietnam. The story of the monk Tuệ Tĩnh, who was sent to Ming China as an emissary in the fourteenth century and never returned, was related in chapter 5 {1: 57}. While not telling us nearly enough about the domestic Vietnamese context, this example reveals that Vietnam was involved in networks of Buddhist medical exchange in the premodern period. It also suggests the important role of Vietnamese monks as cultural mediators, interpreters, and synthesizers of Buddhist medicine. Forthcoming scholarship on the early history of Vietnamese Buddhist medicine will hopefully fill in more details of what is undoubtedly a rich history.[45]

## TRANSLOCATION I: TIBET

I use the word "translocation" to describe the third trajectory of Buddhist medicine, which characterized large parts of Southeast and Central Asia (e.g., Sri Lanka, mainland Southeast Asia, the Himalayan region, Mongolia, and certain areas home to Central Asian ethnic groups that lie within the modern borders of India, China, and Russia). In these areas, Indian ideas about the body, illness, and health did not die out as a result of Islamization, nor did they become absorbed into native linguistic and cultural systems. Rather, cross-culturally transmitted knowledge introduced from India planted seeds here that would grow into culture-specific, Buddhist-inflected medical traditions. These long-lasting local traditions developed and thrived throughout the remainder of the premodern period, and they remain relevant parts of the health care system today.

Many of the cultures in question were also on the receiving end of a fair amount of Chinese and Islamic medical influence. All of these imported concepts and practices were hybridized with native traditions of shamanism, spirit medicine, or other local healing practices. Thus, the medical traditions of each region are characterized by distinct local features. Nevertheless, in the parts of the world affected by the trajectory of translocation, Indian medical ideas tended to have more cultural cachet and social prestige than domestic models. Indian medical knowledge also formed the basis of the medical system promulgated by government institutions, political elites, and other authority structures.

In these areas, Buddhism was the dominant framework through which medicine was learned, practiced, and transmitted. Medical knowledge was directly associated with monasteries and the sangha. Ideas were normally expressed in Sanskrit terminology or in closely equivalent translations. Practitioners' founding myths and rituals revolved around venerating Buddhist deities and heroes as patriarchs of their lineages. Many key medical texts were attributed to famous Buddhist authors. A package of Buddhist therapies imported from India—including talismans, amulets, *sūtra* chanting, *dhāraṇī* and mantra incantations, astrology, exorcisms, empowerments, binding rites, and consecrated water or medicines—were integral parts of the therapeutic repertoire. Further, the language and metaphors used to talk about all of this explicitly and self-assuredly drew upon the Dharma.

The most historically influential example of this sort of translocation is Sowa Rigpa.[46] Indian medical ideas were introduced to Tibet during the Tibetan Empire period (600–850 CE), when a number of Buddhist *sūtras* such as the *Sūtra of Golden Light* were first translated. The medical concepts presented in these texts continued to be elaborated during the so-called Dark Ages (850–950 CE), as evidenced by Tibetan-language manuscripts from Dunhuang, as well as hybrid Sino-Tibetan Buddhist medical texts such as the *Medicine of the Moon King* (Tib. *Menché dawé gyelpo*) {1: 50}.[47] In the Tibetan Renaissance era (950–1250), a number of Āyurvedic treatises were also translated, including Vāgbhaṭa's *Essence of the Eight Branches*.[48] These new teachings were combined with preexisting knowledge from sources such as *Moon King* and the *sūtras* to produce a distinctively Tibetan medical synthesis.

These trends culminated in the twelfth-century composition of the Tibetan medical classic *Secret Essence of Ambrosia in Eight Branches: An Instructional Tantra*, more commonly known as the *Four Tantras* (Tib. *Gyushi*) {1: 60, 61}.[49] The knowledge presented in this seminal treatise was heavily influenced by the *Essence of the Eight Branches*. The fundamental theoretical backbone along which the text's medical practices were organized consisted of the core Indian concepts of the Elements, *tridoṣa*, and Winds. But the text also synthesized a variety of practices and ideas that were coming into Tibet via the exchange networks, such as alchemy, Chinese pulse-reading, and Greco-Roman-Islamic urinoscopy, as well as local healing traditions.[50]

Significantly, the *Four Tantras* repackaged all of this medical material from across Asia within an unmistakably Buddhist wrapping.[51] Calling itself a *tantra*, the text is composed in the style of a Buddhist scripture. It purports to record the words of the buddha Bhaiṣajyaguru, who manifested himself in the form of two sages, Rikpé Yeshé (literally "Gnostic Awareness") and Yilekyé (literally "Mind-Born"), to deliver an authoritative teaching on medicine.[52] In addition to incorporating ideas and practices from various Asian systems of medicine, the *Four Tantras* also recommends Buddhist ritual practices drawn from Vajrayāna Buddhism. Most notable is chapter 31 of the "Explanatory Tantra" section, which lays out the virtues a physician should cultivate and the pitfalls to avoid. Here, the text outlines rituals for worshipping Bhaiṣajyaguru with prayer and mantras and prescribes a set of visualizations the doctor can use to empower his practice. According to this chapter, the path of medicine is not separate from the path

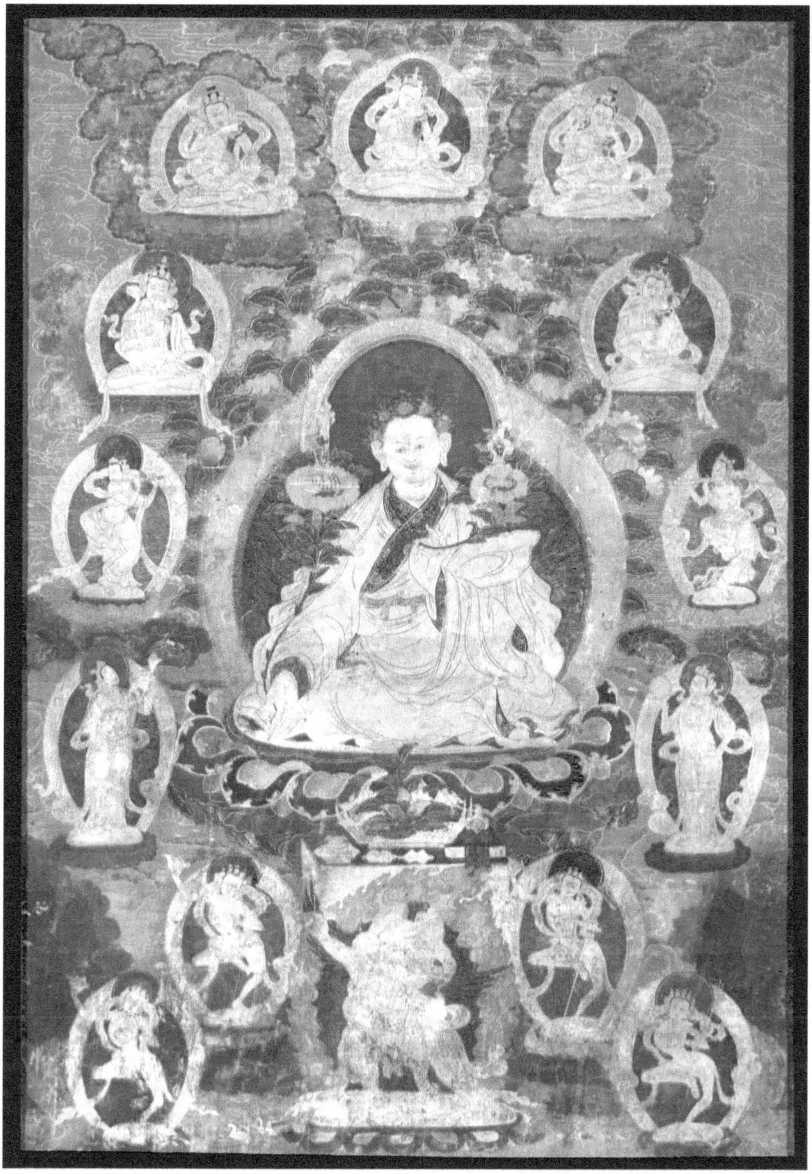

7.3 Seventeenth-century portrait of Yutok Yönten Gonpo, the twelfth-century forefather of Tibetan medicine. The central figure is surrounded by buddhas and other male and female divinities.

From the Rubin Museum of Art. Image courtesy of Wikimedia Commons, public domain.

of the Dharma: the physician who practices with integrity and compassion will ultimately become a buddha.

Modern scholars identify the author of the *Four Tantras* as the twelfth-century Tibetan physician Yutok Yönten Gonpo.[53] Yutok, a nonmonastic practitioner of Vajrayāna, is credited with not only authoring the *Four Tantras* but also founding the system of training known as the "Heart Essence of Yutok" (*Yutok nyingthig*), a Tantric system of self-cultivation combining medical and spiritual elements designed for lay physicians.[54] A biography of Yutok composed at the turn of the eighteenth century says that he began to study medicine at the age of eight and traveled to India six times.[55] It goes on to relate how he received medical texts from Indian sages, his various encounters with deities, and his acquisition of great magical powers. While Yutok was a historical person whose biography was inflated with legendary accounts, he also appears to have served as the inspiration for the creation of an altogether mythological "Yutok the Elder," who also looms large as a forefather of Tibetan medicine.[56]

Tibetan medicine in Yutok's time (that is, in the twelfth century) was largely diffuse and uncodified. However, the synthesis he provided in the *Four Tantras* would change this. By the fourteenth century, physicians associated with the Sakya Monastery had developed a medical lineage and standardized practice of medicine centered around the *Four Tantras*.[57] In the seventeenth century, the *Four Tantras* would be further elevated by the official systematization of medicine undertaken by the fifth Dalai Lama (1617–1682) as part of his efforts to consolidate the Buddhist identity of the new Tibetan state.[58] Desi Sangyé Gyatso (1653–1705), his regent, was a close partner in these efforts. The Desi's most important medical composition, the *Blue Beryl* (*Baidurya ngönpo*), was a four-volume commentary on the *Four Tantras* accompanied by a set of seventy-nine Buddhist-style paintings (see figure 3.2, 3.3) .[59] He also wrote the first comprehensive history of Tibetan medicine, which credits Buddhism as its fundamental influence and framework.[60]

Both the Dalai Lama and Sangyé Gyatso made clear in their writings that they saw the practice of medicine as an integral part of the bodhisattva path. Despite Sowa Rigpa's close connection with Buddhism, however, Tibetan physicians did not defer to religious authority on all points. The *Four Tantras* was never included in the Buddhist canon, and its origin and status as Buddha-word was the subject of discussion and controversy in Tibet for centuries {1: 62}.[61] Physicians and monastic experts continually debated the precedence of scriptural authority versus other sources of knowledge such as empirical observation.[62] But while such debates took place among a cadre of elite physicians, Buddhism continued to play an important role in the transmission, codification, practice, and understanding of Tibetan medicine among most practitioners throughout the remainder of the premodern period, as it has continued to do to this day.[63]

In the eighteenth and nineteenth centuries, Sowa Rigpa spread beyond the Tibetan Plateau. Mongolia became home to a flourishing tradition based on locally authored commentaries on the *Four Tantras*. Diagnostics and therapy combined the Indian Elements and *tridoṣa*, the Chinese Five Phases and *yin-yang* theory, and indigenous Mongol healing practices. However, Buddhist concepts provided the overarching framework by which physicians organized these diverse techniques and bodies of knowledge.[64] Buddhist rituals also remained centrally important healing methods {1: 35; 2: 4}.

In the modern period, the Sowa Rigpa tradition has continued to be practiced not only in Tibet and Mongolia but also in Nepal, Bhutan, and parts of modern India, China, and Russia that are influenced by Tibetan and Mongol culture. Given its historical and contemporary significance across such a huge area, Sowa Rigpa can easily be said to be the most influential translocation of Buddhist medicine in Asia in the second millennium. The contemporary practice of this tradition will be explored further in chapter 9.

## TRANSLOCATION II: SOUTHEAST ASIA

Theravāda Buddhist contexts, of course, were markedly different cultural and intellectual environments than Tibet. However, forms of Buddhist medicine emerging in Sri Lanka, Cambodia, Laos, and Thailand shared many similarities with Sowa Rigpa. These Southeast Asian medical traditions were based on concepts, terminologies, and practices that were introduced to the region via Buddhist texts, that were attributed to Buddhist deities and heroes, and that remained closely connected with monastic power structures.

Archaeological evidence indicates that Buddhist monastics and institutions were heavily involved in the promulgation of medicine in this part of the world from early on. In Sri Lanka, for example, ruins of Buddhist medicinal baths and other medical facilities date from the first millennium. The ninth-century hospital at the Buddhist site of Mihintale, near the city of Anurādhapura, is one of the earliest archaeologically excavated hospitals in the world.[65] In the Khmer Empire a few centuries later, King Jayavarman VII constructed a network of 102 hospitals, as mentioned in a previous chapter {1: 24}.

Despite such tantalizing architectural evidence, owing to the toll taken by the tropical climate in this part of the world, the earliest extant texts date to a later period than elsewhere. Scholars are currently on the lookout for more textual evidence, and efforts have recently begun to digitize and examine a number of caches of manuscripts hidden away in monastic libraries across Cambodia, Laos, and Thailand.[66] We know that across the region, monasteries collected medical texts and served as centers of medical education for monks and the laity alike.[67] Upon investigation, many of these locations will no doubt turn out to contain valuable sources of Buddhist medical knowledge, and it is hoped that more information will become available soon.

Yet, even with limited textual evidence, it is still clear that Buddhism played a critical role in the development of medicine in Southeast Asia. Monks authored a number of important medical texts in Sri Lanka, including the *Casket of Medicine* (Pāli *Bhesajjamañjūsā*), composed in the Pāli language in the thirteenth century.[68] Closely related to Vāgbhaṭa's *Essence of the Eight Branches*, and quoting from about eighty other Āyurvedic medical treatises, the medical system introduced in this text is much indebted to Indian models. Comparable materials from Cambodia and Myanmar, available only in much later editions, give us a similar picture of the central role of Buddhist concepts there as well {1: 59}.[69] In all of these places, diagnosis was based on the theory of the Great Elements, and therapy was based on the flavors. Southeast Asian medical traditions were also clearly influenced by Buddhist ethics and morality and make frequent reference to other Buddhist doctrines.

The most detailed glimpses into premodern medical practice from the region come from Thailand. One early incantation text that still circulates today is the *Verses on the Victor's Armor* (Pāli: *Jinapañjara gāthā*; Thai: *Phra gatha chinabanchon*). When chanted, this spell is thought to shield against illnesses and other dangers {1: 34}. While its history remains vague, the text seems to have originally been authored in the late fifteenth or early sixteenth century in the city of Chiang Mai (in modern-day northwestern Thailand), where it was inscribed onto the city's gate to confer protection to residents. In subsequent centuries, the incantation spread to Burma and Sri Lanka. It is still chanted today in Thai temples around the world.

Even more significant for our analysis are the artifacts and sources from the Wat Phra Chetuphon Temple site in Bangkok. In 1792, the Chakri dynasty took control of territory that had previously been split among a number of separate states to create the first unified Siamese kingdom, the Rattanakosin (1782–1932). In the 1830s, this new line of kings constructed a royal temple complex in the new capital, in which they installed a number of medical artifacts.[70] In a continuation of the long tradition of Buddhist royal largesse discussed in chapter 5, this effort was framed by members of the Siamese royal family as a contribution to the education, benefit, and unity of the population.[71] As in the case of both the fifth Dalai Lama and Jayavarman VII, the collection of these artifacts in the royal temple also signaled the Siamese kings' ambitions to centralize medical policy while consolidating political control over their new territory. These efforts also explicitly tied official medical policy to the seat of Buddhist authority in Siam.

A major part of the systematization at Wat Phra Chetuphon was the compilation of medical knowledge from around the kingdom in both stone inscriptions

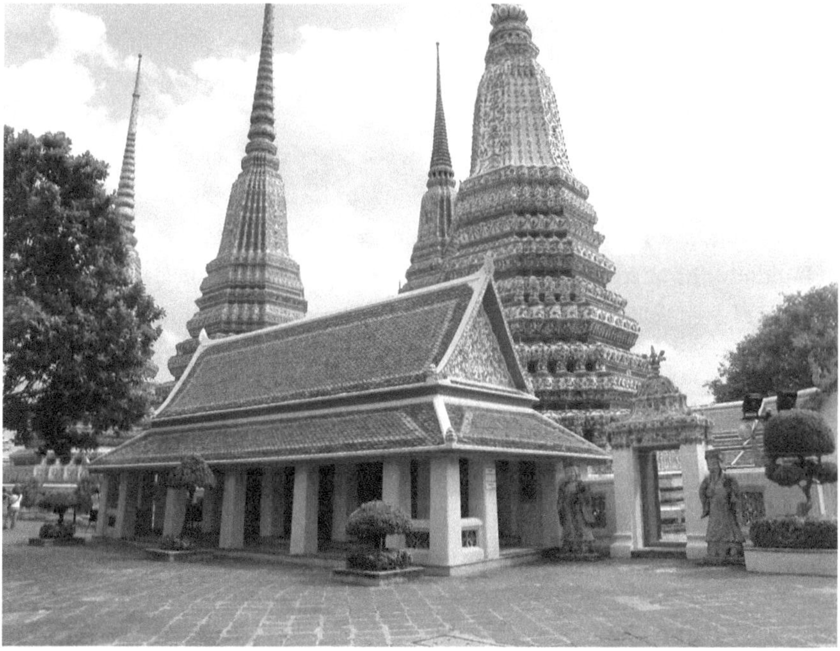

**7.4** This pagoda at the Wat Phra Chetuphon temple in Bangkok, Thailand, houses a number of stone inscriptions of herbal recipes and massage techniques. Inscribed in the 1830s, these were intended to preserve and educate the public on traditional medicine therapies as part of a royal renovation project.
Photo by the author.

and official publications. While a smattering of manuscripts are extant from an earlier period, it is this collection that gives us our first comprehensive overview of a complete medical system from mainland Southeast Asia.[72] Some of these texts hint at the local traditions of medicine prevalent at that time in remoter parts of the kingdom, some of which had nothing to do with Buddhism.[73] Notwithstanding, the synthesis produced at the temple in the nineteenth century was avowedly Buddhist. Its theory hinges on the Elements, *tridoṣa*, and the medicinal flavors, and it copiously uses Sanskrit terminology. Across the corpus, certain volumes (especially those associated with pediatrics) are attributed to the legendary physician Jīvaka, who is celebrated as one of the great founders of the Siamese medical tradition.[74] Other therapies, particularly herbal remedies and yogic exercises, are credited to different Buddhist sages of the forest (Skt. *ṛṣi*; Th. *ruesi*).

Other artifacts compiled at Wat Phra Chetuphon include statues of sages performing health-bestowing yoga postures (see figure 3.4) and diagrams of a Thai system of subtle Wind channels (Th. *sen*; equivalent to Skt. *nāḍī*). Both, in turn, formed the basis of a system of massage and movement therapies not far removed from other traditions of therapeutic movement such as Tibetan *yantra* yoga and Indian *haṭhayoga*.[75]

All of the examples given here are evidence of the central role of the monastic order and temple institutions in preserving and propagating translocated systems of Buddhist medicine. These texts and artifacts are also tangible evidence of Buddhists' intimate involvement in the development of medical knowledge, in matters of medical legitimation and authority, and in the identity and values of healers within Southeast Asia. The continuity of these features in modern times will be addressed in chapters 8 and 9.

* * *

As regional forms of Buddhism began flourishing in Southeast Asia, East Asia, and the Tibetan region, approaches to health and healing underwent accelerated processes of adaptation, transformation, and localization. This chapter has zoomed out to identify three macro-level historical trajectories that took place in different parts of Asia: "displacement" in parts of Asia where Buddhism did not survive over the long term, "domestication" into native medical frameworks in East Asia, and "translocation" in parts of Central and Southeast Asia where Buddhist medicine formed the nucleus of vibrant and long-lasting medical traditions.

These broad patterns can help us to grasp the outlines of the global history of Buddhist medicine. Nevertheless, the reader is reminded that these are generalizations that can provide only a bird's-eye view. This chapter is intended to orient readers to the big picture by bringing diverse local histories into a common overarching narrative that reveals their relationships with one another. However, once we descend from these lofty heights to take a closer look at the histories of Buddhism and medicine in any specific time or place, a much richer picture will emerge than can be captured here. The reader is strongly urged to explore the translations in the anthologies, as well as the citations and further readings in this chapter and throughout all three volumes, to continue the process of finer-grained exploration.

## FURTHER READING

Gyatso, Janet. 2015. *Being Human in a Buddhist World: An Intellectual History of Medicine in Early Modern Tibet*. New York: Columbia University Press. A detailed treatment of a pivotal period in Tibetan medical history, with focus on debates among physicians and religious figures over the relative authority of Buddhist and medical texts.

Kilty, Gavin, trans. 2010. *A Mirror of Beryl: A Historical Introduction to Tibetan Medicine*. Boston: Wisdom. A fascinating Tibetan account of the Buddhist origins of medicine and its development in Tibet, composed by Desi Sangyé Gyatso in the seventeenth century.

Liyanaratne, Jindasa. 1999. *Buddhism and Traditional Medicine in Sri Lanka*. Kelaniya, Sri Lanka: Kelaniya University Press. An overview of the role of Buddhist institutions, practitioners, and texts in the history of traditional medicine in Sri Lanka.

Salguero, C. Pierce, and Andrew Macomber, eds. 2020. *Buddhist Healing in Medieval China and Japan*. Honolulu: University of Hawai'i Press. An analysis of the localization of Buddhist medical ideas and practices in China and Japan.

Suzuki, Yui. 2012. *Medicine Master Buddha: The Iconic Worship of Yakushi in Heian Japan*. Leiden: Brill. A discussion of the emergence of the cult of Bhaiṣajyaguru in medieval Japan.

Triplett, Katja. 2019. *Buddhism and Medicine in Japan: A Topical Survey (500–1600 CE) of a Complex Relationship*. Berlin: De Gruyter. An important in-depth analysis of Buddhist medicine in premodern Japanese society.

CHAPTER 8

# *Modernizations*

Having explored the themes of circulation, translation, and localization in the premodern period over the last three chapters, this one turns to a discussion of the thoroughgoing transformation of Buddhist medicine in the modern era. Modernity is much more than just a period of time, and there is robust and ongoing scholarly debate on precisely how to use this term.[1] While interesting in their own right, these debates are beyond the scope of this book. Here, I employ the concept of modernity loosely, using it as a convenient shorthand to refer to the period of time from the onset of European colonialism and missionary activity in Asia in the early sixteenth century through to the end of the twentieth century. Developments in the twenty-first century will be discussed in the next chapter.

In the modern period, Buddhist approaches to health and healing continued to be widely practiced all over Asia, but understandings of both religion and medicine were rapidly transforming. In the early modern period, Western colonizers and Asian reformers alike criticized Buddhism along with many other aspects of traditional Asian culture as "superstition." As new discoveries and developments transformed the face of modern medicine, the very idea that practicing rituals, chanting *sūtras*, or engaging in mental exercises such as meditation could have real benefits for health seemed to fly in the face of the emerging scientific medical paradigm. However, Buddhist apologists of this period worked hard to resolve the apparent incompatibilities, creating new forms of Buddhism that could be presented as scientific, ecumenical, and international. This movement produced new forms of medical practice that were not only influenced or inspired by Buddhism but also were verifiable by science. Some of these, such as therapeutic meditation, have become highly visible, internationally popular features of Buddhist medicine today.

## COLONIAL RUPTURES

At the end of the fifteenth century, Portuguese ships rounded the Cape of Good Hope at the southern tip of the African continent and burst into the Indian Ocean. By the mid-1500s, thanks to superior military technology and a willingness to use it in pursuit of profit, Portugal had seized coastal trade posts throughout South and Southeast Asia and had begun to exert control over the trade in these strategic waters. The mercenaries aboard these ships were sometimes accompanied by members of the Catholic missionary group known as the Jesuits (or the Society of Jesus). Converting the Asian population to Christianity had been a priority for the Jesuits from the founding of the order in 1540, and one of the original Jesuits, Francis Xavier (1506–1552), traveled widely in Asia to lay the groundwork for this initiative. In the sixteenth century, Jesuit missions were established in Ceylon (modern-day Sri Lanka), China, India, and Japan. In the seventeenth and eighteenth centuries, the society expanded its operations to modern-day Myanmar, Thailand, Tibet, Vietnam, and other parts of the Buddhist world.

Jesuits tended to use the latest developments in Western science to ingratiate themselves with segments of Asian society.[2] Their missionary strategy often included translating Western medical treatises, setting up hospitals, and organizing health-related charities. One place where the Jesuits were involved with such medical missionary work was Japan, where Catholicism enjoyed tremendous success during the so-called Christian century (1550–1650). Ultimately, the Japanese government felt that the church had gained too much power and popularity, and moved to outlaw Christianity in 1614. Correspondence, eyewitness reports, and other historical documents are extant from this period, attesting in both Japanese and Portuguese to the conflicts and competitions over medical theory and practice between Jesuits and Buddhists {2: 1, 2}.

Following the Catholic lead, Protestant missionary activity in Asia began in the seventeenth century with Dutch and British colonialism. Protestants also used European medicine and charitable health-care initiatives to promote their religion and thus entered into confrontations and competitions with local healers and medical authorities similar to those faced by the Jesuits.[3] In contrast to the precariousness of the Portuguese presence in Japan, however, British colonial efforts were more successful in the long term. Britain was eventually able to seize control of whole swathes of Buddhist Asia (including Ceylon in the late eighteenth century and Burma and parts of Nepal and Bhutan in the first half of the nineteenth).

Although the British Empire did not impose Christianity on its colonized populations by force, it did allow Protestant missionaries great leeway to engage in missionary activities in its colonies. In addition to promoting Christianity, these missionary groups also worked hard to dissuade colonized populations from following Buddhism. By the nineteenth century, all over colonized Asia from India to the Philippines, anti-traditional, pro-modern, and pro-Western propaganda was being actively promulgated by missionaries and colonizers.

These efforts periodically targeted Buddhist healing practices as an object of scorn. One illustrative example is a popular booklet written in the Sinhala language produced in 1851 by the Ceylon Religious Tract Society, a Protestant missionary group {2: 6}. Mocking patients who sought out Buddhist ritualists to exorcize illness-causing demons, the tract argued that truly civilized people would pay a visit to "intelligent doctors" who prescribed modern medicine.[4] This tract sold tens of thousands of copies and was still in print more than fifty years later.

Documents composed by Western observers in this era contain some factual information about Buddhist ideas and practices valuable for historians of medicine. However, even those who purported to be providing objective ethnographic information could not disguise their disdain. Their accounts are filled with biased and racist vitriol against the supposed ignorance, gullibility, and inferiority of Asian people. Frequently, these observers saw Asian "backwardness" in matters of religion and medicine as interconnected. For example, a report by Father Sangermano, a Barnabite missionary in colonial Burma between 1783 and 1808, calls attention to the "superstitions and prejudices" of native Burmese medical and religious therapies.[5] Likewise, a short treatise on Burmese medicine by Dr. Keith Norman Macdonald written in 1879 draws a firm line between the religious and medical practices of the "semi-barbarous peoples of the Asiatic" and those of the "more civilised communities of the European continent."[6] Similarly dismissive attitudes are expressed in a number of popular and scholarly publications of the time about Chinese, Indian, and other Asian cultures {2: 7}.[7]

It was not just the Westerners showing disdain, however. Local elites all over Asia often consumed such literature, internalized its messages, and wrote their own anti-traditionalist and anti-Buddhist propaganda.[8] Even if they did not all convert to Christianity, many educated intellectuals joined the European colonists' call for the elimination of "ignorance" and "superstition" from Buddhism.[9] Reformers also frequently called for the suppression of traditional healing methods in favor of modern medicine. Although scientific approaches to healing were only just emerging in Europe and North America in this period, reformers often perceived an enormous gap between the innovations of modern medicine and traditional approaches. Drawing, negotiating, and defending stark lines separating "religion," "superstition," "magic," and "medicine" were key characteristics of modernity.[10]

By the nineteenth century, European missionaries, colonial authorities, and local elites across Asia were taking steps to outlaw, repress, or severely marginalize healers who incorporated religious activities into their repertoires of practice. Modernizers were influential even in countries that never were colonized, and various reform movements along these lines emerged in the second half of the century. The modernizations of Meiji-era Japan (1868–1912), for example, were not directly imposed by colonial powers but rather arose from internal political processes in response to perceived Western superiority. Inspired by European (particularly German) models, these reforms led to the thoroughgoing transformation of Japanese society in a remarkably short period of time. With the prioritization of "Western learning" during this period, critiques of Buddhist medicine intensified among elites. The practice of empowerment rituals, which had become ubiquitous among religious healers of all sects and persuasions, had already come under assault in the first half of the nineteenth century.[11] When, as part of the Meiji reforms, new penal codes were passed in 1874 and 1907, healing using rituals, spells, prayers, charms, holy water, and other Buddhist techniques was outlawed. When soon thereafter Japan itself became a colonizer, its colonial administrators attempted to repress or reform traditional medicine in Taiwan, Korea, and Mongolia as well.[12]

The Rattanakosin kingdom in modern-day Thailand also avoided outright colonization by European powers, but it also did not escape the pressure to abandon traditions. The 1830s royal project at the Wat Phra Chetuphon temple celebrating traditional Siamese medicine was discussed in the previous chapter. The objects collected and installed in and around the medical pagoda suggest an enormous amount of pride in traditional medical knowledge and its Buddhist origins at the time of this construction. Nevertheless, just a few decades later, a string of Siamese kings embarked on a multipronged campaign to modernize the government the army, and society as a whole. These reforms drastically reorganized the relationship between the state and institutions of both Buddhist and traditional medicine.

The fourth Rattanakosin king, Mongkut (also known as Rama IV, r. 1851–1868), began the process by purifying Siamese Buddhism of "superstitious" elements. Practices that deviated from the new orthodoxy—including a wide range of healing meditations, mantras, and other forms of magical healing—began to be

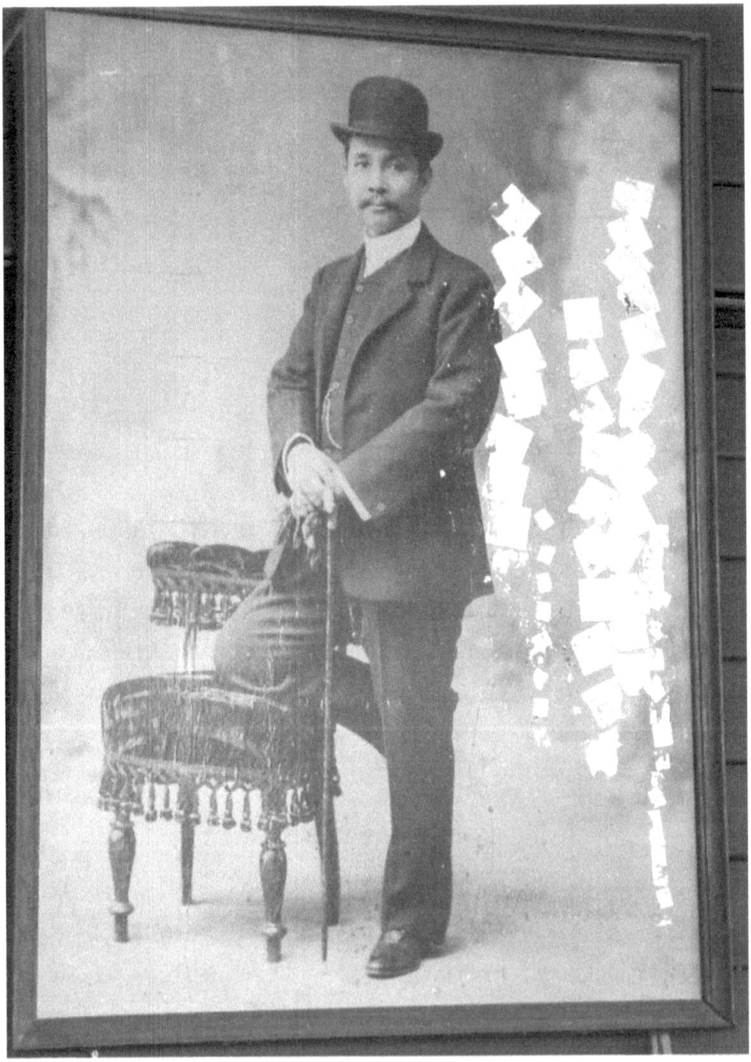

**8.1** King Chulalongkorn, a ruler notable for modernizing Thai society, ironically is frequently worshipped by Thais as a powerful spirit in contemporary times. Here, his portrait has been adorned with gold leaf as an offering for good luck and protection.
Photo by the author.

repressed in Siam from this point onward.[13] The next ruler in the dynasty, Chulalongkorn (also known as Rama V, r. 1868–1910), further consolidated Bangkok's authority over the Thai sangha. Although certain high-profile resistors of this policy rose to fame, such as Khruba Siwichai (1878–1939) in the far northwestern region of the country, the net effect was the disenfranchisement of local Buddhist leaders, organizations, and traditions around the kingdom {2: 30}. Chulalongkorn's repression of local languages in favor of the Bangkok dialect and writing system also meant the loss of oral and written transmissions of traditional medical knowledge.

Chulalongkorn enlisted Western help to develop a European-style healthcare system. Missionaries, engineers, and physicians—often citizens of the United States, Germany, or other countries that were not regional colonial powers and therefore seen as safer—were patronized by the royal family to build and staff hospitals and develop medical and public health services.[14] However, these Western specialists were not neutral. Their ethnocentric attitudes and cultural chauvinism toward native Siamese religion, medicine, and culture are amply recorded in treatises written around the turn of the twentieth century {2: 7}.[15] The Siamese kings after Chulalongkorn were all educated in the West and seem to have shared Western observers' general distaste for traditional medicine. Laws in 1923 and 1936 made the practice illegal, while the government more aggressively implemented a modern (i.e., Western-style) medical and public health system.[16]

## BUDDHIST APOLOGETICS

The authority scientific medicine enjoyed in this period is hard to overstate. Virtually all aspects of public health and medicine were revolutionized through the application of scientific methods. The role of microorganisms in causing disease was established in the 1850s and 1860s, with lifesaving innovations in antiseptic surgery, public sanitation, and nursing care following shortly thereafter. Vaccines for cholera, rabies, tetanus, typhoid fever, and bubonic plague all became available in the late nineteenth century.[17] By century's end, physicians knew the causes of the most deadly infectious diseases affecting humanity and understood how to cure them or greatly mitigate their danger. Such breakthroughs continued at a rapid pace throughout the first half of the twentieth century, including the discovery of a number of antibiotics beginning in 1928. All of these medical innovations were disseminated in Asia by missionaries, by colonial officials, and through the international circulation of scientific publications.

Given the dramatic and immediate lifesaving effects of such measures, it is no mystery that there was such enthusiasm for modern medicine.[18] However, modernist rhetoric and reforms were inspired not only by tangible evidence of progress, but also by the racial hierarchies and social Darwinism that prevailed in Europe and North America in the late nineteenth and early twentieth centuries. These currents of thought were heavily intertwined with the science of the times. Elites fashioned themselves into "modern" people by emphasizing scientism and secularism and distancing themselves from the magic and superstition of the so-called backwards cultures.[19] In a more sinister vein, scientific discoveries in areas as diverse as genetics, evolution, and linguistics were put into the service of "proving" the superiority of Europeans and the inferiority of "the Asian race."

Colonial administrations and Western-influenced governments in Asia promoted not only modernization campaigns but also the narratives that underpinned them. Educated elites across Asia who followed these developments in many cases agreed with the notion that traditional ideas and practices were inferior and deluded. For many who fully adopted a modern Westernized lifestyle, Buddhism no longer seemed to offer much beyond backward-looking superstition.

At the same time, however, many devoted authors and thinkers chose not to abandon Buddhism but to reframe it in ways that would make it more compatible with the changing times. Some of these apologists saw Buddhist institutions and practices as valuable assets supportive of health and hygiene initiatives and coinciding with the priorities of the state.[20] Many began arguing that Buddhism was wholly compatible with (or even superior to) modern science. These authors often cherry-picked certain Buddhist doctrines as "evidence" of this compatibility.[21] For example, Taixu (1890–1947), an influential Buddhist reformer in Republican-era China, argued in a 1923 treatise that the omniscient Buddha had known of the existence of microscopic germs long before the present day. As evidence, he cited certain passages in Buddhist texts from the medieval period that described tens of thousands of tiny, invisible creatures filling the human body and floating in water {2: 9§1}.[22] As discussed in chapter 4, visualizing these creatures was part of a long Buddhist tradition of meditations on the impurities of the human body. For Taixu and other apologists, however, examples like this were used as evidence that the Buddha had known about bacteriology and other medical breakthroughs thousands of years before the dawn of modern science.

Taixu thought that Buddhist teachings held the key to understanding reality and saw modern medicine and other sciences as providing evidence that the Buddha's teachings had been correct all along. In contrast, certain other Buddhist reformers understood modern science and the Dharma as mutually edifying domains of knowledge, each adding important perspectives that were missing from the other. Such thinkers often called for Buddhism and science to be integrated. An early proponent of such an approach was the Japanese author Hara Tanzan (1819–1892), whose 1869 work, "On the Difference Between the Brain and the Spinal Cord," combined traditional East Asian medicine, Daoist inner alchemy, European anatomy, and Buddhist doctrine to create a modern physiological model of the process of enlightenment {2: 5}. A 1920 treatise by the Chinese polymath Ding Fubao similarly argued for synthesis. Laying out a simple rubric that still resonates for many practitioners in the twenty-first century, Ding argued that the health of the material body was the domain of science, whereas spiritual or mental health was the domain of Buddhism {2: 9§2}.

By the mid-twentieth century, such efforts at integration and reconciliation had become commonplace, a fully normalized feature of what scholars usually refer to as "Buddhist modernism."[23] Among both Asian intellectuals and a newly emerging cadre of "Orientalist" Western scholars studying Buddhism in academic centers in the West, the Buddha was increasingly spoken of as something like a proto-scientist or empirical philosopher ahead of his time.[24] While certain superstitious ideas may have crept into the texts because of the misunderstandings of his benighted followers, the argument went, the core of the Dharma was fully compatible with modern science and medicine. This viewpoint continues to shape the contemporary experience of Buddhism around the world today—perhaps most notably among people who identify as "secular," "nontraditional," or "nondenominational" Buddhists.[25]

## MEDICALIZING MEDITATION

If the notion that the Dharma and science are inherently compatible was one of the principal ideological commitments of Buddhist modernism, health has always been one of the main arenas in which Buddhist thought leaders have sought to demonstrate this compatibility. Among all of the health-related topics that Buddhist modernists have weighed in on, however, it is mental health that has received by far the most attention—and it is the mental health benefits of meditation that have gained the lion's share.

The Buddhist tradition has always had much to say about mental well-being. The role of Buddhist contemplations, morality, self-moderation, rituals, and subtle body practices in maintaining healthy mental and emotional states are well elaborated in all of the historical forms of Buddhism. However, in the second half of the nineteenth century, Buddhist thinkers began to draw explicit connections between Buddhism and modern medical disciplines and increasingly came to interpret meditation using modern psychology and psychiatry.

Before the nineteenth century, the serious practice of Buddhist meditation was usually limited outside of monastic circles.[26] In colonial Burma, however, the monk Ledi Sayadaw (1846–1923) began to promote certain types of meditation among the laity. His decision to disseminate this practice to as wide an audience as possible was in large part a response to the threat that it would be eradicated by colonial authorities.[27] As meditation became increasingly laicized in the twentieth century, it became ever more popular in Asia and beyond.

There are several routes by which Buddhist meditation became a secular mental health therapy. In the early 1900s, the internationally recognized Buddhist scholar and popularizer D. T. Suzuki (1870–1966) connected Zen mediation with increased mental vitality, resiliency, and strength.[28] In Japan at this time, Buddhist contemplations and breathing exercises were combined with Shinto healing practices, Western spiritualism, and interventions from the emergent field of psychology as novel treatments for the ailment of "neurasthenia."[29] Characterized by fatigue, headaches, and emotional imbalance, this nervous disorder was commonly considered a symptom of failure to adapt to the rapid pace of modern life. (The resonances with the contemporary understanding of meditation as a tool to reduce stress and anxiety while increasing productivity are clear.)

One of the earliest Buddhist-inspired formal mental health protocols was a Japanese system called Naikan ("introspection"). Naikan originated when Yoshimoto Ishin (1916–1988) modified a contemplative technique developed by adherents of the Jōdo Shinshū sect that combined contemplation of Amitābha Buddha with the practice of asceticism. In 1941, Yoshimoto introduced a system of therapeutic self-examination that he argued would be more accessible to a wider range of people {2: 20}.[30] Working as a prison chaplain in the post-war period, he began offering a version of this technique in prisons. This, in turn, began to be studied by Japanese clinical psychologists in the 1960s. The practice eventually was adopted by therapists and psychiatrists to treat a range of disorders (notably including alcoholism) and went on to become a mainstream mental health intervention in Japan.

Meditation also began to move into the medical mainstream in the United States at the turn of the twentieth century. Americans were inspired to see yoga and meditation practices as compatible with modern spirituality through the translation activities of Buddhist apologists and reformers such as the Sri Lankan Anagārika Dharmapāla (1864–1933), the Hindu swami Vivekananda (1864–1902), and the aforementioned D. T. Suzuki, as well as organizations such as the Theosophical Society and the Pali Text Society. In the first half of the twentieth century, an increasingly diverse range of organizations and individuals—including practitioners of Christian Science, Swedenborgianism, African American spiritualism, and other elements of the so-called Mind Cure movement—became interested in the healing dimensions of meditation.[31] Both Zen and the increasingly popular Hindu practice of Transcendental Meditation caught the eye of some of the founding figures of American psychotherapy in this era, who began to express interest in these techniques for their potential benefits on mental health.[32] Buddhist styles of meditation became more well known in the 1950s and 1960s through the writings of the "Beat Generation" on Zen and the first generation of celebrity Buddhist gurus such as Shunryu Suzuki (1904–1971) and Chögyam Trungpa (1939–1987).[33]

By the 1970s, Buddhist meditation teachers all over the world were repeating the mantra that meditation is good for one's health.[34] For example, the Burmese-Indian lay teacher Satya Narayan Goenka (1924–2013), who may have been the most prolific Buddhist meditation teacher of the modern era, frequently told his students the story of how meditation cured his debilitating migraine headaches.[35] The Burmese teacher Mahāsi Sayadaw, popular among a generation of Western seekers who traveled to Southeast Asia to learn about Buddhism, published a compilation of stories about the healing powers of *vipassana* in 1976.[36] The popular American teacher Jack Kornfield (b. 1945), who learned meditation in Forest Sangha monasteries in Thailand in the 1960s and 1970s and earned a PhD in psychology in the United States in 1977, developed meditation classes and wrote books that closely linked meditation with mental well-being.

This trend eventually led to the creation of the mindfulness-based stress reduction (MBSR) program at the University of Massachusetts Medical Center in 1979 by Jon Kabat-Zinn (b. 1944). Kabat-Zinn had deep personal connections with Buddhism, having studied under Seung Sahn (a Korean Zen master), Thích Nhất Hạnh (a Vietnamese Buddhist meditation teacher), and leading Western Buddhist figures. He also held a PhD in molecular biology and was interested in integrating Buddhist practices into academic medical and scientific settings. The MBSR protocol he developed would for the first time provide the means of standardization necessary for proper clinical research on the psychological and physical benefits of meditation.[37]

The development of MBSR, and eventually several other similar treatments such as mindfulness-based cognitive therapy (MBCT), have enabled a great amount of clinical research to be conducted on the medical benefits of meditation. (A recent search of the PubMed database maintained by the U.S. National Library of Medicine yielded more than sixteen thousand results for the key word "mindfulness.")[38] This research has shown the practice of Buddhist-inspired meditation in general, and mindfulness protocols in particular, to have benefit in certain areas of mental well-being.[39] The verdict is still out on the mechanism by which the practice works to achieve these benefits, although recent research has focused on measuring changes in neurological structures, telomeres, hormones, and other objective physical markers of health.[40] At the same time, contemporary meditation research has been criticized for its biases of commission and omission, as well as the generally poor quality of study design and methodology. We will return to these issues in the next chapter.

## ASIAN MEDICAL REVITALIZATION

While meditation was being reframed as a modern psychological therapy, in the second half of the twentieth century, an analogous process of revitalization was taking place with respect to traditional Asian medicines more broadly. After it had been long denigrated, marginalized, and repressed by colonial authorities and modern reformers, official attitudes toward traditional medicine began shifting.[41]

It must be noted that traditional medicine had never been completely eliminated by the processes of modernization. In fact, even at the height of the fervor for eliminating "superstition," séances, spiritualism, mesmerism, and all kinds of anomalous phenomena were popular across the Western world.[42] Similarly, even at the height of the colonial period in the late nineteenth and early twentieth centuries, many reformers and modernizers in India, China, Siam, Tibet, Vietnam, and elsewhere insisted that practitioners need not abandon traditional treatments. In many places at the time, Buddhist practitioners and institutions were still actively involved in publishing and disseminating traditional medical texts, and with some success despite the changing political and cultural circumstances {1: 58, 59; 2: 9}.

Apologists were also actively advocating entering into dialogue with modern science to improve the efficacy of treatments and restructuring traditional medical institutions to modernize the administration of medicine.[43] For example, Khyenrap Norbu (1883–1962), one of the leading Tibetan physicians of the twentieth century, captured the sentiments of many Buddhist practitioners when he argued that the integration of Tibetan medicine with modern medical and surgical techniques was the only way for one to become the "true manifestation of Bhaiṣajyaguru" {2: 10}. Norbu was named the head of both the Chagpori monastic medical college (mentioned in the previous chapter) and the Mentsikhang, a new lay medical college founded by the thirteenth Dalai Lama in 1916. The Mentsikhang combined traditional Sowa Rigpa methods, Tantric ritual, and astrological medicine with modern medicine modeled after colonial British and Chinese public health efforts.[44]

Calls for the integration of traditional and modern medicine became more common in the middle of the twentieth century, when a series of medical revival movements swept across Asia. These developments were partially fueled by the success of an integrative model developed in China. There in the 1950s, the Communist leadership had begun to officially support practitioners of traditional medicine.[45] Chairman Mao Zedong (1893–1976) himself had called for the restoration of the traditional Buddhist method of couching cataracts.[46] His most influential revival initiative was the "barefoot doctors" program, which was envisioned as a more expansive and much less expensive alternative to biomedical infrastructure.[47] These efforts revived traditional practices, but reinterpreted them for the modern era by combining them with scientific medical approaches.

Similar experiments were ongoing in other Asian countries.[48] The success of these projects in bringing basic health care to impoverished rural populations came to the notice of the World Health Organization (WHO) in the 1970s, as the organization was researching the "health-cost burden and unequal distribution of health resources" in the developing world.[49] The WHO's Alma-Ata Declaration of 1978 called for international cooperation between governments and nongovernmental organizations in achieving "health for all" by the year 2000.[50] As a direct result of the WHO's research into integrative models, the declaration called for the inclusion of traditional practitioners among the health care resources that should be developed and mobilized to achieve that goal.

As a result of the success of the revival movements, and encouraged by the WHO declaration, forms of traditional medicine that had been officially ignored or repressed were now freely mined for effective practices. Medical systems that had been demonized as "superstition" came to be valued and more likely to receive financial support from governments across Asia. To be sure, the forms of "traditional" medicine supported and promoted at this time looked quite different from medicine as practiced in the premodern period. In all cases, they represented not a return to ancient forms of healing but rather hybrids of traditional therapies and modern biomedical approaches.

In no case did governments consider traditional medical frameworks superior to biomedicine or place traditional medicine above biomedicine in administrative hierarchies. Nevertheless, in societies where traditional medicine derived from Buddhist ideas and used Buddhist frames of authority, medical revitalization meant that connections between Buddhism and health care were officially reestablished. In Thailand, for example, the government rebranded Siamese healing traditions as "Thai Traditional Medicine" (Th. *phaet phaen thai*, referred to in official documents as "TTM" in obvious mimicry of "Traditional Chinese Medicine," or "TCM").[51] New, government-sponsored TTM initiatives included the "Monk Doctor" program, which used monastics as frontline public health workers.[52]

While most notably affecting impoverished parts of Asia, traditional medical revitalization also started to receive increasing recognition in Japan. In 1963, after Buddhist healing rites had been outlawed for several generations, the Japanese Supreme Court ruled that these practices were now legal if they served as complements to, not replacements for, modern biomedical therapy.[53] In 1976, the Japanese government added forty-four classical medicine (Jp. *kanpō*) formulas to the list of drugs covered by the national health insurance program, marking a transition in government policy from merely tolerating traditional medicine to officially supporting it for the first time since the Meiji reforms.[54]

In the West, the 1970s and 1980s also saw not only the increasing popularization of meditation, but also rising interest in acupuncture, yoga, and many other aspects of Asian medicine. In contrast to the developing world, where medical revival was a matter of urgent public health necessity, the popularity of Asian medicine in affluent countries was made possible by the near elimination of infectious diseases as causes of death. (In the United States, for example, infectious disease mortality was cut by 99 percent between 1900 and the early 1980s.)[55] As the danger of traditional killers such as smallpox, typhus, typhoid, diphtheria, and tetanus became negligible, people had the luxury to begin exploring the benefits of traditional medicine for chronic diseases such as diabetes, heart disease, and arthritis. It was in the areas of extending the life span and improving quality of life that traditional Asian medicine—now understood as compatible with modern life and even able to be studied through clinical trials—seemed to have the most to contribute.

* * *

Buddhist medicine has never been a static or monolithic tradition. Like Buddhism itself, it defies easy generalizations. While it presents itself as timeless, in actuality it has been continually reinterpreted and reinvented in countless local contexts throughout its history. The encounter between Buddhism and modern science dramatically changed the face of Buddhist medicine around the globe. In the early modern period, most of the practices and beliefs that had been widespread and prestigious for centuries came to be widely seen as superstitious and backward. Faithful devotees, however, sought to recreate the Buddha as an empirical proto-scientist or psychologist. Some traditional Buddhist healing techniques that could be reframed as compatible with science—meditation, in particular—came to be seen internationally as worthy of both popularization and serious scientific study. The laiciziation and medicalization of meditation in the second half of the twenty-first century coincided with the revival of traditional Asian medicine in Asia and abroad. Biomedicine, having achieved its position as the dominant global medical system, now began to make room for traditions it had previously written off as superstitious. Eastern and Western populations alike began to develop an appetite for new hybrid forms of healing.

The period between 1800 and 2000 thus saw both the complete transformation of Buddhist medicine and a reorientation in Western attitudes toward the potential health benefits of Buddhist healing and other Asian medical practices. The processes of modernization, medicalization, and popularization discussed here involved a series of translations of Buddhist medical ideas and practices into new languages, new cultural contexts, and new conceptual worlds. What has been gained and what has been lost in these processes of adaptation remains a frequent topic of debate among practitioners of Buddhist and Buddhist-inspired health interventions today.[56] However, while Buddhist medicine has been fundamentally transformed over the last two centuries, many continuities have persisted across the *longue durée*. Contemporary continuities and ruptures will be discussed in the next chapter, which provides an update on Buddhist medicine in the twenty-first century.

## FURTHER READING

Hammerstrom, Erik J. 2015. *The Science of Chinese Buddhism: Early Twentieth-Century Engagements*. New York: Columbia University Press. An analysis of the efforts of apologists and reformers to make Chinese Buddhism compatible with the modern scientific worldview emerging in the early twentieth century.

Hickey, Wakoh Shannon. 2019. *Mind Cure: How Meditation Became Medicine*. New York: Oxford University Press. A social history of the spread of meditation and yoga to the United States in the nineteenth and twentieth centuries, including a critique of contemporary mindfulness.

Lopez, Donald. 2008. *Buddhism and Science: A Guide for the Perplexed*. Chicago: University of Chicago Press. An analysis and critique of the presumed compatibility between Buddhism and science, from the emergence of the discourse in the nineteenth century to contemporary proponents such as the Dalai Lama.

McMahan, David L. 2008. *The Making of Buddhist Modernism*. New York: Oxford University Press. The definitive book on the twentieth-century emergence of the global phenomenon of "Buddhist modernism."

Wilson, Jeff. 2014. *Mindful America: The Mutual Transformation of Buddhist Meditation and American Culture*. New York: Oxford University Press. A history of the invention and popularization of mindfulness in the United States, with attention paid to its widespread cultural resonances.

## CHAPTER 9

# *Contemporary Buddhist Medicine*

This chapter draws our centuries-long historical exploration to a conclusion by summarizing some of the ways that Buddhism continues to shape health care and health-seeking activities today. The spectrum of healing practices discussed throughout this book—whether traditional, modern, or in between—is still actively used across the world.[1] With an overwhelming amount of data available to study in the present day, this chapter necessarily focuses on just a few major themes. The chapter first examines how Buddhism is playing an increasingly visible and increasingly official role in certain traditions of revitalized Asian medicine. Second, I provide a brief overview of some of the ways that Buddhism continues to intersect with biomedical research, clinical practice, and secular health care institutions in complicated and potentially controversial ways. Third, I explore the increasing complexity of the feedback loops that characterize the contemporary globalization of Buddhist medicine. And finally, I briefly discuss the effects of digital technology on the speed of the diffusion of Buddhist medicine in contemporary global culture.

## BUDDHISM AND ASIAN MEDICINE

Buddhism remains an essential ingredient in folk and popular healing traditions all across Asia {e.g., 2: 14, 19, 26, 28, 30, 31, 33, 34}. However, in the twenty-first century, Buddhism has become closely allied with formal medicine and public health in many places. This is especially true in countries where local governments give official support to revitalized and modernized therapies historically connected with Buddhist ideas and institutions. In Thailand, for example,

Buddhist medicine has become a highly visible aspect of national medical policy. In the mid-2000s, the Thai Ministry of Public Health generated reports for the World Health Organization (WHO) and other international bodies showcasing Buddhist philosophies, ethics, and practices as major elements of the national public health care system.[2]

Wat Phra Chetuphon, the temple that houses the nineteenth-century artifacts discussed in chapter 7, retains its status as most revered among the traditional medical institutions in the country. The texts compiled and codified there under the auspices of the Siamese kings continue to be used in the training of traditional doctors (Th. *mo boran*) across the country. The principal diagnostic techniques and herbal formulas that these practitioners use every day are based on the Elements, *doṣa*, and flavors.[3] The knowledge within the tradition continues to be credited in large part to Jīvaka and the forest sages, and the training of traditional doctors, therapists, and midwives is explicitly and self-consciously Buddhist in orientation.

With the emergence of licensure regulations for a wider range of practitioners beginning in 2004, Thai Traditional Medicine is now controlled by the national government more closely than ever before. Practitioners around the country have had to choose between obtaining licensure to comply with the parameters of the Ministries of Public Health and Education or continuing to practice independently with marginal legal status {2: 30}. Unlicensed folk healers continue to practice a spectrum of Buddhist healing rites. Their blessings, exorcisms, talismans, binding rituals, purification, and invocation of and possession by deities are immensely popular, and most of these practices involve a panoply of Buddhist symbols, incantations, and other elements (see, e.g., {1: 34; 2: 30}).[4] These practitioners remain completely unregulated by the state, although they are periodically subjected to brief but never very effective purges.

Whether licensed or unlicensed, Buddhist legends and rituals continue to figure importantly in the social lives and professional identities of Thai healers. Statues of Jīvaka, the forest sages, other Buddhist deities and spirits, and famous historical monastics can be found on altars in virtually all medical clinics across the country (see, e.g., figure 4.2). Empowering incantations are recited daily by most practitioners to these figures, and they are often ritually called upon to inhabit healing spaces or descend into the bodies of traditional medicine practitioners to empower their work {2: 16}. This is done even at government-licensed schools.[5]

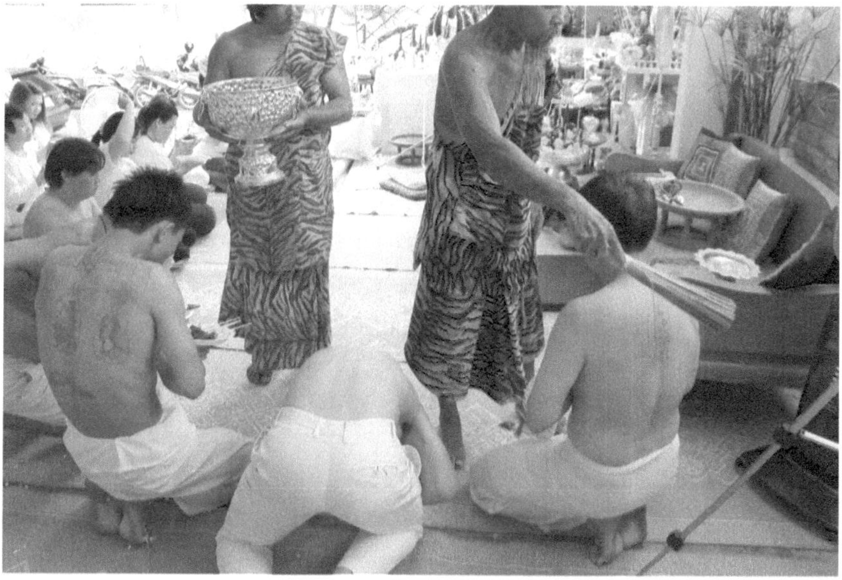

9.1 A Buddhist yogi (Th. *ruesi*) leads a blessing ceremony at a traditional medicine school in Chiang Mai, Thailand. He invokes healing spirits, inviting them to descend and possess his students, the school's practitioners, and other members of the audience in order to recharge their healing abilities for the coming year.
Photo by the author.

Next door to Thailand, Buddhism is also playing a central role in the official health-care system in Myanmar. The traditional Burmese medicine system, called "Knowledge of the Remedies of the Country" (*taing-yin hsay pyinnya*), has four core branches: Buddhist knowledge of the body, Āyurvedic medicine, astrology and astronomy, and alchemy.[6] Regulated by the government since the 1950s, this revived and modernized medical system is similar to Thailand's in that it represents a hybrid of historical and biomedical streams of practice. Also as in Thailand, tensions over what types of healing are legally recognized continue to affect the experience of patients and practitioners. Although government licenses became mandatory for practitioners in 2008, unlicensed healers continue to offer a wide range of therapies. One particular class of healers called "wizards" (*weikza*) continue to command popular attention and patronage for their performance of Buddhist rituals, blessings, alchemy, and other therapies {2: 19, 31}.[7] Often, these legally marginalized practitioners feel the need to marshal scientific evidence or credentials to give their healing techniques a patina of legitimacy. They may also be able to capitalize on fame, charisma, or social connections to gain official favor despite their technically illegal status {2: 31}.[8]

Like both Thai and Burmese traditional medicine, Sowa Rigpa's status as a Buddhist tradition is largely unquestioned by contemporary practitioners, who continue to heavily rely on Buddhist concepts, even as these ideas are being reinterpreted in light of biomedical perspectives and incorporated into new regulatory schemes (see, e.g., {2: 12, 13, 32, 33}).[9] The leading international organization promoting Sowa Rigpa globally today is the Men-Tsee-Khang, established in 1961 as part of the Tibetan government in exile in Dharamshala, India. (This twentieth-century institution is not to be confused with the original Mentsikhang discussed in chapter 8, which is located in Lhasa.) The Men-Tsee-Khang proudly proclaims its Buddhist identity and lineage with an image of Bhaiṣajyaguru on the banner of its website.[10] Its medical recommendations include traditional healing mantras, *yantra* yoga, and meditations. It also continues to recommend the consumption of "precious pills" made and consecrated through traditional rituals.

In Bhutan, although many folk healers continue to operate outside of the official system, both Sowa Rigpa and Buddhist religious values have been incorporated into national health-care policy {2: 33}[11] and into the Ministry of Health's much-touted plan for maximizing the "gross national happiness" of the population {2: 17}.[12] The Bhutanese government also actively promotes connections between Buddhism and health in its international tourism promotions: the official website of the Tourism Council of Bhutan, for example, mentions meditation retreats along with hot spring therapy on a page dedicated to "spirituality and wellness."[13]

Recently, Sowa Rigpa has been recognized by the United Nations Educational, Scientific, and Cultural Organization (UNESCO) as part of the "intangible cultural heritage" of Bhutan. Recently, both India and China have been vying to gain similar recognition—no doubt to profit more from the commercialization of the tradition.[14] Sowa Rigpa continues to be practiced widely by ethnically Tibetan communities in those two countries, and it also has been formally recognized by both the Indian and Chinese national health-care systems. This means that the market for Sowa Rigpa medicines is potentially huge. The industry already is estimated at just under $1 billion in China alone.[15]

Sowa Rigpa also continues to thrive within the boundaries of Nepal and Mongolia and among ethnic Buryats, Kalmyks, Mongols, and Tibetans in neighboring countries.[16] It is increasingly being practiced by diasporic communities in the West, and it is also catching on with a growing number of European and American professionals and enthusiasts.[17] With all of these developments, it appears that this particular form of Buddhist medicine is poised to continue to attract attention, patronage, and controversy in the years to come.

## BUDDHISM AND BIOMEDICINE

In addition to Buddhism's connections with traditional Asian medicine, a number of contemporary articulations between Buddhism and biomedicine are worth following. While it would be impossible to mention all of the relevant examples here, the Tzu Chi Foundation is a particularly high-profile entity that operates on the global stage. Tzu Chi is a transnational nongovernmental organization (NGO) headquartered in Taiwan committed to ensuring universal access to biomedical treatments as a core part of its mission.[18] Focusing on "Buddhist compassionate relief," Tzu Chi is known for building hospitals and organizing mobile health clinics, through which it is able to bring routine health care and disaster assistance to impoverished people both in Taiwan and around the world.[19] While the medical services offered through such efforts are almost exclusively of a biomedical nature, the organization's raison d'être is to give its volunteers the opportunity to enact the Mahāyānic path of compassion in the world. Tzu Chi's volunteer surgeons, ophthalmologists, dentists, and other medical specialists often describe their charitable work as allowing them to embody the "helping hands" of Avalokiteśvara and thus make progress on the bodhisattva path.[20]

Tzu Chi has brought humanitarian aid to people affected by hurricanes in the United States and the Caribbean, earthquakes in China, and the 2004 Indian Ocean tsunami. However, it was Japanese Buddhist organizations that rushed to fill the need after the simultaneous earthquake, tsunami, and nuclear disaster in Japan on March 11, 2011. The disaster, which resulted in around twenty-five thousand casualties, provided fuel for the development of the field of interfaith chaplaincy in that country {2: 18, 21}. Following a model adapted from the West, chaplaincy provided a novel way for Buddhist clergy to engage in "spiritual care" (Jp. *supirichuarukea*, borrowed from the English) in hospitals and other secular environments while also extending the role of Buddhist clergy beyond their traditional association with death in contemporary Japanese culture.[21] This new professional niche has more overtly integrated Buddhist clergy with modern institutions of health and wellness in Japan.[22]

Meanwhile, the most visible connections between Buddhism and mainstream health care globally continue to center on therapeutic meditation. In the twenty-first century, the Buddha continues to be understood by many as a scientist of the mind, and the core practices he taught are often assumed to be fundamentally harmonious with modern psychology and psychiatry.[23] By 2014 mindfulness had become so mainstream in the United States that *Time* magazine dedicated its front cover to the "mindful revolution." Only two years later, the size of the meditation industry was estimated at $1 billion per year.[24]

It is not just mindfulness that is a promising healing modality. Scientists and practitioners are also currently adapting other forms of Buddhist contemplative practice to modern clinical and research settings {2: 21, 23}. Researchers have begun to look into the medical benefits of compassion meditation (Pāli *mettā-bhāvanā*), certain visualization exercises, and Tibetan *yantra* yoga, for example.[25] Buddhist interventions have led to novel approaches to treating psychological trauma and disorders.[26] Such practices are now enthusiastically promoted, supported, and disseminated by high-profile celebrities and popular media outlets across the world.

As it has moved out of the temple into the lab, and from there into new arenas of culture, meditation has continued to be further secularized. It has become increasingly common for therapeutic meditation protocols to be taught by facilitators with little or no knowledge of Buddhism, who interpret this practice and its benefits wholly in terms of biomedical and scientific paradigms. Articles in English-language popular media typically deemphasize the connection between mindfulness and Buddhism.[27] The disassociation of meditation from religion has allowed for its wide acceptance by researchers in the disciplines of psychology, psychiatry, neurology, and medicine. Organizations such as the Foundation for a Mindful Society,[28] the Mindfulness Initiative,[29] the Mindfulness in Schools Project,[30] and various centers for research also promote the benefits of mindfulness in many arenas of modern life without drawing attention to the Buddhist roots of the practice. This process of secularization has made possible the adoption of Buddhist-inspired meditation practices in health-care settings where overtly religious interventions would not be welcome. Mindfulness has been formally integrated, for example, into the National Health Service of the United Kingdom, where it is now prescribed to people experiencing recurrent depressive episodes {2: 22}.[31] It is also being used by various branches of the U.S. Armed Forces to treat mental health conditions and reduce stress.[32]

While enthusiasm for mindfulness and other forms of meditation is undoubtedly on the rise, a backlash has emerged as certain scholars, practitioners, and interpreters of Buddhism have begun to voice concerns.[33] Some feel that, as Buddhist-inspired practices are separated from the larger philosophical and ethical tradition in which they were originally developed, they have become watered down, misguided, or simply less effective.[34] Others have critiqued the commodification of "McMindfulness," which they argue may actually have negative consequences for well-being in the long run {2: 24}. They argue that commercialization of the practice shifts the onus of dealing with anxiety, depression, and malaise onto the individual, causing the practitioner to internalize or psychologize these pressures rather than see their broader social or ethical dimensions.[35] Instead of analyzing structural factors such as oppressive labor policies in the workplace or the ill effects of socioeconomic inequality, for example, unhappiness and stress become individual failures and personal responsibilities.

Another area of controversy is a small but suggestive body of research indicating that there are some mental health risks to intensive participation in Buddhist-style meditation. While investigation is still in a nascent phase, traditional warnings about "meditation illness" {1: 36–38} may prove to be validated, as researchers begin to show that a certain percentage of the participants in meditation programs will predictably experience negative side effects.[36]

Finally, a third strain of resistance suggests that, since therapeutic meditations ultimately derive from Buddhist contexts, they should not be introduced into secular settings without robust processes of informed consent. Such critics fear that meditation teachers are using mindfulness as a Trojan horse to sneak religion into schools, hospitals, and other secular settings.[37] Such concerns may be partially well founded, as entry-level mindfulness courses are indeed often characterized by teachers as "Dharma gates," a way of potentially interesting a large number of people in studying Buddhism more intensively. Even the founder of mindfulness-based stress reduction, Jon Kabat-Zinn, has admitted that his clinical model "was developed as one of a possibly infinite number of skillful means for bringing the Dharma into mainstream settings."[38]

Concerns about how Buddhism does or does not align with modern health care are not unique to the West. Contemporary practitioners and patients in many cultural contexts express feeling stuck in the middle of an opposition between "science" and "religion" (these issues are raised many times in the second volume of the *Anthology*).[39] These tensions are negotiated or articulated in a number of ways depending on personal and political circumstances, but they are a common feature of contemporary Buddhist medicine.

That being said, other people perceive no conflict whatsoever. For them, Buddhist therapies have a relatively stable or established role alongside biomedical interventions as "complementary" or "alternative" approaches.[40] This perceived complementarity makes it possible for such patients to visit a Buddhist healer for a treatment with rituals or other similar interventions while also undergoing biomedical treatment without experiencing cognitive dissonance. For example, a devotee may visualize their cardiologist as a form of Avalokiteśvara, inviting the all-powerful bodhisattva to guide the scalpel during a surgical procedure.[41] Such visualizations—and other informal prayers, meditations, and rituals—represent simple ways of integrating Buddhism and biomedicine that are extremely common among Buddhists around the world {e.g., 2: 34}. Countless people continue to seek solace in Buddhist orientations, doctrines, and practices in these seen and unseen ways, ensuring that Buddhism remains an inseparable companion to biomedicine in the contemporary period.

## GLOBALIZATION

Along with the ongoing interconnection of Buddhist medicine with both traditional and modern medicine, its recognition by governments and international bodies, the popularization of its research, and its ongoing secularization, another of the most significant features of Buddhist medicine in the twenty-first century is its globalization. When scholars speak of "globalization," they tend to mean not only the global spread of a phenomenon but also the multidirectionality and complexity of its circulation.[42] By any definition, it is clear that Asian medicines of all kinds are today are affected by currents of globalization.[43]

In the twenty-first century, the movements of Buddhist medicine are now truly worldwide. Today, people from Nova Scotia to Naples to Nairobi have heard that Buddhism is good for your health. No contemporary form of Buddhist or Buddhist-inspired medicine is isolated from the ramifications of globalization. This book has pushed back numerous times against simplistic one-way models of cross-cultural exchange, arguing that complex multidirectional processes have been at work in forming Buddhist medicine since early in the Common Era. And today, all forms of Buddhist medicine are entangled in complex feedback loops that extend around the world and back again.

Take the case of contemporary Thai Traditional Medicine. Earlier, we focused on the role of local medical revival movements in Southeast Asia in legitimizing and popularizing traditional Buddhist practices and explored how these movements relate to colonialism, modernization, decolonization, and health care policy. However, we must also add to this picture an appreciation that traditional medicine in Thailand today is just as powerfully shaped by complex feedback loops involving Western tourists. In the 2000s, tourists became increasingly interested in Thai medical arts—in particular, healing meditation retreats, Thai massage therapy (Th. *nuad paen thai*), yoga-like therapeutic exercises (Th. *ruesi dat ton*), and certain aspects of ritual healing such as empowered tattoos (Th. *sak yan*).[44]

This interest was inseparable from the Thai government's efforts to promote tourism in general, and medical tourism in particular, in the 1990s and early 2000s.[45] Since that time, Wat Phra Chetuphon's collection of medical artifacts has become a major tourist attraction. A prestigious traditional massage and medicine school is associated with the temple, and countless visitors from around the world cycle through the massage clinic and foot massage stations on the temple grounds.[46] Also as a direct result of this interest, the northwestern city of Chiang Mai has become an important destination for tourists to study traditional massage and medicine.[47] Hundreds of schools have opened across the city in the last two decades, and forms of massage learned in that city are now practiced widely in the West.

In nearly all of these tourist settings, the Buddhist roots of Thai Traditional Medicine are explicitly emphasized. No center is complete without a prominent Buddhist altar. Practices such as meditation, incantations, and empowerment rituals to invoke Jīvaka's blessings are performed by Western students in tourist schools around the country. Emphasizing that traditional medicine is historically intertwined with Buddhism has been commercially advantageous when catering to Western tourists and aficionados.[48] These strong Buddhist resonances are one of the most obvious points of distinction of Thai medicine in the multibillion-dollar international Asian medicine marketplace, and the cachet of such resonances is a major reason certain students seek out this tradition versus other Asian medical systems.[49]

These Buddhist practices are often internalized by Westerners as important parts of Thai Traditional Medicine training and are subsequently taught in massage centers in the West, even by teachers who do not self-identify as Buddhist. Students traveling to Thailand are normally eager to perform a pilgrimage of sorts, seeking a "spiritual" experience studying with Thai teachers. School owners in Chiang Mai then are pressured to further enhance the Buddhist content of their trainings to meet the heightened expectations of their visitors. The notion that learning Thai massage or medicine is a deeply spiritual process closely connected with Buddhism is thus a feedback loop that is mutually constructed and reinforced by both Thai providers and Western consumers of religio-medical tourism.

An equally multifaceted feedback loop can be seen in the activities of the Won Buddhist order. This is a modern, nontraditional form of Buddhism headquartered in Iksan, South Korea.[50] Influenced by Protestant Christian missionary visions of social transformation prevalent in Korea in the early twentieth century, Won Buddhism has since its founding been heavily invested in education and health care. The organization's Wonkwang University is home to medical schools specializing in both biomedicine and traditional Korean medicine. Thus, it is fair to say that Won Buddhism's connections with health are a product of colonialism, Buddhist modernism, biomedicine, and traditional medical revivalism.

To add another wrinkle to the story, the popularity of mindfulness in the English-speaking world is influencing how clinicians at Wonkwang are thinking about meditation these days. Treatment programs such as mindfulness-based stress reduction and mindfulness-based cognitive therapy are now taught in Korea (as they are in Japan, Taiwan, Thailand, and elsewhere in Asia).[51] Just as Korean monastics and clerics have consulted with scientists in the West to develop methodologies for clinical meditation research, they are also beginning to incorporate scientific perspectives and secularized meditation protocols into the meditation trainings offered at their own temples or meditation centers {2: 23}.[52] At Wonkwang, this trend is encouraging faculty in the Korean medicine unit to explore the mental and emotional dimensions of health care and integrate mindfulness and other Buddhist-influenced tools into their curricula.[53]

However, while meditation has moved from East to West and back again, models of proselytism have moved in the opposite direction. Having learned from the Korean experience with Christian evangelical missionaries in the twentieth

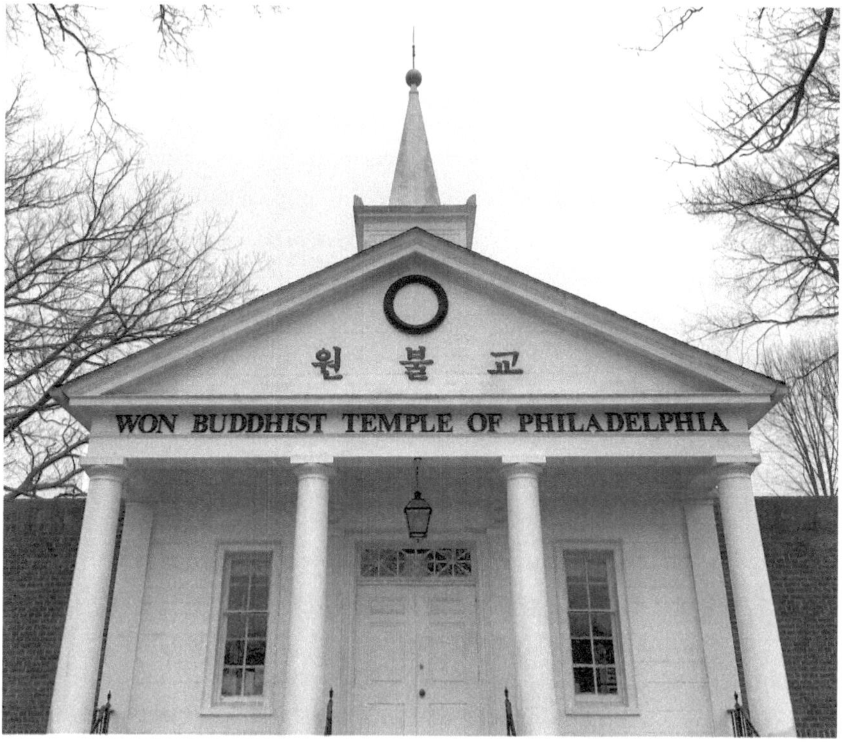


**9.2** Won Temple of Philadelphia, housed in a converted church in Glenside, Pennsylvania, represents a continuation of this modern Korean order's mission to combine Buddhist teachings with charity and medical education.
Photo by the author, courtesy of the Jivaka Project (http://jivaka.net), Creative Commons license.

century, in the twenty-first, Won Buddhism has turned the tables. The organization now maintains a large missionary operation in the United States, which in no way limits itself to spreading Won Buddhism just among Korean Americans. As part of its mission to promote health care and health education, in 2001 it established the Won Institute of Graduate Studies in the suburbs north of Philadelphia.[54] Today the institute offers the only accredited master's degree program in acupuncture in the state of Pennsylvania, as well as certificate courses in herbal medicine, meditation, and Won Buddhism. The institute also organizes a number of charitable medical outreach programs in the Philadelphia area involving acupuncture, including a low-cost clinic for veterans and free treatments for people with opioid addictions and the homeless.[55]

If Won Buddhism in Korea is the product of various cultural syntheses, its development in the United States has been even more complex. To be propagated in this new cultural and regulatory environment, the vision of the founder of the Won Buddhist order is being tailored in unique ways to accommodate local constraints and capitalize on local opportunities.[56] Operating the acupuncture school has required a number of compromises to comply with local legal requirements, for example. The academic affairs of the institute are primarily managed not by Won Buddhists but by a corps of professional administrators focused on maintaining the institute's accreditation. The faculty consists mostly of Western-trained acupuncturists without affiliation to Won Buddhism, because these are the people licensed to practice in the United States. Because of the need to conform to U.S. licensure standards for acupuncture education, the curriculum focuses entirely on Chinese, rather than Korean, acupuncture protocols. Nevertheless, the institute is overseen by the Won Buddhist Temple of Philadelphia and retains close connections with the headquarters in Korea. Won clergy regularly travel between the Philadelphia area and Iksan and have taken American students on trips to Wonkwang University and its environs for study and cultural tourism.

The transnational feedback loops outlined here are specific to Thai medicine and Won Buddhism, but they are also emblematic of the current state of the multidirectional interactions between Buddhism and Asian medicine globally today. The networks through which Buddhist medicine now moves have become impossibly complex, with a virtually infinite number of nodes, interconnections, and feedback loops. Buddhist networks are also entangled with other networks such as transnational organizations, international aid, tourism, capitalism, proselytism, scholarship, and legal and regulatory structures. Enmeshed in this thicket of loops upon loops, diverse aspects of Buddhist medicine are culturally translated back and forth with great rapidity, all while being continually refracted and re-refracted through the vast array of local and global lenses.

## ACCELERATION AND DIGITALIZATION

Given the entangled, globalized circuits that characterize the network of exchange of Buddhist medical knowledge today, it is now easier than ever for individuals to combine a wide range of practices and ideas to create their own individualized practice of Buddhist medicine. One Buddhist leader I interviewed in Philadelphia, for example, reported having grown up in Taiwan in a family that worshipped Avalokiteśvara, then training in Chinese Pure Land, Japanese Zen, and Tibetan mantra practice {2: 35§9}. After moving to Philadelphia, she undertook interfaith chaplaincy training and served patients in that capacity in a major hospital in the city. In other words, this one transnational practitioner's training has spanned Taiwanese, Chinese, Japanese, Tibetan, and Western traditions, and she has freely crossed institutional lines between temples, meditation groups, and biomedical settings. She now is a popular local meditation teacher with her own group of primarily White meditation students, although she periodically volunteers with other Chinese-speaking people through the local Tzu Chi chapter in Philadelphia's Chinatown. She also works at an academic institution where she comes into frequent contact with academic scholars of Buddhist studies. This one individual is thus a perfect encapsulation of the many kinds of intersections, syntheses, and contradictions of contemporary global Buddhism—and she is only one of countless similar figures who live in this particular city.[57]

Such an individual's ability to access information on Buddhist medicine has greatly expanded in the twenty-first century thanks to the intensification and acceleration of information sharing. With the internet, it is now possible for information to be gathered from and transmitted to all corners of the world by innumerable people simultaneously. A meditation teacher in Philadelphia or any other Buddhist practitioner in any other part of the world can just as easily find herself chatting in an online forum with a monk in Taipei or a meditation scientist in New York—or both—instantaneously and at virtually no cost.

While the meditation teacher I mentioned is not well known outside of Philadelphia's Buddhist circles, savvy individuals who have taken advantage of digital communication tools have been able to position themselves as international spokespeople or experts and gather large virtual communities around particular aspects of Buddhist medicine. Nida Chenagtsang (b. 1971), for example, has become one of the most internationally visible proponents of the nexus between Sowa Rigpa and Vajrayāna Buddhism {2: 12}.[58] "Dr. Nida" and his followers use a range of digital resources to promote his ideas, including websites, audio recordings, YouTube videos, and various social media platforms, in addition to more traditional media like books and magazines.

Nida's online presence, however, is dwarfed by that of the fourteenth Dalai Lama, Tenzin Gyatso (b. 1935).[59] One of the most important authorities in

Tibetan Buddhism, he is by far the best known Buddhist in the world and, one could say, the de facto face of contemporary global Buddhism. While he has spoken on many subjects unrelated to health, he has for many years been very involved in popularizing the notion that Buddhist practice has a beneficial effect on mental health. He helped to establish the Mind and Life Institute, an organization dedicated to promoting and funding scientific research in that area.[60] With the "memeification" of his visage on social media, his messages connecting Buddhism and wellness (whether authentic or simply attributed to him) are now seen by millions upon millions of Buddhists and non-Buddhists alike on a daily basis. This has played no small part in Buddhism being indelibly associated with well-being in popular culture the world over.

While the Dalai Lama may be a bona fide global celebrity, there is in fact no central figure or other authority who dictates what does and does not count as Buddhist medicine. The proliferation of online venues and social media outlets

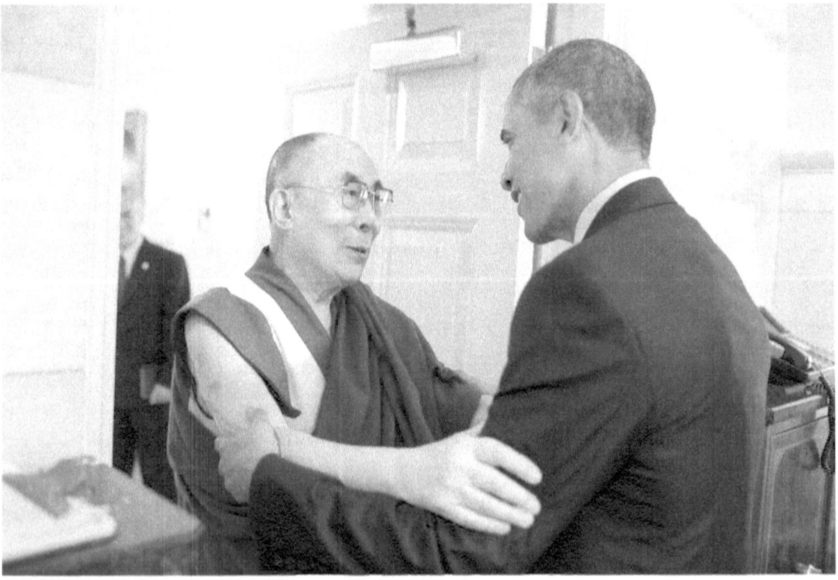

9.3 The fourteenth Dalai Lama, Tenzin Gyatso (b. 1935), meets with President Barack Obama at the entrance to the Map Room of the White House, June 15, 2016. This internationally recognized Buddhist figure has been instrumental in popularizing links between Buddhism and well-being.
Photo by the White House. Image courtesy of Wikimedia Commons, public domain.

today has given practitioners, patients, researchers, enthusiasts, and dabblers the world over countless opportunities to share their ideas, no matter how niche. Buddhist healing techniques from around the world are now easily accessible on YouTube, Instagram, Facebook, Twitter, WeChat, and other platforms in dozens of languages. (To give an example of the scope of this phenomenon, at the time of writing, a Google search for "Buddhist medicine" reveals almost 32 million hits. The same search term in Chinese reveals 14 million, in French 4.8 million, in German 3.6 million, in Spanish 3.2 million, and in Arabic nearly 1 million.)[61] The net result is that knowledge that would have been difficult or impossible to find in previous eras is now freely shared, and interested practitioners can now learn a range of techniques online in many languages {2: 19, 27}.

The "ocean of practice" has always been characterized by hybridity and syncretism. Aspects of Buddhist medicine historically have been unbundled from their original cultural and intellectual contexts and traded along networks of exchange. But, in the Information Age, those packages of information are now atomized into millions of tiny digital pieces: blog posts, podcasts, videos, images, memes, and tweets that are diffused by innumerable people simultaneously, scattered throughout the global culture. As a consequence, contemporary interested parties now can freely draw upon and intermix the whole range of ideas and practices derived from any and all forms of Buddhism, whether Nikāya, Mahāyāna, or Tantric; historical or modern; local or global.

In such an environment, it is no surprise that various aspects of Buddhist medicine have been extracted from Buddhism and incorporated into popular new health interventions or that more such hybrids are emerging every day. Frequently, these innovations involve combinations with other aspects of Asian healing that also have been atomized, memeified, and diffused into the ether, such as Chinese medicine, Āyurveda, various types of yoga, Transcendental Meditation, shamanism, martial arts, and so many others {2: 15, 27, 29}. Practitioners of these new hybrids may embrace the label "Buddhist" for themselves or their teachings and may find a role for Buddhism among other strongly felt religious, cultural, or ethnic identities {2: 28}. Or they may soundly reject the label, preferring to identify as secular, Christian, "spiritual not religious," or anything else {2: 29}.

In the end, Buddhism has become one more source of information in the pluralistic global marketplace of ideas about health and healing—a rich well of material from which ideas and practices are extracted, adapted, recombined, and recirculated across the globe—reaching ever more individuals in ever more unique configurations at an ever quickening pace. Whether individuals use this information to heal themselves, treat others, establish an identity, or just as entertainment, today Buddhist medicine is reaching more people than ever before. It is also being put to many different purposes than ever before and has come to mean many different things to many different people.

* * *

Buddhist medicine has never been one-dimensional. In any given historical time or place, it has been a diffuse body of knowledge at once situated deeply in local sociopolitical and cultural contexts but also characterized by complex transnational flows and counterflows across cultural and spatial boundaries. The second half of this book has traced the cross-cultural circulation of these ideas and practices throughout history. The development of the Silk Road and Indian Ocean maritime routes resulted in the emergence of a pan-Asian network through which Buddhist medical knowledge was transmitted and developed in the premodern period. The colonial era brought Western cultures into sustained contact with Buddhism, and by extension with Buddhist medical ideas and practices, for the first time. By the twentieth century, such encounters were being facilitated and accelerated by international scholarly research, the activity of transnational organizations, and the availability of worldwide communication and travel.

Studying the history of Buddhist medicine in previous historical periods is enormously complex, but the ocean of practice is even more vast and chaotic than ever today. It is a fractal swirl of currents and countercurrents, each leading off into an infinite number of eddies of equal complexity. No one could ever plumb all of its depths or fathom all of its secrets. A short chapter such as this can only outline the shape of the ocean, relate some basic facts about it, and point out some interesting areas that invite more exploration. The four trends discussed here seem poised to continue in the immediate future, and it is hoped that scholars will continue to keep an eye on these developments.

A few final points may be worth mentioning about the effect our own scholarship has on the processes of globalization outlined here. Even if we scholars would like to paint ourselves as neutral observers—looking out from our ivory tower at the ocean of practice below but never getting our feet wet—this of course is never the case. Our work always has an impact on the people we study and on the society and culture we live in. I am thinking in particular of how this very book, and the project of which it is a part, brings work done by an international cast of scholars into common conversation, creating new collaborations and lines of communication that did not exist before. By sculpting a huge amount of disparate knowledge of history and the present into a unified narrative, it provides connections and articulations between historical developments and Buddhist traditions, allowing readers to discover and create new connections that previously may not have been visible. Also, by virtue of being published and distributed by a major university press, this project will inevitably participate in the dissemination of the construct of "Buddhist medicine" around the world. I am also cognizant that all of you are creating ever more fractal, global currents and eddies through your acts of reading, reflecting on, and talking about this material. The ocean churns on!

## FURTHER READING


Adams, Vincanne, Mona Schrempf, and Sienna R. Craig, eds. 2011. *Medicine Between Science and Religion: Explorations on Tibetan Grounds*. New York: Berghahn. A collection of essays by leading scholars of Tibetan medicine on the intersections of Buddhism, medicine, and science in Tibetan cultural areas.

Gleig, Ann. 2019. *American Dharma: Buddhism Beyond Modernity*. New Haven, Conn.: Yale University Press. An ethnographic study of contemporary American Buddhism, focused on the emergence of a postmodern sensibility that has begun overturning many of the conceptions of "Buddhist modernism."

Grieve, Gregory Price, and Daniel Veidlinger. 2015. *Buddhism, the Internet, and Digital Media: The Pixel in the Lotus*. Abingdon-on-Thames: Routledge. A collection of essays about how Buddhism is transforming and being understood by practitioners in the digital age.

Helderman, Ira. 2019. *Prescribing the Dharma: Psychotherapists, Buddhist Traditions, and Defining Religion*. Chapel Hill: University of North Carolina Press. An ethnographic and historical exploration of the relationship between Buddhism and psychotherapy from Freud to the present day.

Patton, Thomas Nathan. 2018. *The Buddha's Wizards: Magic, Protection, and Healing in Burmese Buddhism*. New York: Columbia University Press. An ethnographic exploration of the *weikza*, popular healers, magicians, and ritualists in contemporary Myanmar.

Salguero, C. Pierce. 2016. *Traditional Thai Medicine: Buddhism, Animism, Yoga, Ayurveda*. Revised ed. Bangkok: White Lotus. A short review of the history and contemporary practice of traditional medicine in Thailand. Includes chapters on herbal, yogic, magical, and ritual healing.

# Conclusion

As I finish writing this book in mid-2020, a novel coronavirus, SARS-CoV-2 (COVID-19), has emerged in Wuhan, China, and quickly has developed into a global pandemic.[1] I have been watching as Buddhist organizations have sprung into action around the world to meet this health-care challenge. Buddhists leaders worldwide have called for compassion, generosity, solidarity, calm, and mindfulness in response to the catastrophe.[2] They have moved their religious services online and created resources and teachings to address the crisis. However, they have also mobilized more direct measures to combat the virus and the anxieties and other fallout associated with it. These responses have been diverse, reflecting sectarian and cultural differences, but they have notably echoed many of the themes discussed throughout this book.

For example, in an April 2020 press release, Tzu Chi USA (an affiliate of the transnational Buddhist disaster-relief organization discussed in chapter 9) announced a massive medical charity project, promising to deliver millions of masks and other medical supplies to frontline health-care workers and launching an assistance program for people impacted financially by the pandemic.[3] These U.S. initiatives complement Tzu Chi's extensive international relief efforts to help contain and mitigate the effects of the virus. The organization's headquarters has also disseminated Dharma teachings tailored for these difficult times.[4] These included "daily reminders" for devotees to pray, maintain right mindfulness, purify the mind, cultivate compassion, practice vegetarianism, and treat the disaster as an opportunity for spiritual awakening.

Other large-scale Buddhist responses to the COVID-19 pandemic include that of Soka Gakkai International, an organization headquartered in Tokyo with an estimated twelve million members in 192 countries. In a press release, Soka

Gakkai's president, Minoru Harada, announced that chapters in the United States, Italy, and Malaysia would be donating masks and raising funds to support frontline health-care workers, while youth members in Japan promoted a "stay home" initiative on Twitter.[5] The large Thai Buddhist organization Dhammakaya took to YouTube to call for its estimated three million members across the globe to "meditate against coronavirus," with the goal of accumulating one million minutes of meditation in a collective action to "heal the world."[6]

Meanwhile, the Dalai Lama used his considerable media platform to share his thoughts on COVID-19. In an article on *Time* magazine's website, he interpreted the crisis according to the principles of interdependence, suffering, and impermanence and called for compassion and hope.[7] In an article written for Chinese and Tibetan Buddhists, he called upon devotees to chant mantras to the deity Tārā to offer strength and protection against the virus.[8] Dr. Nida Chenagtsang and other leading voices in Sowa Rigpa and Tibetan Buddhism have also called for the practice of ritual, meditation, and traditional medicine approaches as part of a comprehensive approach to addressing the pandemic.[9]

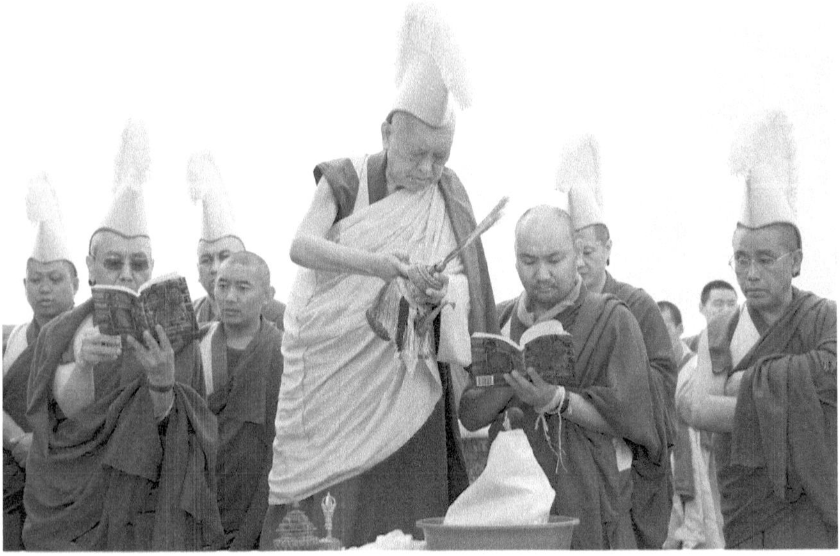

**Con.1** Vajrayāna monks performing a Padmasambhāva incense ritual to benefit those affected by COVID-19 and help mitigate the spread of the virus. Kopan Monastery, Nepal. Photo by Ven. Lobsang Sherab, courtesy of the Foundation for the Preservation of the Mahayana Tradition.

All of these actions are emblematic of the diversity of Buddhist responses to the COVID-19 pandemic. Owing to the size and reach of these organizations, their initiatives are higher in profile and larger in scale than most others. But around the world, Buddhist organizations of all types—whether Theravāda, Mahāyāna, or Vajrayāna; traditional or post-traditional; local or global—are actively involved in supporting their communities in similar ways.

Smaller-scale responses have included local charitable efforts.[10] Thai temples have distributed protective charms and face masks with talismans printed on them.[11] Japanese temples have performed expulsion rites and shared protective images of deities with their followers on Twitter.[12] In Sri Lanka, helicopters have sprinkled blessed water from the sky in an effort to stop the virus from spreading.[13] And the governor of Michigan has worked with Headspace, an online company and maker of a smartphone app, to provide all citizens of Michigan access to free content related to meditation.[14]

Given the centrality of themes such as healing meditations, protective rituals, and medical charity throughout this book, it is not surprising to see such efforts playing starring roles in the Buddhist response to COVID-19. Buddhists have almost always taken such measures seriously as medical and public health interventions. How or why they have thought these measures work is a more complex question, however. Contemporary Buddhists who primarily interpret the tradition through a modern lens may prefer secular and psychological interpretations of these responses—perhaps appealing to stress reduction or the placebo effect (what some scholars have called the "meaning response").[15] Other Buddhists may interpret the threat of the novel coronavirus in terms of demonic influences, karma, or subtle energies.

Culturally diverse, geographically expansive, and always multivocal, the Buddhist tradition as a whole continues to speak in all of theses registers simultaneously. Buddhist responses to COVID-19 and Buddhist interpretations of those responses do not necessarily coincide in their specifics. Nevertheless, these responses can be seen to coalesce around themes that are deeply intertwined with Buddhist doctrine and that have a history that can be traced back to the very beginning of the Buddhist tradition. What makes these various interventions "Buddhist medicine" is not that they agree with one another in matters of detail but that they are all part of the ongoing, millennia-long cross-cultural conversation about Buddhism and health we have been exploring in this book.

This book has demonstrated that Buddhism has always had a lot to say about medicine. Its investigation has shown great variation in the understanding of this relationship across times and places. Sometimes, stark distinctions have been made between religion and medicine. For example, many early Pāli sources argue that healing is a worldly realm of knowledge that has no place among serious practitioners of the Dharma. Much later, in the colonial period, Buddhism seemed to many Western commentators and Asian reformers nothing more than superstition, and they too would have denied that it had any useful role to play in medicine. Today, some commentators have likewise argued that any practices with Buddhist roots (including even the most secular versions of mindfulness) should be expurgated from secular spaces such as hospitals and doctors' offices because of their historical association with religion.

Other people, however, have thought of Buddhism and medicine as overlapping categories. Certain Mahāyāna texts see medical knowledge as crucially important "expedient means" that are part and parcel of the knowledge to be mastered by bodhisattvas in their quest to benefit all sentient beings. Many Mahāyāna and Tantric Buddhist texts take for granted that the human body will be healed through the serious practice of the Buddha's teachings and refer to the Dharma as a "Great Medicine" in a literal, nonmetaphorical sense. At times—say, in the Khmer empire in the twelfth century, in Tibet in the late seventeenth century, or in Siam in the 1830s—ideas, rituals, institutions, and other elements associated with Buddhism were central to the official medical system that was promulgated by the state. Likewise, many contemporary policy-makers, physicians, and medical scientists from Bhutan to Bangkok to Buenos Aires feel that Buddhism has preserved valuable techniques that can benefit patients in the twenty-first century and that it would be unethical not to use them. (Apparently, officials in the government of Michigan agree.)

The point is that there is no one-size-fits-all response to the question of how Buddhists have understood medicine: it is a vast topic that has generated—and continues to generate—much thought, reflection, and argument. This book set out to give a big-picture overview of this 2,400-year-long conversation. It has introduced a wide range of ideas and practices and traced their development across time and space while emphasizing global and comparative frameworks. It has examined how Buddhist perspectives have intersected, intertwined, and blended with other currents of medical thought across Asia and around the world. It has explored how key institutions, social networks, and transnational flows of information between and among them have influenced the implementation of ideas and practices on the ground in distinct times and places. It has asked who has forwarded the position that Buddhist interventions are efficacious, how they have framed these claims, and what are the larger cultural and intellectual trends in which these discourses have taken place. The book has also examined how Buddhist practices came to be thought of as legitimate objects of scientific medical study and how they came to be so widely disseminated in Buddhist and non-Buddhist contexts across the contemporary world. Along the way, I have highlighted the scholarship of many researchers who have contributed to telling this story. And I have pointed out some gaps in the academic study of Buddhist medicine that need to be filled in.

Establishing this new field of inquiry has required a big-picture narrative, both a summary of what we know and a blueprint to be used as a starting point for future study. Now the work of nuancing, refining, and challenging the grand narrative presented here can begin. Despite its inevitable shortcomings, I hope that this book has made the point that Buddhism has provided individuals with intellectual tools to frame and understand illness and health in all periods of time and all locations across the world wherever it has been practiced. It has shaped health-seeking behaviors in conscious and unconscious ways for billions of people and offered a range of popular therapies and institutional structures for dealing with the sick. Whatever the study of Buddhist medicine may bring to light in the future, there can be no doubt that medicine has been a central concern of Buddhism or that Buddhism has been a vitally important part of the history of medicine globally.

Personally, I believe that the Buddhist response to the COVID-19 pandemic and other topics discussed throughout this book have made clear that Buddhist medicine is not just an interesting subject of academic study. It also offers tools for thinking about health care in radically different ways from the individualism, secularism, and scientism of mainstream biomedical and public health discourses.[16] It invites us, for example, to appreciate the interconnectivity between our subjective mental, emotional, or spiritual experience on the one hand and the well-being of our material bodies on the other. It highlights the embeddedness of each individual within humanity and calls upon us to respond compassionately to the health inequities caused by racism, socioeconomic disparities, and other forms of suffering we humans inflict upon one another. Buddhist medicine draws our attention to how our health is interdependent with how we treat non-human beings and the natural environment and how our destruction of the planet is at once a moral and medical catastrophe. Buddhist medicine also holds out the possibility that our well-being is influenced by forces bigger than us—whether we interpret those forces as external entities, internal states of mind, or simply as metaphors.

Whatever stance you might take on these big questions, I hope that this book has presented you with a set of priorities and frameworks that can open up new possibilities for reimagining how you might think about your own well-being. Whether you identify as Buddhist is beside the point: especially in times of global crisis, I believe we need all the help we can get to orient toward healing our bodies, our minds, our communities, and our world.

# Notes

## INTRODUCTION

1. Davies 2015; Kucinskas 2018.
2. See, e.g., Fraser 2013; Goleman and Davidson 2017.
3. On the number of Buddhists globally, see "Buddhists," *Pew Research Center*, December 18, 2012. http://www.pewforum.org/2012/12/18/global-religious-landscape-buddhist/; "Buddhist Countries 2021," *World Population Review*. http://worldpopulationreview.com/countries/buddhist-countries/, accessed August 10, 2021.
4. See, e.g., Hardacre 1982; Palmer 2007; Penny 2012; McCall 2016; Stein 2017. On "Tibetan" singing bowls, see Ben Joffe, "Tripping On Good Vibrations: Cultural Commodification and Tibetan Singing Bowls," *Savage Minds*, October 13, 2015, https://savageminds.org/2015/10/31/tripping-on-good-vibrations-cultural-commodification-and-tibetan-singing-bowls.
5. See, e.g., Gyatso 2017, which is a direct response to my use of the term in light of her research on Tibet. McGrath 2020a takes an alternative position, arguing for the applicability of this term in the Tibetan case but with a narrower range of meaning than my use. An argument against the parallel term "Daoist medicine" is made in Stanley-Baker 2019.
6. An analysis of the history of this term is available in Salguero 2015a. The term "Buddhist medicine" (Ch. *fojiao yixue* or *foyi*; Jp. *bukkyō igaku*) appears not to have been in use until the twentieth century. Its emergence at that time was likely a counterpoint to other terms such as "Chinese medicine" (Ch. *zhongyi*) and "Western medicine" (Ch. *xiyi*) being developed at around the same time.
7. A useful discussion of the entanglement of medicine and religion more generally can be found in Lüddeckens and Schrimpf 2019. This book will not take up the task of rigorously defining the word "medicine" or of distinguishing it from "healing" or other similar words. My position for the present purposes is that any approach to human health whose doctrines and practices are articulated, codified, and institutionalized is worthy of being spoken about as "medicine." As we shall see, Buddhist approaches to health and healing satisfy all of these criteria.
8. Cf. Birnbaum 2016.
9. {2: xvi}.
10. Throughout this book, I have used phonetic transcriptions of Tibetan terminology rather than the Wylie system that is standard in scholarly circles. This is in order to

ensure that all readers are able to approximately pronounce these terms, which I hope will facilitate better conversations in the classroom and among nonspecialists.

11. See, e.g., de Vibe et al. 2012; Goyal et al. 2014; Fox et al. 2014; Goldberg et al. 2018. A critical review of early research in this area between 1980 and 2003 is found in Weaver, Vane, and Flannelly 2008. Goleman and Davidson 2017 is a readable introduction to the scientific research for nonscientists.
12. Didonna 2008; Brown, Creswell, and Ryan 2015.
13. Demiéville 1937, translated in Demiéville 1985.
14. The scholars who have most contributed to this area include Vincanne Adams, Sienna Craig, Barbara Gerke, Stephan Kloos, Geoffrey Samuel, and Mona Schrempf. See entries in the references for these authors.
15. The scholars who have most contributed to this area include Anna Andreeva, Frances Garrett, Robert Kritzer, Amy Paris Langenberg, and Katja Triplett. See entries in the references for these authors. See also Cole 1998: 192 -225; Boisvert 2000; Goble 2016; Kameyama 2016; Lin 2017; Buckelew 2018; Lomi 2018.
16. The scholars who have most contributed to this area include Anna Andreeva, Raoul Birnbaum, Chen Ming, Catherine Despeux, Andrew Goble, Michel Strickmann, Katja Triplett, and me. See entries in the references for these authors.
17. These have included meetings in Tangshan, China (organized by the University of British Columbia and the People's University of China in 2009), at the University of California, Berkeley (organized by the Center for Buddhist Studies in 2012), at the Donghwasa Temple in Daegu, South Korea (organized by Columbia University in 2013), at the University of Leeds (organized by the UK Association for Buddhist Studies in 2014), and at the University of British Columbia (organized by the Program in Buddhism and Contemporary Society in 2015). There also have been numerous panels on this topic at the American Academy of Religion and the Association for Asian Studies over the past decade.
18. See Kleine and Triplett 2012; Salguero and McGrath 2017; Wallace 2019; Salguero and Macomber 2020; {1}; {2}.
19. Beyond the current project, notable exceptions of which I am aware include works cited in the bibliography by Chen Ming and Ronit Yoeli-Tlalim.
20. Some scholars who have forwarded suggestions in this regard include Bushell 2009; Samuel 2014b, 2015; Radich 2016; Cheung 2017; Tidwell 2020.

## 1. NIKĀYA BUDDHISM

1. On Magadha, see Bronkhorst 2007; on controversies surrounding dating the lifetime of the Buddha, see Bechert 1991–1997; Bechert 1995; Cousins 1996.
2. See discussion in Wynne 2019.
3. See, e.g., Robinson, Johnson, and Thanissaro 2011.
4. The Buddhist sources are discussed in further detail in chapter 6.
5. Bareau 2013.
6. See fuller discussion in Salguero 2018a. For points of comparison with other "worldly arts," see Fiordalis 2014 on divination or Kotyk 2017a on astrology.

7. For a discussion of this distinction, see Liyanaratne 1999: 59–71; Ruegg 2008: 131–34; Barrett 2009; Kleine 2013; Fiordalis 2014: 98–101.
8. See also Langenberg 2014.
9. See examples in Demiéville 1985; Kitagawa 1989; Zysk 1998; Ṭhānissaro 2007: ch. 5; Mazars 2008; Fish 2014; Anālayo 2016. This contrasts with Jain and other Indian contemporaries, who seem to have had a much less sanguine opinion of doctors and medical care in general (Granoff 1998a, 1998b).
10. Demiéville 1985: 31–35.
11. *Mahavagga* 8.26.1–8, translated in Horner 2000: 431–34.
12. Shinohara 2007; Salguero 2014a: 123–25, 2015a.
13. See also Demiéville 1929.
14. Zysk 1998: 73–83; Sik 2016: 137–192.
15. The structure of the *vinayas* is discussed in Frauwallner 1956. The medical section of the Pāli Vinaya is translated in full in Horner 2000: 269–350.
16. Stanley-Baker 2019b.
17. Different categories of early Indian healer, such as *cikitsaka*, *bhiṣaj*, and others, are discussed in Olivelle 2017.
18. Salguero 2018a: 11–15.
19. The Pāli version of this biography is found in *Mahāvagga* 8.1.1–36, translated in Horner 2000: 379–97. See discussion in Zysk 1998: 52–61. The Chinese title *yiwang* unambiguously reads "King of Physicians," but this may come from a Chinese misreading of the Sanskrit term *vidya-rāja*, which was intended to identify Jīvaka as the "royal physician" {1: p. 202n36}.
20. Salguero 2009.
21. *Mahāvagga* I.31.
22. See summary of the early Buddhist source materials in Demiéville 1985; Mitra 1985; Mazars 2008.
23. Salguero 2018c.
24. For a general introduction to Āyurveda, see Cerulli 2010; translations in Wujastyk 2003; further resources in Wujastyk 2017.
25. For a recent comparison of Greek and Indian understandings of the Elements, among other concepts, see McEvilley 2002: 300–9. A number of histories of Āyurveda from the early twentieth century and before also contain such comparisons, although they are unreliable in light of more recent historical research. A comprehensive study of Greco-Indian medical exchanges remains a desideratum.
26. See, e.g., MN 28, 62, 140; T 26.30. See discussion and references in Mitra 1985: 40–45; Chinese parallels in Salguero 2018c; For a roundup of Chinese sources on the Elements and *tridoṣa*, see Demiéville 1985: 65–76.
27. Demiéville 1985: 71, 81.
28. On the historical emergence and development of *tridoṣa* in early medical and Buddhist texts, see Scharfe 1999.
29. AN 10.60. This appears to be one of the earliest mentions of the *tridoṣa* in Indian literature, although they are not identified with that word in this passage (see discussion in Scharfe 1999).

30. See discussion of authorship and contents of Indian medical treatises in Meulenbeld 1999–2002; Wujastyk 2003.
31. Salguero 2018c.
32. See also Granoff 1998a: 227; Granoff 2011; Salguero et al. 2017: 291–93.
33. Salguero 2010–2011.
34. This argument is best articulated in Zysk 1998, although the premise has been challenged by some reviewers of the book.
35. See Salguero 2014a: 67–95, especially 67–70.
36. See discussion in Krug 2019.
37. The various inhabitants of the Indian spirit world are discussed in DeCaroli 2004; Smith 2006, especially 471–578.
38. Misra 1981: 73–80; Granoff 1998b: 298–300; DeCaroli 2004. See also DN 32, from the Pāli, which tells of the taming of the *yakṣas* (Pāli *yakkha*).
39. See Peri 1917; Shaw 2005: 110–42.
40. DeCaroli 2004: 82–83; Rees and Yoneda 2013.
41. DeCaroli 2004: 143–72.
42. Granoff 1998b.
43. Granoff 1998b. On relics more generally, see Ruppert 2000.
44. Ohnuma 2004: 140–41. See also Granoff 1998b: 296. Perhaps ironically, the Buddha later died of a gastrointestinal condition usually identified as food poisoning (see Wasson and O'Flaherty 1982; Strong 2012).
45. See discussion and translation of several Jain and Buddhist stories in Granoff 1998a, 1998b.
46. MN 86, translated in https://www.accesstoinsight.org/tipitaka/mn/mn.086.than.html, accessed August 10, 2021.
47. Other Buddhist texts in which truth statements are used to heal snakebites are discussed in Slouber 2017: 34–37.
48. Harvey 2015: 17.
49. See also SN 41.10; 46.14, 46.15, 46.16, 52.10. Healing through contemplation of various qualities of the Dharma is discussed in Anālayo 2015, 2016.
50. AN 10.60. See discussion in Anālayo 2016: 99–109.

## 2. MAHĀYĀNA BUDDHISM

1. For an overview of scholarship on the emergence of Mahāyāna Buddhism, see Drewes 2010a, 2010b.
2. See overview of this literature in Demiéville 1985; Salguero 2014a, 2018d.
3. See Katz 2010.
4. Salguero 2018a.
5. Pye 1978.
6. Salguero 2018a: 18–19. The status of medicine as an expedient means in Tibetan Tantric tradition is discussed in Wallace 2001: 43–55.
7. See, e.g., Salguero 2013.
8. Salguero 2013: 345.
9. See Chen H. 2007: 159–62; Salguero 2014a: 112–16.

10. See, e.g., Scharfe 1999.
11. Many of these instances are collected in Demiéville 1985.
12. Kritzer 2004, 2009, 2012, 2013, 2014a, 2014b; Garrett 2005, 2007b, 2008a, 2008b, 2015; Langenberg 2017. For Nikāya writings on similar topics, see Boisvert 2000. A Hindu parallel is transalted in Kapani 1989. The Āyurvedic medical literature is surveyed in Das 2003.
13. It is also notable that Patañjali's *Yoga Sūtras* were similarly organized into an eight-fold system.
14. Cf. Wezler 1984.
15. Salguero 2010–11. See also Wayman 1957.
16. Some of these discrepancies are discussed in Demiéville 1985; Köhle 2016.
17. On the shifting sex of this deity, see Yü 2001: 407–48.
18. Many chapters in both {1} and {2} feature this bodhisattva. Other highlights in the scholarship of this deity's healing powers include Strikmann 1996: 136–59; Yü 2001: 37–72; Czaja 2005; Orzech, Sørensen, and Payne 2011: 94–99; Salguero 2014a: 130–32; Mai 2018.
19. Birnbaum 1989a: 24–51, 115–48.
20. On Buddhist cosmology, see Sadakata 1997.
21. Gómez 1996.
22. Shinohara 2007.
23. Stone 2008.
24. For general information on this deity, see Birnbaum 1989a; Kuo 1994; Suzuki 2012; Dorje 2014; Salguero et al., 2017: 286–89; Shi 2020. On the translation of his name, see {1: p. 247n8}.
25. Soper and Ōmura 1959: 174–78, 207–10.
26. See discussion in {1: p. 235}.
27. In Southeast Asia, see Woodward 2011.
28. White 1996: 66–77; Mabbett 1998; Young 2014; Walser 2016.
29. See additional sources attributed to Nāgārjuna in Deshpande and Fan 2012.
30. Strickmann 2002: 89–122; McBride 2011; Salguero 2014a: 88–91. On *dhāraṇī* more generally, see McBride 2005; Copp 2014.
31. For translation of the relevant passage of the *Lotus Sūtra*, see Watson 1993: 307–11.
32. Watson 1993: 309–10.
33. See translation in Emmerick 2004: 44.
34. See Okuda, Noro, and Ito 2005; Robson 2014.
35. Salguero et al. 2017: 286–89.
36. Details of the medieval Chinese Bhaiṣajyaguru ritual are discussed in Shi 2020.

## 3. TANTRIC BUDDHISM

1. Samuel 2008 provides a general introduction to the emergence of Tantra in India and its spread abroad. See more focused studies in Snellgrove 1987; Davidson 2002; Orzech, Sørensen, and Payne 2011; Shinohara 2014.
2. Note that the word "Hinduism" was not created until much later and is used here and elsewhere throughout the book as a term of convenience to refer to a range of religious and cultic traditions that would become part of the notion of Hinduism (see Sharma 2002).

3. See Davidson 2002: 336–40; Orzech, Sørensen, and Payne 2011 (especially chapters 1, 2, and 11); Lü 2017.
4. Davidson 2002: 113–68; Samuel 2008.
5. Dowman 1986; Katz 2010.
6. See, e.g., Dowman 1986: 204–6.
7. See overview in Samuel 2008.
8. Gray 2014.
9. A range of East Asian Tantric practices focused on healing is described in Strickmann 1996, 2002; Davis 2001; McBride 2011; Lomi 2014; Salguero 2014a: 86–92; select chapters in {1}.
10. See discussion in Cousins 1997; Crosby 2000, 2013.
11. Birnbaum 1989a: 69–72; Mollier 2008: 134–173.
12. Beyer 1973; Shaw 2005: 306–56.
13. See also Samuel 2012a, 2016; Kapstein 2014. On Uṣṇīṣavijaya, see Shaw 2005: 291–305.
14. Shaw 2005; Samuel 2008: 246–49; Hidas 2012.
15. Strickmann 2002: 151–56; Shaw 2005: 224–33. On other snakebite goddesses in Tantric Buddhism, see Slouber 2017: 35–36, 103, 105–7.
16. See full translation in Greene 2021.
17. Slouber 2017: 41–42. See French translation of this text in MacDonald 1962; discussion in Wallis 2002. Similar practices from a Hindu Tantric milieu are discussed throughout Slouber's book.
18. Slouber 2017: 120–21.
19. Slouber 2017: 121.
20. Slouber 2017: 121.
21. T 848: 20b; translated in Geibel 2005: 82.
22. For a discussion of the importance of Sanskrit letters in Japanese Tantric practice, see Abe 1999: 288–93, 339–40.
23. On the history of mandalas, see Samuel 2008: 224–28; Shinohara 2014.
24. Gray 2007a.
25. See discussion in Wallace 2001: 43–55.
26. On this text's medical contents, see Stablein 1976a; Wallace 2001; Arnold 2009 (see especially contributions by Kilty, Vargas, and Wallace); see also full translation in Wallace 2004. The section that most concerns the use of conventional medicine is "Great Exposition on Elixirs, Midwifery, and the Like," in the "Chapter on the Individual" (Wallace 2004: 163–217).
27. Beyer 1973: 367–75; Wallace 2004: 166.
28. Wallace 2004: 205–17.
29. White 1996; Zysk 2007; Samuel 2008.
30. White 2003; Samuel 2008: 229–70.
31. For a history of possession in Indian religions, see Smith 2006. On healing in particular, see part 4 of that book.
32. See Davis 2001; Strickmann 2002: 204–208; Robson 2011: 251–54.
33. See, e.g., Gray 2006, 2007b; Dalton 2011; Cuevas 2019; Goble 2019: 95–133.
34. Wallace 2004: 180.

35. Wallace 2004: 179. On the consumption of sexual fluids in Tantric rites more generally, see White 2003.
36. Wallace 2004: 179.
37. White 1996; Walter 1980.
38. See Gerke 2013, 2021; Czaja 2013.
39. White 1996: 71–73; Wallace 2004: 186–88.
40. Beyer 1973: 391–92.
41. Garrett 2009; Gerke 2012, 2017a, 2017b, 2019a; Cantwell 2017; Chui 2019. For closely analogous practices among Tibetan practitioners of the Bön religion, see Sehnalova 2017.
42. Beyer 1973: 396–97.
43. On the history of the subtle body, see Snellgrove 1987: 288–94; White 1996; Dalton 2004; Samuel 2008: 285–89, 2013, 2014a; Baker 2019: 86–111. For a broader comparison of divergent views of the body among different Indian religio-medical groups, see Wujastyk 2009a.
44. The evidence for historical connections with China, such that it is, is evaluated in Filliozat 1969; White 1996: 61–66; Samuel 2008: 278–85.
45. T 620. The text is discussed and translated in Greene 2021 but seems largely to have been overlooked by historians of Tantra.
46. See discussion in Samuel 2008.
47. Examples of the localization of the Tantric subtle body in medieval East Asia can be seen in Rambelli 2000; Macomber 2018: 280–333. For remnants persisting in the healing practices of contemporary Thailand, see Salguero 2016: 54–62.
48. Wujastyk 2003: 117–8; Zysk 2007.
49. See, e.g., Wallace 2004: 167–68, 2008: 214–15.
50. Perhaps confusingly, the Elements themselves were each thought to have subtle Winds associated with them. It is also worth noting that Tantric instantiations of the Element theory typically expand the function of the Space or Void Element, *ākāśa*, to encompass much more than merely the empty spaces where the other four Elements are lacking, as was described in earlier Buddhist texts.
51. Extensive discussions of the implications of Winds, *nāḍīs*, and *cakras* for health and healing are found in Wallace 2004; Guarisco 2017.
52. Gyatso 2015: 193–250; Guarisco 2017: 45–51.
53. Snellgrove 1959; Sopa 1983; Wallace 2004: 70–127; Mullin 2006: 23–41; Gray 2007a; Guarisco 2017.
54. See discussion in Garrett and Adams 2008.
55. Notice that the typical Western associations of the moon with femininity and the sun with masculinity are reversed in this model.
56. Lipman 2010: 57.
57. E.g., Guarisco 2017: 244.
58. Wallace 2004: 83–111; 2008. See discussion of medical astrology more generally in Akasoy, Burnett, and Yoeli-Tlalim 2008; Kotyk 2017b, 2019.
59. Wallace 2004: 168–77.
60. Wallace 2001: 52, 163.
61. Baker 2012, 2017, 2019.
62. Loseries-Leick 1997; Chaoul 2007.

63. Samuel 1989: 199; Guarisco 2017: 59–60.
64. Dalton 2004: 293. A full sequence for this type of meditation is outlined in Bangdel and Huntington 2003: 240–51. See also George 1971: 106–30.
65. Gray 2007a: 704.
66. Guarisco 2017: 292.
67. Wallace 2001: 51; 2004: 172.
68. Lipman 2010: 34–35, 66–67. The textual history of this collection is discussed in Germano 1992: 26–38. The texts attributed to Padmasambhava in particular are discussed on pp. 33–35. See also Jacoby 2014; Grimes and Szántó 2018.
69. See, e.g., Schaeffer 2003a; Samuel 2008; Birch 2011; Grimes and Szántó 2018; Mallinson 2019, 2020.

## 4. COMMON QUESTIONS

1. See discussion in Salguero 2018c: 255–58.
2. See also Capitanio 2013; Birnbaum 2017.
3. See, e.g., Barclay, Eliza, "Thich Nhat Hanh's Final Mindfulness Lesson: How to Die Peacefully," *Vox*, October 11, 2019, http://www.vox.com/2019/3/11/18196457/thich-nhat-hanh-health-mindfulness-plum-village. For a biography of Hạnh, see Powers 2016b.
4. Granoff 1998a, 1998b: 287–88.
5. For general overviews of Buddhist concepts of the body, see Wilson 2004; Gardiner 2016; Salguero 2018c.
6. Salguero 2018c: 249–55.
7. Kritzer 2014a; Salguero 2018c: 252–54.
8. Wilson 1995.
9. This cycle of texts has been summarized in Kritzer 2009, 2014b. Examples of the genre are analyzed in more detail in Boisvert 2000; Garrett 2008a; Langenberg 2015. Compare with Tantric visions of the same processes in Lipman 2010: 47–51; Guarisco 2017: 224–30. A Hindu example of the genre is translated in Kapani 1989. Āyurvedic models of conception, gestation, and birth are reviewed in Das 2003.
10. Salguero 2018c: 254.
11. Some of these polemics against the female body are no doubt connected to the primarily male monastic order's desire to promote celibacy among the ordained. See discussion of Buddhist sexuality more generally in Faure 1998; Cabezón 2017.
12. Zysk 2016.
13. Salguero 2020a: 28.
14. See, e.g., Luang Pho Daeng's mummified body at Wat Khunaram in Ko Samui, Thailand.
15. See, e.g., "Rainbow Body 101: Everything You Didn't Know," *Gaia*, March 6, 2020, http://www.gaia.com/article/rainbow-body-101-everything-you-didnt-know. See also Chenagtsang 2014.
16. See Snellgrove 1987: 288–89.
17. See discussion in Mrozik 2007.
18. Strong 2012: 18; Anālayo 2015.
19. The Buddha's final illness is discussed in Strong 2012, and the identification of the food he consumed is discussed in Wasson and O'Flaherty 1982.

20. See partial translation in Blum 2013, especially the chapter "Manifesting Disease." On the difference between the Buddha's body and that of an ordinary human being, see also Radich 2007: 1080–85.
21. See analysis of the Buddha's bodies in Radich 2007, 2016. For a Tantric view of this doctrine, see Wallace 2001: 143–81.
22. Richter 2020 provides a discussion of the influence of the sickbed trope in medieval China.
23. See also Salguero 2016: 33–40; 2017a.
24. See, e.g., Flanagan 2012.
25. See, e.g., Stablein 1980; Deck 2002; Wattanagun 2017.
26. See also MN 135. Such perspectives are discussed in detail in Mrozik 2007.
27. SN 36.21.
28. See discussion in Strong 2012.
29. Strong 2012.
30. Strong 2012: 24.
31. Mather 1981; Greene 2016; Barstow 2019.
32. See Kajiwara 2004.
33. Granoff 1998b, especially p. 294.
34. Dowman 1986: 204–6.
35. Harvey 1993; Hamilton 1996; Ozawa-De Silva and Ozawa-De Silva 2011.
36. Muecke 1979; Clifford 1984; Jacobson 2007; Millard 2007; Yoeli-Tlalim 2010; Deane 2014a, 2014b, 2019a, 2019b.
37. See Britton 2019.
38. See Zysk 1998: 52–61.
39. Demiéville 1985: 49.
40. It is also problematic for contemporary practitioners who hold Jīvaka up as an exemplar that the Pāli version of the story says he was sometimes paid by his patients with slaves.
41. Horner 2000: 384.
42. See, e.g., "Dalai Lama's American Doctor Wants More Compassion in Medicine," *PBS NewsHour*, October 27, 2015, http://www.pbs.org/newshour/show/dalai-lama-2, accessed August 10, 2021.
43. See, e.g., "Everyone Deserves Good Health," *Tzu Chi USA*. August 11, 2015, https://tzuchi.us/blog/everyone-deserves-good-health. See also discussion in Kloos 2019; Craig, Gerke, and Sheldon 2020.
44. Demiéville 1985: 56; Salguero 2013: 346.
45. Sahni 2008.
46. Mather 1981; Greene 2016; Barstow 2019.
47. See also "Advice Book: A Healthy Diet," *Lama Yeshe Wisdom Archive*, May 2014 (posted December 2014), https://www.lamayeshe.com/advice/healthy-diet, accessed August 10, 2021.
48. See also Gyatso 2015: 343–96.
49. See, e.g., Keown 1995, 1999; Florida 1998; Ratanakul 1999a, 2004.

### 5. CIRCULATIONS

1. On the early spread of Buddhism across the Indian subcontinent, see Neelis 2011.

2. While the historical Aśoka's connections with Buddhism are more tenuous (Norman 2006: 147–69), the Aśoka of Buddhist legend was a magnanimous donor to the sangha, often providing gifts of medicine. See translations in Strong 1983; Li 1993.
3. See discussion in Heirman and Bumbacher 2007; Neelis 2011: 289–310; Sen 2014; Wong and Heldt 2014; Meinert 2015; Acri 2016; Heirman 2018; Kellner 2019; Yoeli-Tlalim 2021.
4. On Iranian Buddhism, see Folz 2010; Vaziri 2012; De Chiara and Braarvig 2013.
5. Nguyen 1990.
6. See discussion of the role of epidemics in global history in McNeill 1998. A specific archaeological example from a Silk Road relay station is discussed in Yeh et al. 2016. On the increase of plagues connected to the spread of Buddhist temples across Japan, see Como 2019.
7. Indo-Greek Buddhism is discussed in Narain 1957; Fussman 1993; Behl 2014; Halkias 2014.
8. The quote comes from Horner 2000: 381.
9. Zysk 1998: 55; Naqvi 2011: 54–60.
10. See discussion in Naqvi 2011.
11. However, Gregory Schopen has raised doubts that this Buddha was firmly associated with healing in the Sanskritic tradition {1: p. 235}.
12. Slouber 2017: 36–37.
13. Upasak 1977; Scharfe 2002: 131–65; Kumar 2011.
14. Zysk 1999.
15. See summary discussion in Wujastyk 2003: 194–95.
16. Vogel 1965: 8–10. On Yijing's role in Buddhist networks of exchange, see Sen 2018.
17. Chaudhary 1975.
18. On the notion of "centers of calculation," see Latour 1987; Jöns 2011.
19. Filliozat 1935; Wujastyk 1998a.
20. Chau 1911: part 2; Schafer 1963; Akasoy and Yoeli-Tlalim 2007. A preliminary attempt to trace these networks through a digital database is described in Stanley-Baker 2019b.
21. Akasoy and Yoeli-Tlalim 2007; Akasoy, Burnett, and Yoeli-Tlalim 2016.
22. Schafer 1963: 176–94; Bielenstein 2005; Chen M. 2007, 2013: 114–23.
23. Unschuld 2006: 25; Chen M. 2007.
24. Sen 2001, 2003: 44–53.
25. Several of these medicinals are discussed in more detail in Dash 1974; Sudarshan 2005; Majupuria 2009.
26. Demiéville 1985: 69–71.
27. On the trade of such substances, see Liu 1988: 93–94.
28. Strong 1983: 288.
29. Dash 1974.
30. The medicinal uses of tea are discussed in Liu 2006; Benn 2015.
31. Salguero 2014a: 133–39, 2020a. See the relevant entries in Ha and Mintz 1972; Fu and Ni 1996. On the genre of biographies of eminent monks more generally, see Kieschnick 1997.
32. Translations of this text are available in Takakusu 1966; Li 2000. Information relevant to medicine is found especially in chapters 4–8, 18, 20, 23, and 27–29. Studies on the medical contents of this text include Liétard 1902; Reddy 1938; Devi 1979; Salguero 2014a: 112–16.
33. See discussion in Wujastyk 2009b; translations in Giles 1923: 47–48; Li 1996: 144.

34. Alexander Gardner, "Rinchen Zangpo," *Treasury of Lives*, http://treasuryoflives.org/biographies/view/Rinchen-Zangpo/10199, accessed June 22, 2020.
35. See discussion of this attribution in McGrath 2020a.
36. Lin 1935.
37. On *kaji*, see Winfield 2005; Josephson 2012.
38. On the history of the Bhaiṣajyaguru cult in medieval Japan, see Suzuki 2012.
39. See also Thompson 2014.
40. On "contact zones," see Pratt 1991; Somerville and Perkins 2003. On "trading zones," see Gallison 1997.
41. See discussion of such facilities in Hirakawa 1963: 96; Demiéville 1985: 54–55; Zysk 1998: 44–46, 147–48 n. 41; Despeux 2010: 43–64; Naqvi 2011.
42. Chen H. 2007: 159–62; Salguero 2014a: 112–16.
43. See, e.g., Canton-Alvarez 2019; Despeux 2020.
44. One scholar refers to the "Buddhist international" (Adshead 2000: 102) and another to the "Buddhist world system" (Elverskog 2010: 26).
45. See discussion of Indian models of kingship in Strong 1983: 38–70; Orzech 1998; Gummer 2000.
46. Some such projects are described in Demiéville 1985: 56–63; Liu 2008. See also some theoretical considerations linking kingship and healing in Thompson 2004.
47. Wujastyk 2009b. Xuanzang identified Harṣavardhana as Buddhist, although he actually seems to have been a Śaivite.
48. Needham 2000: 54. Later examples are discussed in Liu 2008.
49. Salguero et al. 2017: 286–89.
50. Ch'en 1973: 297–301; Gernet 1995: 221–23; Liu 2008.
51. Jacques 1968; Thompson 2004; Chhem 2005; Woodward 2011; Sharrock unpublished.
52. Chhem 2006, 2007, 2009.
53. Guarisco 2017: 5. See also Dominique Townsend, "Sakya Paṇḍita Kunga Gyeltsen," *Treasury of Lives*, http://treasuryoflives.org/biographies/view/Sakya-Pandita-Kunga-Gyeltsen/2137, accessed June 22, 2020.
54. McGrath 2017, 2020b.
55. Gyatso 2015: 114–16.
56. Van Vleet 2016.
57. Van Vleet 2015: 204–59.
58. Salguero 2014a: 141–45.

## 6. TRANSLATIONS

1. There has been some debate on what is meant by the term "canon" in reference to Buddhist collections and whether this term is appropriate. For a general overview, see Mizuno 1995; Veidlinger 2010; Silk 2015. On Pāli texts in particular, see Collins 1990. On the Chinese collection, see Wu and Chia 2015; Jones 2019. On the Tibetan, see Stanley 2014.
2. Salomon 1999.
3. Lo and Cullen 2005; Yoeli-Tlalim 2013.
4. Despeux 2010: 43–64, 2020.

5. See, e.g., B. D. Dipananda, "Bringing Ancient Thai Buddhist Manuscripts to the World," *BuddhistDoor Global*, April 8, 2016, https://www.buddhistdoor.net/features/bringing-ancient-thai-buddhist-manuscripts-to-the-world. Toni Huber, "Recently Discovered Ancient Tibetan Manuscripts and What They Reveal About Old Cultures of Ritual and Some Tibetan Buddhist Innovations," *Berkeley Buddhist Studies*, February 28, 2019, https://buddhiststudies.berkeley.edu/news/2019-khyentse-lecture-toni-huber-humboldt-university-berlin-recently-discovered-ancient-tibetan; "*Takaramono no kagaku: minshū sukutta kusuri no genten*," *Yomiuri Shimbun*, October 9, 2020, https://www.yomiuri.co.jp/shosoin/20201009-OYT8T50003/.
6. I have summarized the available Buddhist medical sources in the major Chinese canonical collection in Salguero 2018d.
7. Wood and Barnard 2010.
8. Many of the texts listed in Salguero 2018d are also included in this collection.
9. Mizuno 1995: 164–86.
10. Vipassana Research Institute: http://www.tipitaka.org, accessed August 10, 2021; Sutta Central: http://www.suttacentral.net, accessed August 10, 2021.
11. Göttingen Register of Electronic Texts in Indian Languages: http://gretil.sub.uni-goettingen.de, accessed August 10, 2021.
12. Chinese Buddhist Electronic Texts Association: http://cbeta.org, accessed August 10, 2021; SAT Daizōkyō Text Database: http://21dzk.l.u-tokyo.ac.jp/SAT, accessed August 10, 2021.
13. Buddhist Digital Resource Centre: http://tbrc.org, accessed August 10, 2021; American Institute of Buddhist Studies: http://databases.aibs.columbia.edu, accessed August 10, 2021.
14. Thesaurus Literaturae Buddhicae: http://www2.hf.uio.no/polyglotta/index.php?page=library&bid=2, accessed August 10, 2021.
15. International Dunhuang Project: http://idp.bl.uk, accessed August 10, 2021.
16. Shi and Li 2011, although see critique of the claims this collection makes and its principles of compilation in Burton-Rose 2017.
17. For an extensive discussion of this topic, see Salguero 2014a.
18. On Buddhist languages, see Nattier 1990; Sinor 1995; Boucher 2008: 101–7.
19. For a discussion of apocryphal texts in China, see Buswell 1990.
20. See, e.g., Rambelli 2000.
21. See, e.g., Zysk 1998: 52–61; Chen M. 2005a; Salguero 2009, 2017a.
22. See translation of the Tibetan in Kara 2004 and of a related Chinese text in Unschuld 2010: 314–21. The Dunhuang versions of this text are discussed in Chen M. 2015: 482–87; Despeux 2017: 148–50.
23. On the authorship and contents of this collection, see Hsu 2018. On its influence in defining the contours of Buddhist medicine until the present, see Salguero 2015a.
24. A translation of Zhiyi's longer work on meditation and illness is available in Swanson 2017, vol. 2: 1322–63. For discussion of meditation illness in Japan, see Ahn 2007.
25. The medical section of the Pāli *vinaya* is translated in Horner 2000: 269–350.
26. Bapat and Hirakawa 1970: 205–6, 329–35, 442, 477, 525.
27. See also Heirman and Torck 2012.
28. The Sanskrit is translated in {1: 25}; two Chinese versions in Birnbaum 1989a. See discussion of the textual history in Birnbaum 1989a; Loukota 2019.

29. This chapter is translated from Chinese in Watson 1993: 280–89. Chinese texts and visualizations practices associated with Bhaiṣajyarāja are described in Birnbaum 1989a.
30. See translations from Sanskrit in Emmerick 2004; from Sanskrit, Khotanese, and Chinese in Skjaervø 2004.
31. Translated from Chinese in Watson 1997 or Paul and McRae 2005; from Sanskrit in Thurman 2003. See also comparison of multiple translations in Nattier 2000.
32. Partial translation of this text is in Blum 2013. Relevant excerpts of this and other texts are discussed in Demiéville 1985.
33. Translated in Snellgrove 1959; Wallace 2004; Gray 2007a.
34. Translated from the Sanskrit in Emmerick 2004: 44–49; comparison of Sanskrit, Khotanese, and Chinese in Skjaervø 2004.
35. See also Kara 2004; Unschuld 2010: 314–21.
36. Translation in MacDonald 1962; discussion in Wallis 2002; Slouber 2017: 41–42.
37. Mullin 2006.
38. Guarisco 2017.
39. See also selected translations in Orzech and Sanford 2000; Rambelli 2000; Slouber 2017.; G. Goble 2017; Salguero et al. 2017.
40. See translations in Anālayo 2016, especially chapters 4, 5, 6, 17, 19.
41. See also AN 10.60; SN 41.10; 46.14, 46.15, 46.16, 52.10. All are available in a number of translations in print and online.
42. Translated in Birnbaum 1989a: 115–48.
43. Translation in Woodward and Rhys Davids 2003.
44. See also translation in Mettanando 1999; discussion of connections with medicine in Crosby 2013: 90–92, 97–100.
45. For analysis and complete translation of this text, see Greene 2021.
46. The longer text is translated in Swanson 2017, vol. 2: 1322–63.
47. See translation of Jīvaka's biography from Pāli in Horner 2000: 379–97; from Tibetan in von Schiefner 1906; from Sanskrit in {1: 20}; from Chinese into French in Chavannes 1962: 325–61.
48. See discussion and translation of some of these narratives in Wright 1948; Ohnuma 2004; Shinohara 2007; Campany 2012; Salguero 2014a: 133–39, 2020b.
49. Translated in Rhys Davids 1965; see discussion in Sengupta 1989.
50. MN 28, 62; SN 36.21.
51. See, e.g., Ehara, Soma, and Kheminda 1961; Ñāṇamoli 1999.
52. See discussion in Lusthaus 2013.
53. Cordier 1903; Dash 1985: 9–16.
54. See discussion of text and partial translations in Vogel 1965; Wujastyk 2003: 193–251; Czaja 2019. On an extant Uighur version of the text, see Maue 2008.
55. See translation in Emmerick 1982; discussion in Emmerick 1971, 1974; Chen M. 2002; Zieme 2007.
56. See Filliozat 1979; Dash 1985.
57. Translated in Bagchi 2011, 1941. See discussion in Filliozat 1935, 1937; Wujastyk 1998a; 1998b; 2003: 163–89; Triplett 2019a.
58. See translation and discussion of various versions of this text in Garrett 2008a; Kritzer 2009, 2014b; Langenberg 2017; Pāli equivalents in Boisvert 2000; Tibetan in Guarisco 2017: 224–30.

59. See Saha 1985; Hoernle 1987; Wujastyk 2003: 147–60; Naqvi 2011: 83–92; Slouber 2017: 85.
60. Hoernle 1893, 1902.
61. See Hoernle 1917; Emmerick 1979; Chen M. 2005a.
62. Partially translated in Clark 1995; Men-Tsee-Khang 2011a, 2011b. A structural outline of this text is available in Gerke 2014.
63. While the text is not translated, the painting captions have been. See Parfionovitch et al. 1992; discussion in Czaja 2007; Gyatso 2014.
64. Translated in Kilty 2010.
65. See Liyanaratne 2002–2009.
66. See also translations in Hsia et al. 1986; Deshpande and Fan 2012.

## 7. LOCALIZATIONS

1. The relevant source text is T 1508.
2. This section's outline of the relations between Islam and Buddhism is heavily indebted to Elverskog 2010.
3. See, e.g., Cruijsen, Griffiths, and Klokke 2013.
4. Elverskog 2010: 98.
5. Again, Elverskog 2010 is the best source on these exchanges.
6. Wujastyk 2016.
7. Nappi 2009; Lo 2007.
8. Buell and Anderson 2000; Buell 2007; Goble 2009, 2011: 46–66; Shinno 2016: 138–40.
9. Akasoy and Yoeli-Tlalim 2007; Yoeli-Tlalim 2013, 2021; Blezer 2019.
10. Beckwith 1979; Garrett 2007a; Martin 2008; Yoeli-Tlalim 2012, 2019.
11. Perhaps the best-known example of this phenomenon is the Muslim retelling of the biography of the Buddha in the form of a legend about Bilawar and Budasaf. This tale, in turn, became Christianized as the tale of Saints Barlaam and Josaphat. See Elverskog 2010: 72–73.
12. Elverskog 2010: 104–15.
13. See also Hatley 2007.
14. See Lloyd and Sivin 2002. A general history of Chinese medicine is available in Hinrichs and Barnes 2013.
15. Salguero 2014a: 44–51.
16. Salguero 2014a: 116–19.
17. Schafer 1963: 176–94; Chen M. 2013: 114–223.
18. Salguero 2014a: 39–40.
19. Faxian's comments are translated in Giles 1923: 47–48. Xuanzang's comments are translated in Li 1996: 144.
20. Of particular interest are *Kāśyapa's Compendium* (T 1691) and the *Tantra of Rāvaṇakumāra* (T 1330), both translated at the beginning of the eleventh century.
21. On these governmental efforts, see Goldschmidt 2009.
22. See discussion in Ch'en 1973; Gregory 1991.
23. Salguero 2014a: 141–45.
24. See, e.g., Davis 2001; Teiser 2009; Mai 2018.

25. See also Scheid 2020.
26. On the history of this temple, see Shahar 2008. On the temple's recently published compilation of Buddhist medical texts, see Burton-Rose 2017.
27. See, e.g., Chen Y. 2008; Wu 2000.
28. On the influence of *The Vimalakīrti Sūtra* on medieval poetry, for example, see Richter 2020.
29. Scheid 2020 raises an important counterexample.
30. Baker 1994; Lee 2011; summary in Salguero and Macomber 2020: 6–8.
31. Lee, Ahn, and Kim 2019.
32. Jeong 2013; Lim 2013.
33. On Buddhist medicine in Japan, see Triplett and Kleine 2012; Shinmura 2013; Triplett 2019b. For a general history of Japanese medicine in English, see Fujikawa 1934.
34. Drott 2010.
35. See partial translation in Hsia, Veith, and Geertsma 1986.
36. For a description of this collection in Japanese, see "*Takaramono no kagaku: minshū sukutta kusuri no genten*," *Yomiuri Shimbun*, October 9, 2020, https://www.yomiuri.co.jp/shosoin/20201009-OYT8T50003/. I am indebted to Bryan Lowe for pointing out this article in a tweet.
37. Andreeva 2014, 2015, 2017a, 2018a, 2019a, 2019b.
38. See Goble 2011.
39. See, e.g., Williams 2004a, 2005: 86–116, 178–90; Goble 2016.
40. See, e.g., de Visser 1935: 293–308, 533–571; Abe 1999: 160–62, 341; Williams 2004a; Okuda, Noro, and Ito 2005; Suzuki 2012; Lomi 2014.
41. Triplett 2013, 2019c.
42. On *kaji* more generally, see Winfield 2005; Josephson 2012.
43. See also Rambelli 2000.
44. Miyazaki and Williams 2001; Williams 2004b; Moerman 2015.
45. While finalizing this manuscript, I was glad to find out about C. Michele Thompson's forthcoming book, *The Gardens of Tranquil Wisdom: Tuệ Tĩnh, Vietnamese Buddhism, and Health Care in Trần Dynasty Vietnam*.
46. Samuel 2014a provides an accessible introduction to this system, emphasizing its connections with Buddhism. Note that when I refer to "Tibet" in the premodern context, I am referring to the cultural area centering on the Tibetan Plateau, which includes the modern-day Tibetan Autonomous Zone, the independent country of Bhutan, and parts of neighboring Chinese provinces.
47. On Dunhuang texts, see Yoeli-Tlalim 2013.
48. Van Vleet 2015: 45–49; McGrath 2020b.
49. Clark 1995; Men-Tsee-Khang 2011a, 2011b.
50. Some of these connections are highlighted in, e.g., Akasoy and Yoeli-Tlalim 2007; Yoeli-Tlalim 2013, 2021; Blezer 2019.
51. See discussion in Garrett 2007a; Czaja 2019; McGrath 2020a.
52. See McGrath 2017: 297–304.
53. The textual history of the *Four Tantras* is discussed in detail in Fenner 1996; Schaeffer 2003b; Yang 2010, 2014; Gyatso 2015; McGrath 2020a.

54. Erhard 2007. A modern version of this system is being promoted by Nida Chenagtsang {2: 12}.
55. Kilty 2010: 206–8.
56. Kilty 2010: 193–205. See discussion in Yang 2019.
57. McGrath 2017.
58. See discussion in Schaeffer 2003b; Gyatso 2015: 81–139; Van Vleet 2015: 100–203.
59. Czaja 2007; Gyatso 2014. See reproductions of *thangkas* with translations of textual content in Parfionovitch, Dorje, and Meyer 1992; Williamson and Young 2009.
60. Kilty 2010.
61. See, e.g., Martin 2003; Schaeffer 2003b; Czaja 2005–2006; Garrett 2007a; Gyatso 2014, 2015; McGrath 2017.
62. Gyatso 2015.
63. Further connections between medicine and Tantric practice are discussed in various chapters in McGrath 2019. For the contemporary context, see discussion in chapter 9.
64. Wallace 2012.
65. Mueller-Dietz 1996.
66. See, e.g., the Digital Library of Northern Thai Manuscripts, available at http://lannamanuscripts.net/en, accessed August 10, 2021, and the list of digitized Thai, Lao and Cambodian manuscripts available at http://blogs.bl.uk/asian-and-african/thai.html, accessed August 10, 2021. For a description of the manuscript recovery project, see B. D. Dipananda, "Bringing Ancient Thai Buddhist Manuscripts to the World," *BuddhistDoor Global*, April 8, 2016, https://www.buddhistdoor.net/features/bringing-ancient-thai-buddhist-manuscripts-to-the-world.
67. Blackburn 2001: 58.
68. Translated in Liyanaratne 2002–2009. Various aspects of the history of Sri Lankan Buddhism and medicine are discussed in Liyanaratne 1999.
69. See also Chhem 2004.
70. The artifacts and texts produced at Wat Phra Chetuphon are discussed in Nivat 1933; Griswold 1965; Mulholland 1987: 7–19; summarized in Salguero 2016: 10–17.
71. Nivat 1933.
72. See summary in Salguero 2016: 3–17.
73. For non-Buddhist systems of medicine in a remoter part of Thailand, see also Brun and Schumacher 1994.
74. See Salguero 2016: 101–2.
75. Salguero 2016: 10–16, 53–64.

## 8. MODERNIZATIONS

1. The Japanese historian Naitō Torajirō, for example, famously argued that the Song dynasty (960–1279) marked the beginning of the modern period in China (discussion in Miyakawa 1955). Most other historians have preferred to limit use of the term to much later periods. Such distinctions are also relevant to the argument in Gyatso 2015.
2. Elman 2007; Asen 2009; Puente-Ballesteros 2011.
3. Barnes 2005.
4. On exorcism and ritual healing in Sri Lanka, see Wirz 1954; Yalman 1964; Obeyesekere 1969, 1970; Kapferer 1991; Carbine 2000.

5. Jardine 1893: 166–74. The quote comes from p. 173.
6. Macdonald 1879: iii–iv.
7. For example, on China, see Taylor 1887; on India, see Winternitz 1898.
8. It is helpful to distinguish between "push" and "pull" models of modernization, the former suggesting that modernity is imposed on a society by external forces such as colonialism, and the latter prioritizing the agency of internal actors (see Ritzinger 2017: 7–11). I am suggesting that a combination of push and pull forces was at play in the modernization of Buddhist medicine.
9. See Streicher and Hermann 2019.
10. Josephson-Storm 2017.
11. Josephson 2012; Schrimpf 2019: 62–64.
12. Liu 2009; Duoer 2019: 5–6; Flowers 2021.
13. Laohavanich 2012; Crosby 2013, especially 120–25.
14. Lord 1969; Popp 1985.
15. See also Hofbauer 1943.
16. See discussion in Puaksom 2007; Muksong and Chuengsatiansup 2011; Crosby 2013: 18–45.
17. The first vaccine, for the smallpox virus, was developed in 1796. For a Buddhist text on smallpox inoculation, the prevailing preventive therapy before vaccination was widely available, see {2: 4}.
18. To quote just one statistic from this period, historical data from the U.S. census show that the rate of infant mortality for white children in the United States fell from 216.8 per 1,000 in 1850 to 26.8 per 1,000 in 1950 (Haines 2008).
19. Josephson-Storm 2017.
20. See also Johnston 2016; Norov 2019.
21. Lopez 2008; Hammerstrom 2014, 2015.
22. See also Hammerstrom 2015: 96.
23. On this term, see McMahan 2008.
24. Lopez 2012; McMahan 2008: 89–116. For an introduction to the Orientalists, see Lopez 2013; App 2015.
25. Some contemporary attempts to purify Buddhism from magic and superstition can be seen in Flanagan 2011, 2012; "Superstition Has No Place in Buddhism," *Nation Thailand*, January 13, 2016, https://www.nationthailand.com/opinion/30276824. See also discussion in McMahan 2017; Schrimpf 2019.
26. Some exceptions are noted in Sharf 2015.
27. Jordt 2007; Braun 2013.
28. See, e.g., Jaffe 2015: 1–10.
29. Wu 2012.
30. See also Chilson 2018.
31. Harrington 2008; Singleton 2010; Hickey 2019.
32. Wilson 2014: 23–31; Hickey 2019: 100–36; Helderman 2019.
33. On the role of celebrity in popularizing Buddhism in the West, see Cusack 2011.
34. See Wilson 2014, especially 31–41.
35. See discussion of Goenka in Stuart 2017, 2020.
36. Mahasī 2009.

37. Previous studies conducted on Transcendental Meditation for the most part never gained wide acceptance as reliable scientific research.
38. Search conducted on May 16, 2020: http://www.ncbi.nlm.nih.gov/pmc/?term=mindfulness.
39. See, e.g., the broad meta-analyses in de Vibe et al. 2012; Goyal et al. 2014; Goldberg et al. 2018. See review of previous research in Weaver, Vane, and Flannelly 2008.
40. See, e.g., Fox et al. 2014; Goleman and Davidson 2017.
41. Connor and Samuel 2001.
42. Josephson-Storm 2017.
43. See, e.g., Leslie 1999: 341–67; Monnais, Thompson, and Wahlberg 2012; Andrews 2015.
44. Van Vleet 2015: 260–335.
45. Taylor 2005.
46. Chan 2010.
47. Zhang and Unschuld 2008.
48. See, e.g., Duoer 2019; Coderey 2020.
49. World Health Organization 2008.
50. World Health Organization, "Declaration of Alma-Ata," *World Health Organization Publications*, September 1978, http://www.who.int/publications/almaata_declaration_en.pdf.
51. A summary of medical revival in Thailand is available in Iida 2017.
52. Gosling 1985.
53. Josephson 2012: 134.
54. Messner et al. 2018: 9. See also Schrimpf 2019: 65–66.
55. Fries 2005: 801.
56. See, e.g., discussion in Hickey 2019: 187–218.

## 9. CONTEMPORARY BUDDHIST MEDICINE

1. Highlights in the scholarship on Buddhist healing practices in the late twentieth and early twenty-first centuries not mentioned elsewhere include the following: For Central Asia, the Tibetan Plateau, and Nepal, see Stablein 1973, 1976b; Dietrich 1996; Samuel 1999; Gellner 2001: 221–50; Deck 2002; Litis 2002; Vargas-O'Bryan 2011; Ramble and Roesler 2015; Schrempf and Schneider 2015. For Southeast Asia, see Salgado 1997; Carbine 2000; Souk-Aloum 2001; Tomecko 2009; Chamchoy 2013; Salemink 2015; Elliott 2021. For East Asia, see Arai 2003; Zhao 2016.
2. Chokevivat and Chuthaputti 2005; Wibulbolprasert 2005; Chokevivat, Chuthaputti, and Khumtrakul 2005. For scholarly work advocating turning to Thai Buddhism for insights and resources related to present-day health-care issues, see, e.g., Ratanakul 1999b; Paonil and Sringernyuang 2002; Mettanando 2007.
3. Mulholland 1979; Ratarasarn 1989; Salguero 2016: 41–50.
4. Details of these practices are given in Saowapa 2010; Kitiarsa 2012; Chamchoy 2013; Conway 2014; Salguero 2016: 65–88.
5. See, e.g., Salguero 2017.
6. Coderey 2019, 2020.
7. See also Pranke 1995; Coderey 2012, 2019; Rozenburg 2012; Brac de la Perriere, Rozenberg, and Turner 2014; Rozenberg and Tanabe 2015; Cooler 2016; Patton 2016, 2018.

8. Similar healers in Cambodia are described in Eisenbruch 1992; Bertrand 2005; Ovesen and Trankell 2010: 129–68.
9. Cantwell 1995; Samuel 2001; Pordié 2003, 2007; Kloos 2010, 2016; Gerke 2012, 2017a; Deane 2014a, 2014b, 2019a, 2019b; Blaikie 2016, 2019; Sodargye and Yü 2017.
10. Official website of the Men-Tsee-Khang Tibetan Medical and Astro-science Institute, http://www.men-tsee-khang.org, accessed June 26, 2020.
11. McKay and Wangchuk 2005; Wangchuk, Wangchuk, and Aagaard-Hansen 2007.
12. Wangmo and Valk 2012.
13. "Spirituality and Wellness," *Bhutan Travel*, http://www.tourism.gov.bt/activities/spirituality-wellness, accessed June 26, 2020.
14. Mike Ives, "China and India File Rival Claims Over Tibetan Medicine," *New York Times*, July 27, 2017, http://www.nytimes.com/2017/07/27/world/asia/unesco-tibetan-medicine-india-china.html.
15. "The Asian Context," *Ratimed*, http://www.ratimed.net/field/, accessed March 10, 2020.
16. Dietrich 1996; Wallace 2012; Chudakova 2017, 2021.
17. Janes 2002; Sulek 2006; Kloos et al. 2020. The Ratimed Project (http://www.ratimed.net, accessed August 10, 2021), headed by Stephan Kloos, is an important source of information on the globalization of Sowa Rigpa.
18. Huang 2009, 2017; Jones 2009; Yao 2012; Gombrich and Yao 2013.
19. For a summary of Tzu Chi's disaster relief efforts, see "Tzu Chi," *Wikipedia*. http://en.wikipedia.org/wiki/Tzu_Chi, accessed August 10, 2021. A sense of the organization's involvement in medicine can also be gained from its journal, *Tzu Chi Medical Care*, and other organizational publications. As of March 2019, the Tzu Chi International Medical Association claimed to have completed 13,940 "medical outreaches," mobilized 267,567 medical professionals and 487,557 supporting volunteers, and helped 2.8 million people in more than fifty countries (personal email from organization spokesperson, March 2, 2019).
20. While the sentiment is generalizable, this quote comes from an ethnographic interview I conducted at Tzu Chi's Los Angeles center in 2015. Similar perspectives are explored in Huang 2017.
21. For a history of Japanese monastic involvement with death in Japan, see Stone 2016, especially pp. 272–76.
22. Samuels 2016; Kasai 2016; Benedict 2018; Schrimpf 2019.
23. Wallace 2003; López 2008; Goleman and Davidson 2017; McMahan and Braun 2017.
24. David Gelles, "The Hidden Price of Mindfulness Inc.," *New York Times*, March 19, 2016, http://www.nytimes.com/2016/03/20/opinion/sunday/the-hidden-price-of-mindfulness-inc.html.
25. See, e.g., Chaoul 2007; Bushell 2009; Ozawa-de Silva et al. 2012.
26. See, e.g., Agger 2015; Myers, Lewis, and Dutton 2015. Influence going in the other direction—i.e., the incorporation of psychoanalytic developmental theory and neuroscience into Buddhist teachings—is discussed in Gleig 2016.
27. On June 2, 2021, a Google search for "mindfulness -Buddhist" returned 228 million results, while a search for "mindfulness AND Buddhist" returned only 26.7 million. Searching for "mindfulness AND Buddha" or "mindfulness AND Buddhism" gave even fewer results.
28. Foundation for a Mindful Society: https://www.mindfulsociety.org/, accessed August 10, 2021.

29. The Mindfulness Initiative: https://www.themindfulnessinitiative.org/, accessed August 10, 2021.
30. Mindfulness in Schools Project: http://mindfulnessinschools.org, accessed August 10, 2021.
31. See also Cook 2016, 2018.
32. Grant Hindsley, "The Latest in Military Strategy: Mindfulness," *New York Times*, April 5, 2019, https://www.nytimes.com/2019/04/05/health/military-mindfulness-training.html.
33. In addition to the sources cited in the next few paragraphs, a range of critiques and perspectives are introduced in Williams and Kabat-Zin 2011; Eifring 2015; Purser, Forbes, and Burke 2016. See also Pierce Salguero, "A Roundup of Critical Perspectives on Meditation," *Patheos*, May 11, 2017, http://www.patheos.com/blogs/americanbuddhist/2017/05/a-roundup-of-critical-perspectives-on-meditation.html.
34. Stanley 2012; Monteiro, Musten, and Compson 2015; Samuel 2015; Toneatto 2018; Cheung 2017, 2018.
35. This argument seems to have first been formulated in Žižek 2001 but is now widely associated with Ron Purser (see, e.g., Purser 2019). See also related critiques in Hickey 2019: 187–218 and a response from a Buddhist monastic in Anālayo 2020.
36. Compson 2014; Hanley et al. 2016; Britton 2019.
37. Brown 2013, 2019.
38. Kabat-Zinn 2011: 281. I have capitalized "Dharma" in the quote to match this book's usage.
39. Such issues are raised many times in {2} and are also explored in Schrempf 2007; Adams, Schrempf, and Craig 2011; Gerke 2012; McMahan and Braun 2017; Sodargye and Yü 2017; Taee 2017.
40. See, e.g., Wu 2002; Numrich 2005.
41. This comment is based on a story told to me during an interview with a monk at the Tonghwasa Temple in South Korea in 2013.
42. This is not the place to enter into larger theoretical questions concerning the globalization of Buddhism. For insightful discussion of some these issues, see e.g., Obadia 2015; Starkey and Coward-Gibbs 2018; Kellner 2019; and Gleig 2019, particularly her conclusion.
43. Alter 2005.
44. See discussion in Salguero 2016.
45. See Noree, Hanefeld, and Smith 2016.
46. Wat Pho: http://www.watpho.com, accessed August 10, 2021.
47. As an indication of its current popularity, a Google search for "Thai massage in Chiang Mai" conducted May 10, 2021, returned 5.5 million results.
48. See Kogiso 2012; Iida 2013.
49. This comment is based on my many years of involvement with Thai massage education in North America.
50. While scholars have debated whether to consider Won Buddhism a form of Buddhism or a New Religion (Pye 2002; Baker 2012), the Won Buddhist leaders and members I have extensively interviewed in both Iksan and Philadelphia consider themselves adherents of a modern, reformed Buddhist order. For this reason, I unhesitatingly include Won in my studies of Buddhist medicine. On Won Buddhism more generally, see Chung 2003.

51. For ethnographic data on many types of mindfulness in Thailand, Myanmar, and Sri Lanka, see, e.g., Cassaniti 2018.
52. See, e.g., Kim 2016. These kinds of adaptation are described in Joo 2011. Similar dynamics are afoot in China; see Lau 2017, 2021.
53. Salguero 2020b.
54. Won Institute of Graduate Studies: http://www.woninstitute.edu, accessed August 10, 2021.
55. For further information, see C. Pierce Salguero and research students, "Won Buddhism in Philadelphia," January 2, 2021, *Jivaka Project*, http://www.jivaka.net/philadelphia/won-buddhism.
56. Such issues are discussed in Salguero 2019: 18–19.
57. On the diversity of Buddhist healing practices in Philadelphia, see Salguero 2019 and the Jivaka Project: http://www.jivaka.net/philly, accessed August 10, 2021.
58. See also Joffe 2019: 372–428.
59. A Google search for "Dalai Lama" retrieved more than 47 million results. For comparison, a search for "Nida Chenagtsang" retrieved less than fifty-four thousand. Few other Asian health and spirituality celebrities have an online presence as large as the Dalai Lama, although Deepak Chopra has 38.5 million Google hits and Andrew Weil has 25.4 million (all searches conducted on January 13, 2020). A biography of the Dalai Lama is available in Powers 2016c.
60. His longtime enthusiasm for science is highlighted in Dawn Engle's 2019 film *The Dalai Lama: Scientist* (PeaceJam Productions).
61. Searches conducted January 13, 2020.

## CONCLUSION

1. A version of the content of this section appeared on *Buddhistdoor Global* on August 20, 2020: https://www.buddhistdoor.net/features/buddhist-responses-to-the-covid-19-pandemic-in-historical-perspective.
2. For a collection of materials on Buddhist responses to the COVID-19 pandemic, see "Buddhism in Pandemic," *Jivaka Project*, http://www.jivaka.net/pandemic/, accessed August 10, 2021.
3. "Flatten the Curve with Tzu Chi USA," press release, *Tzu Chi USA*, April 7, 2020. http://tzuchi.us/blog/flatten-the-curve-press-release, accessed August 10, 2021.
4. Tzu Chi Foundation: http://tw.tzuchi.org/en, accessed August 20, 2020.
5. Soka Gakkai: http://www.sgi.org/in-focus/press-releases/response-to-covid-19-pandemic.html, accessed August 20, 2020.
6. World Peace Initiative Foundation, "Meditate Against COVID 19," YouTube video, 2:16. Posted April 3, 2020. http://www.youtube.com/watch?v=TWMrgrhbhOk, accessed August 10, 2021.
7. Dalai Lama, "'Prayer Is Not Enough.' The Dalai Lama on Why We Need to Fight Coronavirus With Compassion," *Time*, April 14, 2020, https://time.com/5820613/dalai-lama-coronavirus-compassion/. See also "A Special Message from His Holiness the Dalai Lama," *DalaiLama.com*, March 30, 2020. http://www.dalailama.com/news/2020/a-special-message-from-his-holiness-the-dalai-lama.

8. "Chanting Tara Mantra Helpful in Containing the Spread of Epidemics Like Coronavirus: His Holiness the Dalai Lama to Chinese Devotees," *Central Tibetan Administration*, January 28, 2020, http://tibet.net/chanting-dolma-mantra-helpful-in-containing-the-spread-of-epidemics-like-coronavirus-his-holiness-the-dalai-lama-to-chinese-devotees.
9. Erik Jampa Andersson, "Tibetan Medicine and Covid-19," *Shrīmālā*, March 11, 2020, http://www.shrimala.com/post/tibetan-medicine-and-covid-19; Carolyn Chan, "Tibetan Medicine and the Coronavirus," *Tibetan Medicine Education Center*, March 2020, http://www.tibetanmedicine-edu.org/n-articles/tibetan-medicine-and-the-coronavirus, accessed August 10, 2021; "Lama Zopa Rinpoche Offers Advice to Protect from the Coronavirus," *Foundation for the Preservation of the Mahayana Tradition*, January 25, 2020, http://fpmt.org/lama-zopa-rinpoche-news-and-advice/advice-from-lama-zopa-rinpoche/lama-zopa-rinpoche-offers-advice-to-protect-from-the-coronavirus.
10. E.g., "Coronavirus: City of Ten Thousand Buddhas in Mendocino County Donates Medical Supplies to Hospitals," *Ukiah Daily Journal*, April 30, 2020, http://www.ukiahdailyjournal.com/2020/04/30/coronavirus-city-of-ten-thousand-buddhas-in-mendocino-county-donates-medical-supplies-to-hospitals.
11. "Thai Buddhist Monks Give Lucky Charms to Devotees to Protect Them from Covid-19," *Yahoo!tv*, April 30, 2020, https://au.tv.yahoo.com/autv-viral/thai-buddhist-monks-lucky-charms-090000110.html.
12. Levi McLaughlin, "Japanese Religious Responses to COVID-19: A Preliminary Report," *Asia-Pacific Journal: Japan Focus*, May 1, 2020, http://apjjf.org/2020/9/McLaughlin.html.
13. "Blessings from the Sky! Sri Lanka Fights Coronavirus with Buddhist Holy Water Sprinkled from Helicopters," *News 18*, March 27, 2020, http://www.news18.com/news/world/blessings-from-the-sky-sri-lanka-fights-coronavirus-with-buddhist-holy-water-sprinkled-from-helicopters-2554127.html.
14. "Governor Whitmer and Headspace Launch 'Stay Home, Stay Mindful' website to Offer Free Mental Health Resources During COVID-19 Pandemic," press release, Office of Governor Gretchen Whitmer, April 17, 2020, http://www.michigan.gov/whitmer/0,9309,7-387-90487-526216--,00.html.
15. Pierce Salguero, "How Do Buddhists Handle Coronavirus? The Answer Is Not Just Meditation," *The Conversation*, May 15, 2020, http://theconversation.com/how-do-buddhists-handle-coronavirus-the-answer-is-not-just-meditation-137966.
16. See also Kloos 2019; Craig, Gerke, and Sheldon 2020.

# *References*

## ABBREVIATIONS

| | |
|---|---|
| {1} | Salguero, C. Pierce, ed. 2017. *Buddhism and Medicine: An Anthology of Premodern Sources*. New York: Columbia University Press |
| {2} | Salguero, C. Pierce, ed. 2019. *Buddhism and Medicine: An Anthology of Modern and Contemporary Sources*. New York: Columbia University Press |
| AN | *Aṅguttara Nikāya*. Translated in Bodhi 1999 and at http://www.accesstoinsight.org |
| *Asian Medicine* | *Asian Medicine: Traditional and Modernity* (2005–2016) or *Asian Medicine: Journal of the International Association for the Study of Traditional Asian Medicine* (2016–present) |
| *BEFEO* | *Bulletin de l'École française d'Extrême-Orient* |
| *BSOAS* | *Bulletin of the School of Oriental and African Studies* |
| *Budd St Rev* | *Buddhist Studies Review* |
| DN | *Dīgha Nikāya*. Translated in Walsche 1995 |
| *EASTM* | *East Asian Science, Technology, and Medicine* |
| *Hist Sci SA* | *History of Science in South Asia* |
| *HJAS* | *Harvard Journal of Asian Studies* |
| *J Budd Eth* | *Journal of Buddhist Ethics* |
| *J Burma St* | *Journal of Burma Studies* |
| *J Glo Budd* | *Journal of Global Buddhism* |
| *J Ind Phil* | *Journal of Indian Philosophy* |
| *J Jap Rel St* | *Japanese Journal of Religious Studies* |
| *JAAR* | *Journal of the American Academy of Religion* |
| *JAOS* | *Journal of the American Oriental Society* |
| *JCBS* | *Journal of Chinese Buddhist Studies* |
| *JIABS* | *Journal of the International Association for Buddhist Studies* |
| *Kailash* | *Kailash: Journal of Himalayan Studies* |
| MN | *Majjhima Nikāya*. Translated in Ñanamoli and Bodhi 1995 and at http://www.accesstoinsight.org |

| | |
|---|---|
| *Oxford Biblio* | Payne, Richard K., ed. *Oxford Bibliographies Online: Buddhism.* Available at http://www.oxfordbibliographies.com |
| *Pacific World* | *Pacific World: Journal of the Institute of Buddhist Studies* |
| SN | *Saṃyutta Nikāya.* Translated in Bodhi 2000 and at http://www.accesstoinsight.org. |
| T | *Taishō Tripitaka.* Takakusu & Watanabe 1924–1935 |

## SOURCES


Abe, Ryuichi. 1999. *The Weaving of Mantra: Kūkai and the Construction of Esoteric Buddhist Discourse.* New York: Columbia University Press.

Abu-Lughod, Janet L. 1989. *Before European Hegemony: The World System A.D. 1250–1350.* New York: Oxford University Press.

Acri, Andrea, ed. 2016. *Esoteric Buddhism in Mediaeval Maritime Asia.* Singapore: ISEAS.

Adams, Vincanne, and Dashima Dovchin. 2000. "Women's Health in Tibetan Medicine and Tibet's 'First' Female Doctor." In *Women's Buddhism, Buddhism's Women: Tradition, Revision, Renewal,* ed E. B. Findly, 433–50. Boston: Wisdom.

Adams, Vincanne, Mona Schrempf, and Sienna R. Craig, eds. 2011. *Medicine Between Science and Religion: Explorations on Tibetan Grounds.* New York: Berghahn.

Adshead, Samuel Adrian M. 2000. *China in World History,* 3rd ed. New York: Palgrave Macmillan.

Aggacitta, Bhikkhu (trans.). 1984 [1976]. *Dhamma Therapy: Cases of Healing Through Vipassanā.* Unique: Penang.

Agger, Inger. 2015. "Calming the Mind: Healing After Mass Atrocity in Cambodia." *Transcultural Psychiatry* 52 (4): 543–60.

Ahn, Jun. 2007. "Malady of Meditation: A Prolegomenon to the Study of Illness and Zen." PhD dissertation. University of California, Berkeley.

Akasoy, Anna, Charles Burnett, and Ronit Yoeli-Tlalim, eds. 2008. *Astro-Medicine: Astrology and Medicine, East and West.* Florence, Italy: Sismel Edzioni del Galluzzo.

—, eds. 2013. *Rashīd al-Dīn: Agent and Mediator of Cultural Exchanges in Ilkhanid Iran.* London: Warburg Institute.

—, eds. 2016 [2011]. *Islam and Tibet: Interactions Along the Musk Routes.* Abingdon: Routledge.

Akasoy, Anna, and Ronit Yoeli-Tlalim. 2007. "Along the Musk Routes: Exchanges Between Tibet and the Islamic World." *Asian Medicine* 3 (2): 217–40.

Alter, Joseph. 2005. *Asian Medicine and Globalization.* Philadelphia: University of Pennsylvania Press.

—. 2009. "Yoga in Asia—Mimetic History: Problems in the Location of Secret Knowledge." *Comparative Studies of South Asia, Africa and the Middle East* 29 (2): 213–29.

Anālayo. 2015. "Healing in Early Buddhism." *Budd St Rev* 32 (1): 19–33.

—. 2016. *Mindfully Facing Disease and Death: Compassionate Advice from Early Buddhist Texts.* Cambridge: Windhorse.

Anālayo, Bhikkhu. 2020. "The Myth of McMindfulness." *Mindfulness* 11: 472–79.

Andreeva, Anna. 2014. "Childbirth in Aristocratic Households in Heian Japan." *Dynamis* 34 (2): 357–76.

—. 2015. "Chūsei Nihon ni okeru osan to josei no kenkō—Sanshō Ruijūshō no bukkyōteki, igakuteki chisiki wo chūshin to shite." In *Hikaku shisō kara mita Nihon bukkyō,* ed. Sueki Fumihiko, 13–36. Tokyo: Sankibō busshōrinkan.

—. 2016. "Embryology in Buddhist Thought." *Oxford Biblio.* https://doi.org/10.1093/OBO/9780195393521-0228.

—. 2017a. "Explaining Conception to Women? Buddhist Embryological Knowledge in the *Sanshō ruijūshō* (*Encyclopedia of Childbirth*, ca. 1318)." *Asian Medicine* 12: 170–202.

—. 2017b. "Childbirth in Early Medieval Japan: Ritual Economies and Medical Emergencies in Procedures During the Day of the Royal Consort's Labor." In {1}, 336–50.

—. 2018a. "Devising the Esoteric Rituals for Women: Fertility and the Demon Mother in the *Gushi nintai sanshō himitsu hōshū*." In *Women, Rites, and Ritual Objects in Premodern Japan*, ed. Karen Gerhart, 53–88. Leiden: Brill.

—. 2018b. "Buddhism and Medicine in Japan." *Oxford Biblio.* https://doi.org/10.1093/obo/9780195393521-0255.

—. 2019a. "Childbirth and the 'Arts of Judgment' in Medieval Japan." In preprint no. 496, *Accounting for Uncertainty: Prediction and Planning in Asia's History*, ed. Dagmar Schäfer, Zhao Lu, and Michael Lackner, 27–41. Berlin: Max Planck Institute for the History of Science.

—. 2019b. "Empowering the Pregnancy Sash in Medieval Japan." In Salguero and Macomber 2020: 160–93.

Andreeva, Anna, and Dominic Steavu. 2015. *Transforming the Void: Embryological Discourse and Reproductive Imagery in East Asian Religions*. Leiden: Brill.

Andrews, Bridie. 2015. *The Making of Modern Chinese Medicine, 1850–1960*. Honolulu: University of Hawai'i Press.

App, Urs. 2015. *Birth of Orientalism*. Philadelphia: University of Pennsylvania Press.

Arai, Paula. 2003. "The Dead as 'Personal Buddhas': Japanese Ancestral Rites as Healing Rites." *Pacific World* 5: 3–17.

—. 2014. "Healing Zen: The Brain on Bowing." In *Disease, Religion and Healing in Asia: Collaborations and Collisions*, ed. Ivette Vargas-O'Bryan and Zhou Xun, 155–69. New York: Routledge.

Arnold, Edward A. 2009. *As Long as Space Endures: Essays on the Kālacakra Tantra in Honor of H. H. the Dalai Lama*. Ithaca, N.Y.: Snow Lion.

Asen, Daniel. 2009. "'Manchu Anatomy': Anatomical Knowledge and the Jesuits in Seventeenth- and Eighteenth-Century China." *Social History of Medicine* 22 (1): 23–44.

Bagchi, Prabodh Chandra. 1941. "New Materials for the Study of the Kumāratantra." *Indian Culture* 7 (3): 269–86.

—. 2011 [1942–43]. "A Fragment of the Kāśyapa-saṁhitā in Chinese." In *India and China: A Collection of Essays by Professor Prabodh Chandra Bagchi*, ed. Bangwei Wang and Tansen Sen, 75–85. London, New York, Delhi: Anthem.

Baker, Donald. 1994. "Monks, Medicine, and Miracles: Health and Healing in the History of Korean Buddhism." *Korean Studies* 18: 50–75.

Baker, Ian. 2017. "Yoga and Physical Culture in Vajrayāna Buddhism and Dzogchen, with special reference to Tertön Pema Lingpa's 'Secret Key to the Winds and Channels.'" In *Mandala of 21st Century Perspectives: Proceedings of the International Conference on Tradition and Innovation in Vajrayana Buddhism*, ed. Dasho Karma Ura, Dorji Penjore, and Chhimi Dem, 54–101. Thimphu: Centre for Bhutan Studies.

—. 2019. *Tibetan Yoga: Principles and Practices*. Rochester, Vt.: Inner Traditions.

Baker, Ian A. 2012. "Embodying Enlightenment: Physical Culture in Dzogchen as Revealed in Tibet's Lukhang Murals."*Asian Medicine* 7 (1): 225–64.

Bangdel, Dina, and John C. Huntington. 2003. *The Circle of Bliss: Buddhist Meditational Art*. Chicago: Serindia.

Bapat, P. V., and A. Hirakawa. 1970. *Shan-chien-p'i-p'o-sha: A Chinese Version by Sanghabhadra of Samantapāsādikā, Commentary on Pali Vinaya*. Poona: Bhandarkar Oriental Research Institute.

Bareau, André. 2013 [1955]. *The Buddhist Schools of the Small Vehicle*. Honolulu: University of Hawai'i Press.

Barnes, Linda L. 2005. *Needles, Herbs, Gods and Ghosts: China, Healing and the West to 1848*. Cambridge, Mass., and London: Harvard University Press.

Barrett, T. H. 2009. "The Advent of the Buddhist Conception of Religion in China and Its Consequences for the Analysis of Daoism." *Sungkyun Journal of East Asian Studies* 9 (2): 149–65.

Barstow, Geoffrey, ed. 2019. *The Faults of Meat: Tibetan Buddhist Writings on Vegetarianism*. Somerville, Mass.: Wisdom.

Batchelor, Martine. 2000. "Tokwang Sunim: A Korean Nun as Medical Practitioner." In *Women's Buddhism, Buddhism's Women: Tradition, Revision, Renewal*, ed. Ellison Banks Findly, 403–4. Boston: Wisdom.

Bechert, Heinz, ed. 1991–1997. *Die Datierung des historischen Buddha* [*The Dating of the Historical Buddha*]. 3 vols. Göttingen, Germany: Vandenhoeck & Ruprecht.

—. 1995. "Introductory Essay: The Dates of the Historical Buddha—A Controversial Issue." In *When Did the Buddha Live? The Controversy on the Dating of the Historical Buddha*, ed. Heinz Bechert, 11–36. Delhi: Sri Satguru.

Beckwith, Christopher I. 1979. "The Introduction of Greek Medicine into Tibet in the Seventh and Eighth Centuries." *JAOS* 99: 297–313.

—. 2011. *Empires of the Silk Road: A History of Central Eurasia from Bronze Age to the Present*. Princeton, N.J.: Princeton University Press.

Behl, Benoy K. 2014. *Northern Frontiers of Buddhism: Buddhist Heritage of Afghanistan, Uzbekistan, Kalmykia, Tibet, China, Mongolia and Siberia*. Delhi: Motilal Banarsidass.

Benedict, Timothy O. 2018. "Practicing Spiritual Care in the Japanese Hospice." *J Jap Rel St* 45 (1): 175–99.

Benn, James A. 2015. *Tea in China: A Religious and Cultural History*. Honolulu: University of Hawai'i Press.

Bertrand, Didier. 2005. "The Therapeutic Role of Khmer Mediums (*kru borameï*) in Contemporary Cambodia." *Mental Health, Religion & Culture* 8 (4): 309–27.

Beyer, Stephan. 1973. *The Cult of Tara: Magic and Ritual in Tibet*. Berkeley: University of California Press.

Bhattacarya, D. C. 1972. "The Five Protective Goddesses of Buddhism." In *Aspects of Indian Art: Papers Presented in a Symposium at the Los Angeles County Museum of Art, October 1970*, ed. Pratapaditya Pal, 85–92. Leiden: Brill.

Bielenstein, Hans. 2005. *Diplomacy and Trade in the Chinese World, 589–1276*. Leiden: Brill.

Biernacki, Richard, and Victoria E. Bonnell. 2008. *Beyond the Cultural Turn: New Directions in the Study of Society and Culture*. Berkeley: University of California Press.

Birch, Jason. 2011. "The Meaning of *Haṭha* in Early Haṭhayoga." *JAOS* 131 (4): 527–54.

Bird, Chloe E., Peter Conrad, Allen M. Fremont, and Stefan Timmermans. 2010. *Handbook of Medical Sociology*, 6th ed. Nashville, Tenn.: Vanderbilt University Press.

Birnbaum, Raoul. 1989a. *The Healing Buddha*. Revised ed. Boulder, Colo.: Shambhala.

—. 1989b. "Chinese Buddhist Traditions of Healing and the Life Cycle." In *Healing and Restoring: Health and Medicine in the World's Religious Traditions*, ed. Lawrence E. Sullivan, 33-57. New York: Macmillan.

—. 2016. "When Is a 'Chinese Landscape Painting' Also a 'Chinese Buddhist Painting'? Approaches to the Works of Kuncan (1612–1673) and Other Enigmas." In *17th-Century Chinese Paintings from the Tsao Family Collection*, ed. Stephen Little, 94–129. Los Angeles: Los Angeles County Museum of Art.

—. 2017. "Two Turns in the Life of Master Hongyi, a Buddhist Monk in Twentieth-Century China." In *The Making of Saints in Modern China*, ed. David Ownby, Vincent Goossaert, and Ji Zhe, 161–208. New York: Oxford University Press.

Bizot, François. 1981. "Notes sur les yantra bouddhiques d'Indochine." In *Tantric and Taoist Studies in Honour of R. A. Stein*, ed. Michel Strickmann, 155–91. Brussels: Institut belge des Hautes Études chinoises.

Blackburn, Anne M. 2001. *Buddhist Learning and Textual Practice in Eighteenth-Century Lankan Monastic Culture*. Princeton, N.J.: Princeton University Press.

Blaikie, Calum. 2016. "Positioning Sowa Rigpa in India: Coalition and Antagonism in the Quest for Recognition." *Medicine Anthropology Theory* 3 (2): 50–86.

—Blaikie, Calum. 2019. "Traditional Medicine and Primary Healthcare in Himalayan India." *Asian Medicine* 14 (1): 145–72.

Blezer, Henk. 2019. "A New Sense of (Dark) Humor in Tibet: Brown Phlegm and Black Bile." In McGrath 2019, 3–58.

Blum, Mark, ed., trans. 2013. *The Nirvana Sutra (Mahāparinirvāṇa-sūtra)*, vol. 1. Berkeley, Calif.: BDK America.

Bodhi, Bhikkhu. 1999. *The Numerical Discourses of the Buddha: A Translation of the Aṅguttara Nikāya*. Boston: Wisdom.

—. 2000. *The Connected Discourses of the Buddha: A Translation of the Samyutta Nikāya*. Boston: Wisdom.

Boisvert, Mathieu. 2000. "Conception and Intrauterine Life in the Pāli Canon." *Studies in Religion/Sciences Religieuses* 29 (3): 301–11.

Boucher, Daniel. 2008. *Bodhisattvas of the Forest and the Formation of the Mahāyāna: A Study and Translation of the Rāṣṭrapālaparipṛcchā-sūtra*. Honolulu: University of Hawai'i Press.

Bowie, Fiona. 2005. *The Anthropology of Religion: An Introduction*. Malden, Mass.: Blackwell.

Brac de la Perrière, Bénédicte, Guillaume Rozenberg, and Alicia Marie Turner. 2014. *Champions of Buddhism: Weikza Cults in Contemporary Burma*. Singapore: National University of Singapore Press.

Bragazzi, Nicola Luigi, Lorenzo Ballico, and Giovanni Del Puente. 2019. "Mental Health Among Italian Nichiren Buddhists: Insights from a Cross-Sectional Exploratory Study." *Religions* 10 (5): 316.

Braun, Eric. 2013. *The Birth of Insight: Meditation, Modern Buddhism, and the Burmese Monk Ledi Sayadaw*. Chicago: University of Chicago.

Britton, Willoughby B. 2019. "Can Mindfulness Be Too Much of a Good Thing? The Value of a Middle Way." *Current Opinion in Psychology* 28: 159–165.

Bronkhorst, Johannes. 2007. *Greater Magadha: Studies in the Culture of Early India*. Leiden: Brill.

Brown, Candy Gunther. 2013. *The Healing Gods: Complementary and Alternative Medicine in Christian America*. New York: Oxford University Press.

—. 2019. *Debating Yoga and Mindfulness in Public Schools: Reforming Secular Education or Reestablishing Religion?* Chapel Hill: University of North Carolina Press.
Brown, Kirk Warren, J. David Creswell, and Richard M. Ryan, eds. 2015. *Handbook of Mindfulness: Theory, Research, and Practice*. New York: Guilford.
Brun, Viggo, and Trond Schumacher. 1994 [1987]. *Traditional Herbal Medicine in Northern Thailand*. Bangkok: White Lotus.
Brun, Viggo, Trond Schumacher, and Terje Bjørnland. 1994. *Traditional Herbal Medicine in Northern Thailand*. Bangkok: White Lotus.
Buckelew, Kevin. 2018. "Pregnant Metaphor: Embryology, Embodiment, and the Ends of Figurative Imagery in Chinese Buddhism." *HJAS* 78 (2): 371–411.
Buell, Paul D. 2007. "How Did Persian and Other Western Medical Knowledge Move East, and Chinese West? A Look at the Role of Rashīd Al-Dīn and Others." *Asian Medicine* 3 (2): 79–95.
Buell, Paul D., and Eugene N. Anderson. *A Soup for the Qan: Introduction, Translation, Commentary, and Chinese Text*. London: Routledge 2000.
Burke, Peter. 2005. *History and Social Theory*, 2nd ed. Ithaca, N.Y.: Cornell University Press.
Burton-Rose, Daniel. 2017. "Desiderata for the Principles of Compilation of a Canon of Buddhism and Medicine: A Consumer's Guide to the *Zhongguo Fojiao yiyao quanshu* (*Complete Works of Chinese Buddhist Medicine and Pharmacopeia*, 2011)," *Asian Medicine* 12: 203–32.
Bushell, William C. 2009. "Integrating Modern Neuroscience and Physiology with Indo-Tibetan Yogic Science." In Arnold 2009, 385–98.
Buswell, Robert E., ed. 1990. *Chinese Buddhist Apocrypha*. Honolulu: University of Hawai'i Press.
—, ed. 2004. *Encyclopedia of Buddhism*. 2 vols. New York: MacMillan.
Bynum, William F., Anne Hardy, Stephen Jacyna, Christopher Lawrence, and E. M. Tansey. 2013. *The Western Medical Tradition: 1800 to 2000*. Cambridge: Cambridge University Press.
Cabezón, José Ignacio. 2017. *Sexuality in Classical South Asian Buddhism: Studies in Indian and Tibetan Buddhism*. Sommerville, Mass.: Wisdom.
Campany, Robert Ford. 2012. *Signs from the Unseen Realm: Buddhist Miracle Tales from Early Medieval China*. Honolulu: University of Hawai'i Press.
Canton-Alvarez, Jose A. 2019. "A Gift from the Buddhist Monastery: The Role of Buddhist Medical Practices in the Assimilation of the Opium Poppy in Chinese Medicine During the Song Dynasty (960–1279)." *Medical History* 63 (4): 475–93.
Cantwell, Cathy. 1995. "The Tibetan Medical Tradition, and Tibetan Approaches to Healing in the Contemporary World." *Kailash* 17 (3/4): 157–84.
—. 2017. "Reflections on Rasāyana, Bcud Len and Related Practices in Nyingma (Rnying Ma) Tantric |Ritual." *Hist Sci SA* 5 (2): 181–203.
Capitanio, Joshua. 2013. "Health, Illness, and the Body in Buddhist and Daoist Self-Cultivation." In *Brahman and Dao: Comparative Studies of Indian and Chinese Philosophy and Religion*, ed. Ithamar Theodor and Yao Zhihua, 181–94. Lanham, Md.: Lexington.
Carbine, Jason A. 2000. "Cosmology and Healing (Sri Lanka)." In *The Life of Buddhism*, ed. Frank E. Reynolds and Jason A. Carbine. Berkeley: University of California Press.
Cassaniti, Julia. 2018. *Remembering the Present: Mindfulness in Buddhist Asia*. Ithaca, N.Y.: Cornell University Press.
Cerulli, Anthony. 2010 [revised online edition 2013]. "Āyurveda." In *Brill's Encyclopedia of Hinduism*, vol. 2, *Texts, Rituals, Arts, and Concepts*, ed. K. A. Jacobsen, H. Basu, A. Malinar, and V. Narayanan, 267–80. Leiden: Brill.

Chaithavuthi, Jan, and Kanchanoo Muangsiri. 2005. *Thai Massage the Thai Way in Theory and Practice*. Chiang Mai, Thailand: Thai Massage Book Press.

Chamchoy, Paveena. 2013. "The Efficacies of Trance-Possession Ritual Performances in Contemporary Thai Theravada Buddhism." PhD dissertation. University of Exeter. https://ore.exeter.ac.uk/repository/bitstream/handle/10871/15758/ChamchoyP_TPC.pdf?sequence=3&isAllowed=y.

Chan, Chi-Chao. 2010. Couching for Cataract in China. *History of Ophthalmology* 55.4: 393–98.

Chaoul, M. Alejandro. 2007. " 'Magical Movements' ('Phrul 'Khor) in the Bon Tradition and Possible Applications as a CIM Therapy." In Schrempf 2007: 285–304.

Chau, Ju-kua. 1911. *On the Chinese and Arab Trade in the Twelfth and Thirteenth Centuries*. Translated by Friederich Hirth and W. W. Rockhill. St. Petersburg: Imperial Academy of Sciences.

Chaudhary, Radhakrishna. 1975. *The University of Vikramaśīla*. Patna: Bihar Research Society.

Chavannes, Edouard. 1962. *Cinq cents contes et apologues: Extraits du Tripitaka chinois et traduits en français*. Paris: Libraire d'Amerique et d'Orient.

Cheah, Joseph. 2011. *Race and Religion in American Buddhism: White Supremacy and Immigrant Adaptation*. Oxford: Oxford University Press.

Chen Huaiyu. 2007. *The Revival of Buddhist Monasticism in Medieval China*. New York: Peter Lang.

Chen, Janet Y. 2014. *The Search for Modern China: A Documentary Collection*. New York: Norton.

Chen Jidong. 2017. "The Dawn of Modern Buddhism: Contacts Between Chinese and Japanese Buddhism in the Late Nineteenth Century." *Studies in Chinese Religions* 3 (1): 1–25.

Ch'en, Kenneth. 1973. *The Chinese Transformation of Buddhism*. Princeton, N.J.: Princeton University Press.

Chen Ming. 2002. *Yindu fanwen yidian 'Yili jinghua' yanjiu*. Beijing: Zhonghua shuju.

—. 2005a. *Dunhuang chutu huhua yidian 'Qipo shu' yanjiu*. Hong Kong: Xinwenfeng chuban.

—. 2005b. *Shufang yiyao: Chutu wenshu yu xiyu yixue*. Beijing: Peking University Press.

—. 2007. "The Transmission of Foreign Medicine via the Silk Roads in Medieval China: A Case Study of the *Haiyao bencao*." *Asian Medicine* 3 (2): 241–64.

—. 2013. *Zhonggu yiliao yu wailai wenhua*. Beijing: Peking University Press.

—. 2015. "Silu chutu mijiao yixue wenxian chuyi." *Dunhuang Tulufan yanjiu* 15: 473–96.

—. 2017. *Silu yiming*. Guandong: Guandong Jiaoyu chubanshe.

—. 2018. *Dunhuang de yiliao yu shehui*. Beijing: Zhongguo dabaike quanshu chubanshe.

Chen Yunü. 2008. "Buddhism and the Medical Treatment of Women in the Ming Dynasty: A Research Note." *Nan Nü* 10: 279–303.

Chenagtsang, Nida. 2014. *Path to Rainbow Body: Introduction to Yuthok Nyingthig*. n.p.: Sorig.

Chenagtsang, Nida, and Ben Joffe. 2018. *Karmamudra: The Yoga of Bliss: Sexuality in Tibetan Medicine and Buddhism*. Portland, Ore.: Sky.

Cheung, Kin. 2017. "Meditation and Neural Connections: Changing Sense(s) of Self in East Asian Buddhist and Neuroscientific Descriptions." PhD dissertation. Temple University. https://scholarshare.temple.edu/handle/20.500.12613/963.

—. 2018. "Implicit and Explicit Ethics in Mindfulness-Based Programs in a Broader Context." In *Handbook of Ethical Foundations of Mindfulness*, ed. Steven Stanley, Ronald E. Purser, and Nirbhay N. Singh, 305-321. n.p.: Springer.

Chhem, Rethy Kieth. 2004. "A Khmer Medical Text: 'The Treatment of the Four Diseases' Manuscript." *Siksācakr: Journal of the Center for Khmer Studies* 6: 33–42.

—. 2005. "Bhaiṣajyaguru and Tantric Medicine in Jayavarman VII Hospitals." *Siksācakr: Journal of the Center for Khmer Studies* 7: 8–18.

—. 2006. "La médecine angkorienne sous Jayavarman VII (1181–1220 de n.è.)." *Comptes rendus des séances de l'Académie des Inscriptions et Belles-Lettres* 4: 1977–1998.

—. 2007. "La médecine au service du pouvoir angkorien: Universités monastiques, transmission du savoir et formation médicale sous le règne de Jayavarman VII (118–1220 A.D.)." *Canadian Journal of Buddhist Studies* 3: 95–124.

—. 2009. "Médecine et santé à Angkor: pouvoir royal, compassion et offre médicale sous le règne de Jayavarman VII (1181–1220)." PhD dissertation. Université de Montréal. https://papyrus.bib.umontreal.ca/xmlui/handle/1866/6663.

Chilson, Clark. 2018. "Naikan: A Meditation Method and Psychotherapy." *Oxford Research Encyclopedia of Religion*. https://doi.org/10.1093/acrefore/9780199340378.013.570.

Chokevivat, Vichai, and Anchalee Chuthaputti. 2005. "The Role of Thai Traditional Medicine in Health Promotion." Paper presented at the *6GCHP* conference, Bangkok, Thailand, August 7–11, 2005. http://asianmedicinezone.com/wp-content/uploads/2014/09/THE-ROLE-OF-THAI-TRADITIONAL-MEDICINE-IN-HEALTH-PROMOTION1.pdf.

Chokevivat, Vichai, Anchalee Chuthaputti, and Pavana Khumtrakul. 2005. "The Use of Traditional Medicine in the Thai Health Care System." World Health Organization http://asianmedicinezone.com/wp-content/uploads/2014/09/The-Use-of-Traditional-Medicine-in-the-Thai-Health-Care-System.pdf.

Chudakova, Tatiana. 2017. "Plant Matters: Buddhist Medicine and Economies of Attention in Postsocialist Siberia." *American Ethnologist* 44 (2): 341–54.

—. 2021. *Mixing Medicines: Ecologies of Care in Buddhist Siberia*. New York: Fordham University Press.

Chui, Tony. 2019. "Conceptualization of 'Taking the Essence' (bcud len) as Tantric Rituals in the Writings of Sangye Gyatso: A Tradition or Interpretation?" *Religions* 10 (4): 231.

Chung, Bongkil. 2003. *The Scriptures of Won Buddhism: A Translation of the Wŏnbulgyo Kyojŏn with Introduction*. Honolulu: University of Hawai'i Press.

Chuthaputti, Anchalee, and Benjama Boonterm. 2010. "Traditional Medicine in Kingdom of Thailand: Integration of Thai Traditional Medicine in the National Health Care System of Thailand." In *Traditional Medicine in ASEAN: Based on Country Report Presentations in the "Conference on Traditional Medicine in ASEAN Countries," 31 August–2 September 2009 Bangkok, Thailand*. Bangkok: Bangkok Medical Publisher. http://asianmedicinezone.com/wp-content/uploads/2015/03/Traditional-Medicine-in-Kingdom-of-THAILAND1.pdf.

Clark, Barry. 1995. *The Quintessence Tantras of Tibetan Medicine*. Ithaca, N.Y.: Snow Lion.

Clifford, Terry. 1984. *Tibetan Buddhist Medicine and Psychiatry: The Diamond Healing*. York Beach, Maine: Samuel Weiser.

Coderey, Céline. 2012. "The Weikza's Role in Arakanese Healing Practices." *J Burma St* 16 (2): 181–211.

—. 2019. "Immortal Medicine: Understanding the Resilience of Burmese Alchemic Practice." *Medical Anthropology* 38 (4): 412–24.

—. 2020. "Myanmar Traditional Medicine: The Making of a National Heritage." *Modern Asian Studies* 55 (2): 514–51. https://doi.org/10.1017/S0026749X19000283.

Cohen, Alvin P. 2002. *Introduction to Research in Chinese Source Materials*. New Haven, Conn.: Yale University Press.

Cole, Alan. 1998. *Mothers and Sons in Chinese Buddhism*. Stanford, Calif.: Stanford University Press.

Collins, Steven. 1990. "On the Very Idea of the Pali Canon." *Journal of the Pali Text Society* 15: 89–126.

Como, Michael. 2019, October 17. "Roadways, Shrines and Spirits in Ancient Japan." Lecture presented at Stanford University, Stanford, Calif.

Compson, Jane. 2014. "Meditation, Trauma and Suffering in Silence: Raising Questions About How Meditation Is Taught and Practiced in Western Contexts in the Light of a Contemporary Trauma Resilience Model." *Contemporary Buddhism* 15 (2): 274–97.

Connor, Linda H., and Geoffrey Samuel, eds. 2001. *Healing Powers and Modernity: Traditional Medicine, Shamanism and Science in Asian Societies*. Westport, Conn.: Bergin & Garvey.

Conrad, Lawrence I. 2011. *The Western Medical Tradition: 800 B.C.–1800 A.D.* Cambridge: Cambridge University Press.

Conway, Susan. 2014. *Tai Magic: Arts of the Supernatural in the Shan States and Lan Na*. Bangkok: River Books.

Cook, Joanna. 2016. "Mindful in Westminster: The Politics of Meditation and the Limits of Neoliberal Critique." *HAU: Journal of Ethnographic Theory* 6 (1): 69–91.

—. 2018. "Paying Attention to Attention." *Anthropology of This Century*, 22. http://aotcpress.com/articles/paying-attention-attention.

Cooler, Richard M. 2016. "A Buddha Image for Exorcism." *J Burma St* 20 (2): 335–72.

Copp, Paul. 2014. *The Body Incantatory: Spells and the Ritual Imagination in Medieval Chinese Buddhism*. New York: Columbia University Press.

Cordier, Palmyr. 1903. "Introduction a l'étude des traités médicaux sanscrits inclus dans le Tanjur tibetain." *BEFEO* 3 (4): 604–29.

Cousins, L. S. 1996. "The Dating of the Historical Buddha: A Review Article." *Journal of the Royal Asiatic Society* 6: 57–63.

—. 1997. "Aspects of Esoteric Southern Buddhism." In *Indian Insights: Buddhism, Brahmanism and Bhakti*, ed. Peter Connolly and Sue Hamilton, 185–208. London: Luzac Oriental.

Craig, Sienna R. 2012. *Healing Elements: Efficacy and the Social Ecologies of Tibetan Medicine*. Berkeley: University of California Press.

Craig, Sienna R., Barbara Gerke, and Victoria Sheldon. 2020. "Sowa Rigpa Humanitarianism: Local Logics of Care Within a Global Politics of Compassion." *Medical Anthropology Quarterly* 34 (2): 174–91.

Crosby, Kate. 2000. "Tantric Theravada: A Bibliographic Essay on the Writings of François Bizot and Others on the Yogāvacara Tradition." *Contemporary Buddhism* 1 (2): 141–98.

—. 2013. *Traditional Theravada Meditation and Its Modern-Era Suppression*. Hong Kong: Buddha Dharma Centre of Hong Kong.

Crow, David. 2000. *In Search of the Medicine Buddha: A Himalayan Journey*. New York: Jeremy P. Tarcher/Putnam.

Cruijsen, Thomas, Arlo Griffiths, and Marijke J. Klokke. 2013. "The Cult of the Buddhist Dhāraṇī Deity Mahāpratisarā Along the Maritime Silk Route: New Epigraphical and Iconographic Evidence from the Indonesian Archipelago." *JIABS* 35 (1/2): 71–157.

Cuevas, Bryan J. 2019. "The Politics of Magical Warfare." In *Faith and Empire: Art and Politics in Tibetan Buddhism*, ed. Karl Debreczeny, 171–89. New York: Rubin Museum of Art.

Cusack, Carole M. 2011. "The Western Reception of Buddhism: Celebrity and Popular Cultural Media as Agents of Familiarisation." *Australian Religious Studies Review* 24 (3): 297–316.

Czaja, Olaf. 2005–2006. "Zurkharwa Lodro Gyalpo (1509–1579) on the Controversy of the Indian Origin of the *rGyud bzhi*." *Tibet Journal* 30/31 (4/1): 131–53.

—. 2007. "The Making of *The Blue Beryl*—Some Remarks on the Textual Sources of the Famous Commentary of Sangye Gyatsho (1653–1705)." In Schrempf 2007, 345–71.

—. 2013. "On the History of Refining Mercury in Tibetan Medicine." *Asian Medicine* 8: 75–105.

—. 2015. "The Eye-Healing Avalokiteśvara: A National Icon of Mongolia and Its Origin in Tibetan Medicine." In Ramble and Roesler 2015, 125–39.

—. 2019. "Mantras and Rituals in Tibetan Medicine." *Asian Medicine* 14 (2): 277–312.

Dalton, Jacob. 2004. "The Development of Perfection: The Interiorization of Buddhist Ritual in the Eighth and Ninth Centuries." *J Ind Phil* 32: 1–30.

Dalton, Jacob P. 2011. *The Taming of the Demons: Violence and Liberation in Tibetan Buddhism*. New Haven, Conn.: Yale University Press.

Das, Rahul Peter. 2003. *The Origin of the Life of a Human Being: Conception and the Female According to Ancient Indian Medical and Sexological Literature*. Delhi: Motilal Banarsidass.

Dash, Vaidya Bhagwan. 1974. "Harītakī: A Comparative Study of Literature in Ayurveda and Tibetan Medicine." *Bulletin of the Indian Institute of History of Medicine* 4 (1): 1–8.

—. 1985. *Tibetan Medicine: With Special Reference to Yoga Śataka*. Dharamsala: Library of Tibetan Works and Archives.

Davidson, Ronald M. 2002. *Indian Esoteric Buddhism: A Social History of the Tantric Movement*. New York: Columbia University Press.

—. 2005. *Tibetan Renaissance Tantric Buddhism in the Rebirth of Tibetan Culture*. New York: Columbia University Press.

Davies, William. 2015. *The Happiness Industry: How Government and Big Business Sold Us Well-Being*. London: Verso.

Davis, Edward L. 2001. *Society and the Supernatural in Song China*. Honolulu: University of Hawai'i Press.

de Chiara, Matteo, and Jens E. Braarvig. 2013. *Buddhism Among the Iranian Peoples of Central Asia*. Vienna: Verlag der Österreichische Akademie der Wissenschaften.

de Silva, Lily. 1993. "Ministering to the Sick and Counseling the Terminally Ill." In *Studies on Buddhism in Honour of Professor A. K. Warder*, ed. N. K. Wagle and F. Watanabe, 29–39. Toronto: University of Toronto Press.

de Vibe, Michael, Arild Bjørndal, Elizabeth Tipton, and Krystyna Kowalski. 2012. "Mindfulness Based Stress Reduction (MBSR) for Improving Health, Quality of Life and Social Functioning in Adults." *Campbell Systematic Reviews* 8 (1): 1–127.

de Visser, M. W. 1935. *Ancient Buddhism in Japan: Sutras and Ceremonies in Use in the Seventh and Eighth Centuries AD and Their History in Later Times*. Leiden: Brill.

Deane, Susannah. 2014a. "Sowa Rigpa, Spirits and Biomedicine: Lay Tibetan Perspectives on Mental Illness and Its Healing in a Medically-pluralistic Context in Darjeeling, Northeast India." PhD dissertation. Cardiff University. https://orca.cf.ac.uk/73236/1/2015deanesphd.pdf.

—. 2014b. "From Sadness to Madness: Tibetan Perspectives on the Causation and Treatment of Psychiatric Illness." *Religions* 5 (2): 444–58.

—. 2019a. "rLung, Mind, and Mental Health: The Notion of 'Wind' in Tibetan Conceptions of Mind and Mental Illness." *Journal of Religion and Health* 58 (3): 708–24. https://doi.org/10.1007/s10943-019-00775-0.

—. 2019b. "Madness and the Spirits: Examining the Role of Spirits in Mental Illness in the Tibetan Communities of Darjeeling." In McGrath 2019, 309–36.

DeCaroli, Robert. 2004. *Haunting the Buddha*. New York: Oxford University Press.

Deck, Christina. 2002. "Health, Karma, and Practice: Well-Being and Purification in Tibetan Buddhism." http://www.pluralism.org/affiliates/sered/Deck.pdf.

Delaini, Paolo. 2013. *Medicina del corpo, medicina dell'anima: La circolazione delle conoscenze medico-filosofiche nell'Iran sasanide*. Milan: Mimesis.

Demiéville, Paul. 1929. "Chinkiyaku." In *Hōbōgirin: Dictionnaire encyclopédique du Bouddhisme d'après les sources chinoises et japonaises*, vol. 4, ed. Lévi Sylvain, Junjirō Takakusu, Paul Demiéville, and Jacques May, 330–35. Tokyo: Maison Franco-Japonaise.

—. 1985 [1937]. *Buddhism and Healing: Demiéville's Article 'Byō' from Hōbōgirin*. Translated by Mark Tatz. Lanham, Md.: University Press of America.

Deshpande, Vijaya, and Fan Ka-wai. 2012. *Restoring the Dragon's Vision: Nagarjuna and Medieval Chinese Ophthalmology*. Hong Kong: City University of Hong Kong.

Despeux, Catherine. 2010. "Institutions médicales et thérapeutes à Dunhuang et à Turfan." In *Médecine, religion, et société dans la Chine médiévale: Étude de manuscrits chinois de Dunhuang et de Turfan*, ed. Catherine Despeux, 43–63. Paris: Collège de France, Institut des Hautes Études Chinoises.

—. 2017. "Chinese Medical Excrement: Is There a Buddhist Influence on the Use of Animal Excrement-Based Recipes in Medieval China?" *Asian Medicine* 12 (1/2): 139–69.

—. 2020. "Buddhist Healing Practices at Dunhuang in the Medieval Period." In Salguero and Macomber 2020, 118–59.

Devi, Bibha. 1979. "I-Tsing's Observation on Bathing and Its Medical Appraisal." In *Chikitsa: Collection of Research Articles on Ayurveda*, vol. 1, ed. Shyam Kishore Lal and Arun M. Parkhe, 55–57. Shivapuri-Akalkot, Maharashtra: Dharmatma Tatyajimaharaj Memorial Medical Relief Trust.

Didonna, Fabrizio, ed. 2008. *Clinical Handbook of Mindfulness*. New York: Springer.

Dietrich, Angela. 1996. "Research Note: Buddhist Healers in Nepal, Some Observations." *Contributions to Nepalese Studies* 23 (2): 473–80.

Dorje, Gyurme. 2014. "The Buddhas of Medicine." In Hofer 2014, 128–53.

Dowman, Keith. 1986. *Masters of Mahamudra: Songs and Histories of the Eighty-Four Buddhist Siddhas*. Albany, N.Y.: SUNY Press.

Drewes, David. 2010a. "Early Indian Mahāyāna Buddhism I: Recent Scholarship." *Religion Compass* 4: 55–65.

—. 2010b. "Early Indian Mahāyāna Buddhism II: New Perspectives." *Religion Compass* 4: 66–74.

Drott, Edward R. 2010. "Gods, Buddhas, and Organs: Buddhist Physicians and Theories of Longevity in Early Medieval Japan." *J Jap Rel St* 37 (2): 247–73.

Du Bois, Thomas. 2011. *Religion and the Making of Modern East Asia*. Cambridge: Cambridge University Press.

Duoer, Daigengna. 2019. "From 'Lama Doctors' to 'Mongolian Doctors': Regulations of Inner Mongolian Buddhist Medicine Under Changing Regimes and the Crises of Modernity (1911–1976)." *Religions* 10 (6): 373. https://doi.org/10.3390/rel10060373.

Ehara, N. R. M., Soma Thera, and Kheminda Thera. 1961. *The Path of Freedom, by the Arahant Upatissa, Translated Into Chinese (Gedatsu do ron) by Tipitaka Sanghapala of Funan*. Colombo, Ceylon: D. Roland D. Weerasuria.

Eifring, Halvor. 2015. "Meditative Practice and Cultural Context." In *Meditation and Culture: The Interplay of Practice and Context*, ed. Halvor Eifring, 3–8. London: Bloomsbury.

Eisenbruch, Maurice. 1992. "The Ritual Space of Patients and Traditional Healers in Cambodia." *BEFEO* 79 (2): 283–316.

Elliott, Elizabeth M. 2021. "Potent Plants, Cool Hearts: A Landscape of Healing in Laos." PhD dissertation. University College London.

Elman, Benjamin. 2007. "Global Science and Comparative History: Jesuits, Science, and Philology in China and Europe, 1550–1850." *EASTM* 26: 9–16.

Elverskog, Johan. 2010. *Buddhism and Islam on the Silk Road*. Philadelphia: University of Pennsylvania Press.

Emmerick, R. E. 1971. "The Sanskrit Text of the Siddhasāra." *BSOAS* 34 (1): 91–112.

—. 1974. "New Light on the 'Siddhasāra'." *BSOAS* 37 (3): 628–54.

—. 1979. "Contributions to the Study of the *Jīvaka-Pustaka*." *BSOAS* 42 (2): 235–43.

—. 1982. *The Siddhasāra of Ravigupta*. Wiesbaden: Steiner.

—. 2004. *The Sūtra of Golden Light (Suvarṇabhāsottamasūtra)*. 3rd ed. Oxford: Pali Text Society.

Erhard, Franz-Karl. 2007. "A Short History of the *g.Yu thog snying thig*." In *Indica et Tibetica: Festschrift fur Michael Hahn zum 65. Geburtstag von Freunden und Schülern Ciberreicht*, ed. Konrad Klaus and Jens-Uwe Hartman. Vienna: University of Vienna.

Fan, Fa-ti. 2012. "The Global Turn in the History of Science." *East Asian Science, Technology and Society* 6: 249–58.

Faure, Bernard. 1998. *The Red Thread: Buddhist Approaches to Sexuality*. Princeton, N.J.: Princeton University Press.

Fenner, Todd. 1996. "The Origin of the *rGyud bzhi*: A Tibetan Medical Tantra." In *Tibetan Literature: Studies in Genre*, ed. José Ignacio Cabezon and Roger R. Jackson, 458–69. Ithaca, N.Y.: Snow Lion.

Filliozat, Jean. 1934. "La médecine indienne et l'expansion bouddhique en Extrême-Orient." *Journal Asiatique* 224: 301–7.

—. 1935. "Le Kumāratantra de Rāvaṇa." *Journal Asiatique* 226: 1–66.

—. 1937. *Étude de démonologie indienne: Le Kumaratantra de Râvana et les textes parallèles indiens, tibétains, chinois, cambodgien et arabe*. Paris: Imprimerie Nationale.

—. 1969. "Taoïsme et yoga." *Journal Asiatique* 257 (1/2): 41–87.

—. 1979. *Yogaśataka: Texte médical attribué à Nāgārjuna: Textes sanskrit et tibétain, traduction française, notes, indices*. Pondicherry, India: Institut Français d'Indologie.

Fiordalis, David. 2014. "On Buddhism, Divination and the Worldly Arts: Textual Evidence from the Theravāda Tradition." *Indian International Journal of Buddhist Studies* 15: 79–108.

Fish, Jessica. 2014. "Health Care in Indian Buddhism: Representations of Monks and Medicine in Indian Monastic Law Codes." Master's thesis. McMaster University. https://macsphere.mcmaster.ca/handle/11375/16281.

Flanagan, Owen. 2011. *The Bodhisattva's Brain: Buddhism Naturalized*. Cambridge, Mass.: MIT Press.

—. 2012. "Buddhism Without the Hocus-Pocus." *Chronicle of Higher Education* 58 (19). http://www.chronicle.com/article/buddhism-without-the/130203/.

Florida, Robert E. 1998. "The *Lotus Sūtra* and Health Care Ethics." *J Budd Eth* 5: 170–89.

Flowers, James. 2021. "*Hanbang* Healing for the World: The Eastern Medicine Renaissance in 1930s Japan-Ruled Korea." *Social History of Medicine* 34 (2): 650–71.

Folz, Richard. 2010. "Buddhism in the Iranian World." *Muslim Word* 100 (Apr/Jul): 204–14.

Forbes, David. 2019. *Mindfulness and Its Discontents: Education, Self, and Social Transformation.* Black Point, N.S.: Fernwood.

Fox, Kieran C. R., Savannah Nijeboer, Matthew L. Dixon, James L. Floman, Melissa Ellamil, Samuel P. Rumak, Peter Sedlmeier, and Kaline Christoff. 2014. "Is Meditation Associated with Altered Brain Structure? A Systematic Review and Meta-analysis of Morphometric Neuroimaging in Meditation Practitioners." *Neuroscience & Biobehavioral Reviews* 43: 48–73. https://doi.org/10.1016/j.neubiorev.2014.03.016.

Fraser, Andy, ed. 2013. *The Healing Power of Meditation: Leading Experts on Buddhism, Psychology, and Medicine Explore the Health Benefits of Contemplative Practice.* Boston: Shambhala.

Frauwallner, Erich. 1956. *The Earliest Vinaya and the Beginnings of Buddhist Literature.* Rome: Instituto italiano per il Medio ed Estremo Oriente.

Fries, James F. 2005. "The Compression of Morbidity." *The Milbank Quarterly* 83 (4): 801–23. https://doi.org/10.1111/j.1468-0009.2005.00401.x.

Fu Fang, and Ni Qing, eds. 1996. *Zhongguo foyi renwu xiaozhuan.* Xiamen: Lujiang chubanshe.

Fujikawa Yū. 1934. *Japanese Medicine.* New York: Hoeber.

Fussman, G. 1993. "Taxila: The Central Asian Connection." In *Urban Form and Meaning in South Asia: The Shaping of Cities from Prehistoric to Precolonial Times*, ed. Howard Spodek and Doris Srinivasan, 83–100. Washington, D.C.: National Gallery of Art.

Gallison, Peter. 1997. *Image and Logic: A Material Culture of Microphysics.* Chicago: University of Chicago Press.

Gardiner, David. 2016. "Body." In Powers 2016a, 248–60.

Garrett, Frances. 2005. "Ordering Human Growth in Tibetan Medical and Religious Embryologies." In *Textual Healing: Essays on Medieval and Early Modern Medicine*, ed. Elizabeth Furdel, 31–52. Leiden: Brill.

——. 2007a. "Buddhism and the Historicizing of Medicine in Thirteenth-Century Tibet." *Asian Medicine* 2 (2): 204–24.

——. 2007b. "Embryology and Embodiment in Tibetan Literature: Narrative Epistemology and the Rhetoric of Identity." In Schrempf 2007, 411–25.

——. 2008a. *Religion, Medicine and the Human Embryo in Tibet.* London: Routledge.

——. 2008b. "Tibetan Buddhist Narratives of the Forces of Creation." In *Imagining the Fetus: The Unborn in Myth, Religion and Culture*, ed. Jane Marie Law and Vanessa R. Sasson, 107–20. Oxford: Oxford University Press.

——. 2009. "The Alchemy of Accomplishing Medicine (sman sgrub): Situating the Yuthok Heart Essence Ritual Tradition. *J Ind Phil* 37 (3): 207–30.

——. 2010. "Shaping the Illness of Hunger: A Culinary Aesthetics of Food and Healing in Tibet." *Asian Medicine* 6 (1): 33–54.

——. 2015. *Religion, Medicine and the Human Embryo in Tibet.* London: Routledge.

——. 2019. "The Food of Meditation: Dietary Healing and Power in Tibetan Buddhism." *Asian Medicine* 14 (1): 56–80.

Garrett, Frances, and Vincanne Adams. 2008. "The Three Channels in Tibetan Medical and Religious Texts, Including a Translation of Tsultrim Gyaltsen's 'Treatise on the Three Channels in Tibetan Medicine.'" *Traditional South Asian Medicine* 8: 86–115.

Geibel, Rolf W. 2005. The *Vairocanābhisaṃbodhi Sutra*. Berkeley, Calif.: BDK America.

Gellner, David. 2001. *The Anthropology of Buddhism and Hinduism: Weberian Themes*. New Delhi: Oxford University Press.

George, Christopher Starr. 1971. *The Caṇḍamahāroṣaṇa Tantra: Chapters I–VIII*. PhD dissertation. University of Michigan.

Gerke, Barbara. 2007. "Engaging the Subtle Body: Re-approaching *Bla* Rituals Among Himalayan Tibetan Societies." In Schrempf 2007: 191–212.

—. 2011. *Long Lives and Untimely Deaths: Life-Span Concepts and Longevity Practices Among Tibetans in the Darjeeling Hills, India*. Leiden: Brill.

—. 2012. "Treating Essence with Essence: Re-inventing *bcud len* as Vitalising Dietary Supplements in Contemporary Tibetan Medicine." *Asian Medicine* 7: 196–224.

—. 2013. "Mercury in Ayurveda and Tibetan Medicine." Special issue, *Asian Medicine* 8 (1).

—. 2014. "The Art of Tibetan Medical Practice." In Hofer 2014, 16–31.

—. 2017a. "Tibetan Precious Pills as Therapeutics and Rejuvenating Longevity Tonics." *Hist Sci SA* 5 (2): 204–33.

—. 2017b. "Buddhist Healing and Taming in Tibet." In *The Oxford Handbook of Contemporary Buddhism*, ed. Michael Jerryson, 576–90. New York: Oxford University Press.

—. 2019a. "The Buddhist-Medical Interface in Tibet: Black Pill Traditions in Transformation." *Religions* 10 (4): 282.

—. 2019b. "Material Presentations and Cultural Drug Translations of Contemporary Tibetan Precious Pills." In McGrath 2019: 337–67.

—. 2021. *Taming the Poisonous: Mercury, Toxicity, and Safety in Tibetan Medical Practice*. Heidelberg: Heidelberg University Publishing. https://doi.org/10.17885/heiup.746.

Germano, David F. 1992. "Poetic Thought, the Intelligent Universe, and the Mystery of Self: The Tantric Synthesis of Ofrdzogs Chen in Fourteenth Century Tibet." PhD dissertation, University of Wisconsin, Madison. https://philpapers.org/rec/GERPTT.

Gernet, Jacques. 1995 [1956]. *Buddhism in Chinese Society: An Economic History from the Fifth to the Tenth Centuries*. Translated by Franciscus Verellen. New York: Columbia University Press.

Giles, H. A., trans. 1923. *The Travels of Fa-Hsien (399–414 A.D.), or Record of the Buddhistic Kingdoms, by Faxian*. Cambridge: Cambridge University Press.

Girón, Corinne Pruvost. 2002. *Palakkad Pass and the Cattle Trail: An Example of a Territory of Reference in South-India*. Pondichéry: French Institute of Pondicherry.

Gleig, Ann. 2016. "External Mindfulness, Secure (Non)-Attachment, and Healing Relational Trauma: Emerging Models of Wellness for Modern Buddhists and Buddhist Modernism." *J Glo Budd* 17: 1–21.

—. 2019. *American Dharma: Buddhism Beyond Modernity*. New Haven, Conn.: Yale University Press.

Goble, Andrew Edmund 2009. "Kajiwara Shozen (1265–1337) and the Medical Silk Road: Chinese and Arabic Influences on Early Medieval Japanese Medicine." In *Tools of Culture: Japan's Cultural, Intellectual, Medical, and Technological Contacts in East Asia, 1000s–1500s*, ed. Andrew Edmund Goble, Kenneth R. Robinson, and Haruko Wakabayashi, 231–57. Ann Arbor, Mich.: Association for Asian Studies.

—. 2011. *Confluences of Medicine in Medieval Japan: Buddhist Healing, Chinese Knowledge, Islamic Formulas, and Wounds of War*. Honolulu: University of Hawai'i Press.

—. 2012. *Confluences of Medicine in Medieval Japan: Buddhist Healing, Chinese Knowledge, Islamic Formulas, and Wounds of War*. Honolulu: University of Hawai'i Press.

—. 2016. "Women and Medicine in Late 16th Century Japan: The Example of the Honganji Religious Community in Ōsaka and Kyoto as Recorded in the Diary of Physician Yamashina Tokitsune." *Asia Pacific Perspectives* 14 (1): 50–74.

Goble, Geoffrey C. 2017. "Three Buddhist Texts from Dunhuang: *The Scripture on Healing Diseases*, the *Scripture Urging Goodness*, and the *New Bodhisattva Scripture*." *Asian Medicine* 16 (1-2): 265–78.

Goble, Geoffrey C. 2019. *Chinese Esoteric Buddhism: Amoghavajra, the Ruling Elite, and the Emergence of a Tradition*. New York: Columbia University Press.

Goldberg, Simon B., Raymond P. Tucker, Preston A. Greene, Richard J. Davidson, Bruce E. Wampold, David J. Kearney, and Tracy L. Simpson. 2018. "Mindfulness-Based Interventions for Psychiatric Disorders: A Systematic Review and Meta-analysis." *Clinical Psychology Review* 59: 52–60.

Goldschmidt, Asaf Moshe. 2009. *The Evolution of Chinese Medicine: Song Dynasty, 960–1200*. London: Routledge.

Goleman, Daniel, and Richard Davidson. 2017. *Altered Traits: Science Reveals How Meditation Changes Your Mind, Brain, and Body*. New York: Penguin.

Gombrich, Richard, and Yu-Shuang Yao. 2013. "A Radical Buddhism for Modern Confucians: Tzu Chi in Socio-Historical Perspective." *Budd St Rev* 30 (2): 237–59.

Gómez, Luis O. 1996. *Land of Bliss: The Paradise of the Buddha of Measureless Light*. Honolulu and Kyoto: University of Hawai'i Press and Higashi Honganji Shinshu Otani-ha.

Gosho Translation Committee. 1999–2003. *The Writings of Nichiren Daishonin*. Tokyo: Soka Gakkai.

Gosling, David. 1985. "Thailand's Bare-Headed Doctors." *Modern Asian Studies* 19 (4): 761–96.

Goyal, Madhav, Sonal Singh, Erica M. S. Sibinga, Neda F. Gould, Anastasia Rowland-Seymour, Ritu Sharma, Zackary Berger, et al. 2014. "Meditation Programs for Psychological Stress and Well-Being." *Comparative Effectiveness Review* 124.

Granoff, Phyllis. 1998a. "Cures and Karma: Healing and Being Healed in Jain Religious Literature." In *Self, Soul and Body in Religious Experience*, ed. Albert I. Baumgartner, 218–55. Leiden: Brill.

—. 1998b. "Cures and Karma II: Some Miraculous Healings in the Indian Buddhist Story Tradition." *BEFEO* 85: 285–304.

—. 2011. "The Buddha as the Greatest Healer: The Complexities of a Comparison." *Journal Asiatique* 299 (1): 5–22.

Gray, David B. 2006. "Skull Imagery and Skull Magic in the Yoginītantras." *Pacific World* 3 (8): 21–39.

—. 2007a. "The Cakrasamvara Tantra: Its History, Interpretation, and Practice in India and Tibet." *Religion Compass* 1 (6): 695–710.

—. 2007b. "Compassionate Violence? On the Ethical Implications of Tantric Buddhist Ritual." *Journal of Buddhist Ethics* 17: 239–71.

—. 2014. "Tibetan Formulations of the Tantric Path." In Poceski 2014: 185–98.

Greene, Eric Matthew. 2012. "Meditation, Repentance, and Visionary Experience in Early Medieval Chinese Buddhism." PhD dissertation. University of California, Berkeley. https://escholarship.org/uc/item/92v7t1cg.

—. 2016. "A Reassessment of the Early History of Chinese Buddhist Vegetarianism." *Asia Major* 29 (1): 1–43.

—. 2021. *The Secrets of Buddhist Meditation: Visionary Meditation Texts from Early Medieval China*. Honolulu: University of Hawai'i Press.

Gregory, Peter N. 1991. *Tsung-mi and the Sinification of Buddhism*. Princeton, N.J.: Princeton University Press.

Grimes, Samuel, and Péter-Dániel Szántó. 2018. "Mahāsukhavajra's *Padmāvatī* Commentary on the Sixth Chapter of the *Caṇḍamahāroṣaṇatantra*: The Sexual Practices of a Tantric Buddhist Yogī and His Consort." *J Ind Phil* 46 (14): 1–45.

Griswold, A. B. 1965. "The Rishis of Wat Pō." In *Felicitation Volumes of Southeast-Asian Studies Presented to His Highness Prince Dhaninivat Kromamun Bidyalabh Brindhyakorn*, compiled by the Siam Society, 319–28. Bangkok: Siam Society.

Guarisco, Elio, trans. 2017. *Secret Map of the Body: Visions of the Human Energy Structure*, ed. Judith Chasnoff. n.p.: Shang Shung.

Gummer, Natalie. 2000. "Articulating Potency: A Study of the *Suvarṇa[pra]bhāsottamasūtra*." PhD dissertation, Harvard University. https://www.semanticscholar.org/paper/Articulating-potency-%3A-a-study-of-the-Gummer/232d5525c9b4dcaf2e890abb69b509960c2162f1.

Gyatso, Janet. 2014. "Buddhist Practices and Ideals in Desi Sangye Gyatso's Medical Paintings." In Hofer 2014, 198–220.

—. 2015. *Being Human in a Buddhist World: An Intellectual History of Medicine in Early Modern Tibet*. New York: Columbia University Press.

—. 2017. "Review of C. Pierce Salguero, *Translating Buddhist Medicine in Medieval China*," *History of Religions* 57 (1): 99.

Ha, Tae-Hung, and Grafton K. Mintz, trans. 1972. *Samguk yusa: Legends and History of the Three Kingdoms of Ancient Korea*. Seoul: Yonsei University Press.

Haines, Michael. 2008, March 19. "Fertility and Mortality in the United States." *EH.Net Encyclopedia*, ed. Robert Whaples. http://eh.net/encyclopedia/fertility-and-mortality-in-the-united-states/.

Halkias, Georgios. 2014. "When the Greeks Converted the Buddha: Asymmetrical Transfers of Knowledge in Indo-Greek Cultures." In *Religions and Trade: Religious Formation, Transformation and Cross-Cultural Exchange Between East and West*, ed. Peter Wick and Volker Rabens, 65–116. Leiden: Brill.

Hamilton, Sue. 1996. *Identity and Experience: The Constitution of the Human Being According to Early Buddhism*. London: Luzac Oriental.

Hammerstrom, Erik. 2014. "A Buddhist Critique of Scientism." *JCBS* 27: 35–57.

Hammerstrom, Erik J. 2015. *The Science of Chinese Buddhism: Early Twentieth-Century Engagements*. New York: Columbia University Press.

Hanley, Adam W., Neil Abell, Debra S. Osborn, Alysia D. Roehrig, and Angela I. Canto. 2016. "Mind the Gaps: Are Conclusions About Mindfulness Entirely Conclusive?" *Journal of Counseling & Development* 94 (Jan.): 103–13.

Hansen, Valerie. 2017. *The Silk Road: A New History with Documents*. New York: Oxford University Press.

Hanson, Marta E. 2007. "Jesuits and Medicine in the Kangxi Court (1662–1722)." *Pacific Rim Report* 43: 1–10.

Hardacre, Helen. 1982. "The Transformation of Healing in the Japanese New Religions." *History of Religions* 21 (4): 305–20.
Harrington, Anne. 2008. *The Cure Within: A History of Mind-Body Medicine*. New York: Norton.
Harvey, Peter. 1993. "The Mind-Body Relationship in Pāli Buddhism: A Philosophical Investigation." *Asian Philosophy* 3 (1): 29–41.
—. 2015. "Introductory Reflections on Buddhism and Healing." *Budd St Rev* 32 (1): 13–18.
Hatley, Shaman. 2007. "Mapping the Esoteric Body in the Islamic Yoga of Bengal." *History of Religions* 46 (4): 351–68.
Heinze, Ruth-Inge. 1997. *Trance and Healing in Southeast Asia Today*. Bangkok: White Lotus.
Heirman, Ann. 2018. *Buddhist Encounters and Identities Across East Asia*. Leiden: Brill.
Heirman, Ann, and Stephan Peter Bumbacher, eds. 2007. *The Spread of Buddhism*. Leiden: Brill.
Heirman, Ann, and Mathieu Torck. 2012. *A Pure Mind in a Clean Body: Bodily Care in the Buddhist Monasteries of Ancient India and China*. Ghent, Belgium: Academia.
Helderman, Ira. 2019. *Prescribing the Dharma: Psychotherapists, Buddhist Traditions, and Defining Religion*. Chapel Hill: University of North Carolina Press.
Hickey, Wakoh Shannon. 2019. *Mind Cure: How Meditation Became Medicine*. New York: Oxford University Press.
Hidas, Gergely. 2012. *Mahāpratisarā-Mahāvidyārājñī, The Great Amulet, Great Queen of Spells. Introduction, Critical Editions and Annotated Translation*. New Delhi: International Academy of Indian Culture and Aditya Prakashan.
Hinderling, Paul. 1980. *The Thai Village Doctor as a Mediator Between Traditional and Modern Medicine, from Thai-European Seminar on Social Change in Contemporary Thailand*. Amsterdam: University of Amsterdam.
Hinnells, John R., and Roy Porter, eds. 1999. *Religion, Health and Suffering*. London: Kegan Paul.
Hinrichs, T. J., and Linda L. Barnes, eds. 2013. *Chinese Medicine and Healing: An Illustrated History*. Cambridge, Mass.: Belknap.
Hirakawa, Akira. 1963. "The Rise of Mahāyāna Buddhism and Its Relationship to the Worship of Sūpas." *Memories of the Research Department of the Toyo Bunko* 22: 57–106.
Hoernle, A. F. Rudolf. 1893. "The Weber Mss.—another Collection of Ancient Manuscripts from Central Asia." *Journal of the Asiatic Society of Bengal* 62 (1): 1–40.
—. 1902. *Facsimile Reproduction of Weber Mss., Part IX and Macartney Mss., Set I with Roman Transliteration and Indexes*. Calcutta: Baptist Mission.
—. 1917. "An Ancient Medical Manuscript from Eastern Turkestan." In *Commemorative Essays Presented to Sir Ramkrishna Gopal Bhandarkar*, 415–32. Poona: Bhandarkar Oriental Research Institute.
—. 1987. *The Bower Manuscript*. New Delhi: Aditya Prakashan.
Hofbauer, Rudolf. 1943. "A Medical Retrospect of Thailand." *Journal of the Thailand Research Society* 34: 183–200.
Hofer, Teresia, ed. 2014. *Bodies in Balance: The Art of Tibetan Medicine*. Seattle: University of Washington Press.
Horner, I. B., trans. 2000. *The Book of the Discipline (Vinaya-Piṭaka)*, vol. 4. Oxford: Pali Text Society.
Hsia, Emil C. H., Ilza Veith, and Robert H. Geertsma. 1986. *The Essentials of Medicine in Ancient China and Japan: Yasuyori Tamba's Ishimpō*. Leiden: Brill.

Hsu, Alexander O. 2018. "Practices of Scriptural Economy: Compiling and Copying a Seventh-Century Chinese Buddhist Anthology." PhD dissertation. University of Chicago. https://knowledge.uchicago.edu/record/395?ln=en.

Huang, C. Julia. 2009. *Charisma and Compassion: Cheng Yen and the Buddhist Tzu Chi Movement*. Cambridge, Mass.: Harvard University Press.

—. 2017. "Scientific and Sacramental: Engaged Buddhism and the Sacrilization of Medical Science in Tzu Chi (Ciji)." *J Glo Budd* 18: 72–90.

Huisman, Frank, and John Harley Warner. 2006. *Locating Medical History: The Stories and Their Meanings*. Baltimore, Md.: Johns Hopkins University Press.

Hureau, Sylvie. 2010. "Translations, Apocrypha, and the Emergence of the Buddhist Canon." In *Early Chinese Religion*, part 2, *The Period of Division (220–589 AD)*, ed. John Lagerwey and Lü Pengzhi, 741–74. Leiden: Brill.

Iida, Junko. 2013. "Holism as Whole-Body Treatment: The Transnational Production of Thai Massage." *European Journal of Transnational Studies* 5 (1): 81–111.

—. 2017. "The Invention of Medical Tradition in Thailand: Thai Traditional Medicine and Thai Massage." In Pols, Thompson, and Warner 2017, 273–94.

Jackson, Mark P. C. 2013. *The Oxford Handbook of the History of Medicine*. Oxford: Oxford University Press.

Jacobson, Eric. 2007. "'Life-Wind Illness' in Tibetan Medicine: Depression, Generalised Anxiety, and Panic Attack." In Schrempf 2007, 225–45.

Jacoby, Sarah H. 2014. *Love and Liberation: Autobiographical Writings of the Tibetan Buddhist Visionary Sera Khandro*. New York: Columbia University Press.

Jacques, Claude. 1968. "Les édites des hôpitaux de Jayavarman VII." *Études Cambodgiennes* 13: 14–17.

Jaffe, Richard, trans. 2015. *Selected Works of D. T. Suzuki*, vol. 1, *Zen*. Berkeley: University of California Press.

Janes, Craig R. 2002. "Buddhism, Science, and Market: The Globalisation of Tibetan Medicine." *Anthropology & Medicine* 9 (3): 267–89.

Jardine, John, ed. 1893. *The Burmese Empire a Hundred Years Ago, as Described by Father Sangermano*. Westminster: Archibald Constable.

Jaworski, Jan. 1927. "La section des remèdes dans le Vinaya des Malūśāsaka et dans le Vinaya Pali." *Rocznik orjentalistyczny* 5: 92–101.

Jeong Byeong-sam. 2013. "The Characteristics of the Cult of Bhaiṣajyaguru in Silla: On Its Doctrinal Interpretations and Cultic Practices." In *The Cult of the Healing Buddha in East Asia: Donghwasa Temple and Columbia Center for Buddhism and East Asian Religions (C-BEAR) International Conference (May 29–30, 2013)*. Daegu, South Korea: Donghwasa Temple.

Jing, Anning. 1991. "The Yuan Buddhist Mural of the Paradise of Bhaiṣajyaguru." *Metropolitan Museum Journal* 26: 147–66.

Joffe, Ben. 2019. "White Robes, Matted Hair: Tibetan Tantric Householders, Moral Sexuality, and the Ambiguities of Esoteric Buddhist Expertise in Exile." PhD dissertation. University of Colorado.

Johnston, William D. 2016. "Buddhism Contra Cholera: How the Meiji State Recruited Religion Against Epidemic Disease." In *Science, Technology, and Medicine in the Modern Japanese Empire*, ed. David G. Wittner and Philip C. Brown, 62–78. London and New York: Routledge.

Jones, Charles B. 2009. "Modernization and Traditionalism in Buddhist Almsgiving: The Case of the Buddhist Compassion Relief Tzu-chi Association in Taiwan." *J Glo Budd* 10: 291–319.

—. 2019. "Is a *Dazang jing* a Canon? On the Nature of Chinese Buddhist Textual Anthologies." In *Methods in Buddhist Studies: Essays in Honor of Richard K. Payne*, ed. Scott A. Mitchell and Natalie Fisk Quli, 129–43. London: Bloosmbury.

Jöns, Heike. 2011. "Centre of Calculation." In *The SAGE Handbook of Geographical Knowledge*, ed. John A. Agnew and David N. Livingstone, 158–70. London: SAGE.

Joo, Ryan Bongseok. 2011. "Countercurrents from the West: 'Blue-Eyed' Zen Masters, Vipassanā Meditation, and Buddhist Psychotherapy in Contemporary Korea," *JAAR* 79 (3): 614–38.

Jordt, Ingrid. 2007. *Burma's Mass Lay Meditation Movement: Buddhism and the Cultural Construction of Power*. Athens: Ohio University Press.

Josephson, Jason Ā. 2012. "An Empowered World: Buddhist Medicine and the Potency of Prayer in Meiji Japan." In *Deus in Machina: Religion, Technology, and the Things in Between*, ed. Jeremy Stolow, 117–41. New York: Fordham University Press.

Josephson-Storm, Jason Ā. 2017. *The Myth of Disenchantment: Magic, Modernity, and the Birth of the Human Sciences*. Chicago: University of Chicago Press.

Kabat-Zinn, Jon. 2011. "Some Reflections on the Origins of MBSR, Skillful Means, and the Trouble with Maps." *Contemporary Buddhism* 12 (1): 281.

Kajiwara Keiichi. 2004. "Buddhism and Hansen's Disease." *Eastern Buddhist* 36 (1/2): 40–45.

Kameyama, Takahiko. 2016. "Arising of Faith in the Human Body: The Significance of Embryological Discourses in Medieval Shingon Buddhist Tradition" *Pacific World* 18: 41–51.

Kapani, Lakshmi. 1989. "Upanishad of the Embryo/Note on the Garbha-Upanishad." In *Fragments for a History of the Human Body*, vol. 3, ed. Michel Feher, Ramona Naddaff, and Nadia Tazi, 177–96. New York: Zone.

Kapferer, Bruce. 1991. *A Celebration of Demons: Exorcism and the Aesthetics of Healing in Sri Lanka*. 2nd ed. Providence, R.I.: Berg.

Kapstein, Matthew T. 2014. "Textualizing the Icon: The Three Deities of Longevity in Art and Ritual." In Ramble and Roesler 2015, 383–403.

Kara, György. 2004. "An Old Tibetan Fragment on Healing from the Sutra of the Thousand-Eyed and Thousand-Handed Great Compassionate Bodhisattva Avalokiteśvara in the Berlin Turfan Collection." In *Turfan Revisited: The First Century of Research Into the Arts and Cultures of the Silk Road*, ed. Desmond Durkin-Meisterernst, 141–46. Berlin: Reimer.

Kasai, Kenta. 2016. "Introducing Chaplaincy to Japanese Society." *Journal of Religion in Japan* 5 (2/3): 246–62.

Katz, Nathan. 2010. *Buddhist Images of Human Perfection: The Arahant of the Sutta Pitaka Compared with the Bodhisattva and the Mahasiddha*. Delhi: Motilal Banarsidass.

Kellner, Birgit, ed. 2019. *Buddhism and the Dynamics of Transculturality: New Approaches*. Berlin: De Gruyter.

Keown, Damien. 1995. *Buddhism and Bioethics*. New York: Palgrave Macmillan.

Keown, Damien, ed. 1999. *Buddhism and Abortion*. Honolulu: University of Hawai'i Press.

Kieschnick, John. 1997. *The Eminent Monk: Buddhist Ideals in Medieval Chinese Hagiography*. Honolulu: University of Hawai'i Press.

Kilty, Gavin, trans. 2010. *Mirror of Beryl: A Historical Introduction to Tibetan Medicine*. Boston: Wisdom.

Kim Sejung. 2016. "A Study on the Generalized Direction of Mindfulness in Won Buddhism with Special Reference to MBSR." PhD dissertation. Wonkwang University.

Kirby, James N., Cassandra L. Tellegen, and Stanley R. Steindl. 2017. "A Meta-analysis of Compassion-Based Interventions: Current State of Knowledge and Future Directions." *Behavior Therapy* 48 (6): 778–92.

Kitagawa, Joseph Mitsuo. 1989. "Buddhist Medical History." In *Healing and Restoring: Health and Medicine in the World's Religious Traditions*, ed. Lawrence E. Sullivan, 9–32. New York and London: Macmillan.

Kitiarsa, Pattana. 2012. *Mediums, Monks, and Amulets: Thai Popular Buddhism Today*. Seattle: University of Washington Press.

Kleine, Christoph. 2013. "Religion and the Secular in Premodern Japan from the Viewpoint of Systems Theory." *Journal of Religion in Japan* 2: 1–34.

Kleine, Christoph, and Katja Triplett, eds. 2012. "Religion and Healing in Japan." Special issue, *Japanese Religions* 37 (1/2).

Kloos, Stephan. 2010. "Tibetan Medicine in Exile: The Ethics, Politics and Science of Cultural Survival." PhD dissertation. University of California, San Francisco. https://escholarship.org/uc/item/3207476k.

——. 2013. "How Tibetan Medicine in Exile Became a 'Medical System.'" *East Asian Science, Technology and Society* 7: 381–95.

——. 2016. "The Recognition of Sowa Rigpa in India: How Tibetan Medicine Became an Indian Medical System." *Medicine Anthropology Theory* 3 (2): 19–49.

——. 2019. "Humanitarianism from Below: Sowa Rigpa, the Traditional Pharmaceutical Industry, and Global Health." *Medical Anthropology* 39 (2): 167–81. https://doi.org/10.1080/01459740.2019.1587423.

Kloos, Stephan, Harilal Madhavan, Tawni Tidwell, Calum Blaikie, and Mingji Cuomu. 2020. "The Transnational Sowa Rigpa Industry in Asia: New Perspectives on an Emerging Economy." *Social Science & Medicine* 245: 112617.

Kogiso, Kohei. 2012. "Thai Massage and Health Tourism in Thailand: Tourism Acculturation Process of 'Thai Massage.'" *International Journal of Sport and Health Science* 10: 65–70.

Köhle, Natalie. 2016. "A Confluence of Humors: Āyurvedic Conceptions of Digestion and the History of Chinese 'Phlegm' (*tan*)." *JAOS* 136 (3): 465–93.

Kotyk, Jeffrey. 2017a. "Can Monks Practice Astrology? Astrology and the Vinaya in China." In *Rules of Engagement: Medieval Traditions of Buddhist Monastic Regulation*, ed. Susan Andrews, Jinhua Chen, and Cuilan Liu, 503–17. Bochum and Freiburg: ProjektVerlag.

——. 2017b. "Buddhist Astrology and Astral Magic in the Tang Dynasty." PhD dissertation. Leiden University. https://archive.org/details/buddhistastrologykotyk.

——. 2019. "Indo-Iranian and Islamicate Sources of Astrological Medicine in Medieval China." *Asian Medicine* 14 (1): 30–55.

Krishna, Ramachandra Rao Saligrama, and S. R. Sudarshan. 1985. *Encyclopaedia of Indian Medicine*. Bombay: Popular Prakashan.

Kritzer, Robert. 2004. "Childbirth and the Mother's Body in the *Abhidharmakośabhāsya* and Related Texts." In *Indo tetsugaku bukkyō shisō ron shū: Mikogami Eshō kyōju shōju kinen ronshū*, 1085–1109. Kyoto: Nagatabunshodō.

—. 2009. "Life in the Womb: Conception and Gestation in Buddhist Scripture and Classical Indian Medical Literature." In *Imagining the Fetus: The Unborn in Myth, Religion, and Culture*, ed. Jane Marie Law and Vanessa R. Sasson, 73–89. Oxford: Oxford University Press.

—. 2012. "Tibetan Texts of Garbhāvakrāntisūtra: Differences and Borrowings." *Annual Report of the International Research Institute for Advanced Buddhology* 15: 131–45.

—. 2013. "Garbhāvakrāntau ('In the Garbhāvakrānti'): Quotations from the *Garbhāvakrāntisūtra* in Abhidharma Literature and the *Yogācārabhūmi*." In *The Foundation for Yoga Practitioners: The Buddhist Yogācārabhūmi Treatise and Its Adaptation in India, East Asia, and Tibet*, ed. Ulrich Timme Kragh, 738–71. Cambridge, Mass.: Harvard University Press.

—. 2014a. "Affliction and Infestation in an Indian Buddhist Embryological Sutra." In *Scripture:Canon::Text:Context: Essays Honoring Lewis Lancaster*, ed. Richard K. Payne, 181–202. Berkeley, Calif.: Institute of Buddhist Studies and BDK America.

—. 2014b. *Garbhāvakrāntisūtra: The Sūtra on Entry Into the Womb.* Tokyo: International Institute for Buddhist Studies.

Krug, Adam C. 2019. "Buddhist Medical Demonology in the *Sūtra of the Seven Buddhas*." *Religions* 10 (4): 255.

Kucinskas, Jaime. 2018. *The Mindful Elite: Mobilizing from the Inside Out.* New York: Oxford University Press.

Kumar, Pintu. 2011. "The Ancient Nālandā Mahāvihāra: The Beginning of Institutional Education." *Journal of the World Universities Forum* 4 (1): 65–79.

Kuo Li-ying. 1994. *Confession et contrition dans le Bouddhisme chinois du Ve au Xe siècle.* Paris: École française d'Extrême-Orient.

Lancaster, Lewis R. 2012 [1999]. "The Movement of Buddhist Texts from India to China and the Construction of the Chinese Buddhist Canon." *Sino-Platonic Papers* 222: 226–38.

Langenberg, Amy Paris. 2014. "Female Monastic Healing and Midwifery: A View from the Vinaya Tradition." *J Budd Eth* 21. http://blogs.dickinson.edu/buddhistethics/2014/02/22/female-monastic-healing-and-midwifery/.

—. 2015. "Buddhist Blood Taboo: Mary Douglas, Female Impurity, and Classical Indian Buddhism." *JAAR* 84 (1): 157–91.

—. 2017. *Birth in Buddhism: The Suffering Fetus and Female Freedom.* Abingdon-on-Thames: Routledge.

—. 2020. "Love, Unknowing, and Female Filth: The Buddhist Discourse of Birth as a Vector of Social Change for Monastic Women in Premodern South Asia." In *Transdisciplinary Perspectives on Primary Sources in the Premodern World*, ed. Elizabeth Cecil and Peter Bisschop. Berlin: De Gruyter.

—. 2021. "On Reading Vinaya: Feminist History, Hermeneutics, and Translating the Female Body." In *Translating Buddhism: Historical and Contextual Perspectives*, ed. Alice Collett. Albany, N.Y.: SUNY Press.

Laohavanich, Mano Mettanando. 2012. "Esoteric Teaching of Wat Phra Dhammakaya." *J Budd Eth* 19: 483–513. http://blogs.dickinson.edu/buddhistethics/2012/07/17/esoteric-teaching-of-wat-phra-dhammakaya/.

Latour, Bruno. 1987. *Science in Action: How to Follow Scientists and Engineers Through Society.* Cambridge, Mass.: Harvard University Press.

Lau, Ngar-sze. 2017. "Desire for Self-Healing: Lay Practice of Satipaṭṭhāna in Contemporary China." *Asian Medicine* 12 (1/2): 317–35.

—. 2021. "Teaching Transnational Buddhist Meditation with Vipassanā (*neiguan*) and Mindfulness (*zhengnian*) for Healing Depression in Contemporary China." *Religions* 12.3, https://doi.org/10.3390/rel12030212.

Lee Hyunsook. 2011. "The Medicine of Silla in East Asia." *Papers of the British Association for Korean Studies* 13: 1–16.

Lee, U-Jin, Sang-Woo Ahn, and Dong-Ryul Kim. 2019. "An Aspect of Buddhist Medicine in Korea Studied Through *The Sūtra of Great Dhāraṇī of the Uṣṇīṣa-cittā*." *Journal of Korean Medical History* 32 (1): 63–76.

Leslie, Julia. 1999. "The Implications of the Physical Body: Health, Suffering and Karma in Hindu Thought." In Hinnells and Porter 1999, 23–45.

Lewis, Mark Edward. 2009. *China's Cosmopolitan Empire: The Tang Dynasty*. Cambridge, Mass.: Belknap.

Li, Ling, and De Ma. 2017 "Avalokiteśvara and the Dunhuang Dhāraṇī Spells of Salvation in Childbirth." In *Chinese and Tibetan Esoteric Buddhism*, ed. Yael Bentor and Meir Shahar, 338–52. Leiden: Brill.

Li Rongxi. 1993. *The Biographical Scripture of King Aśoka*. Berkeley, Calif.: Numata Center.

—. 1996. *The Great Tang Dynasty Record of the Western Regions*. Berkeley, Calif.: Numata Center.

—. 2000. *Buddhist Monastic Traditions of Southern Asia: A Record of the Inner Law Sent Home from the South Seas*. Berkeley, Calif.: Numata Center.

Liétard, G. A. 1902. "Le pèlerin bouddhiste choinois I-Tsing et la médecine de l'Inde au VIIe siècle." *Bulletin de la Société française d'Histoire de la médecine* 1: 472–87.

Lim Nam-su. 2013. "The Iconography and the Tradition of the Bhaiṣajyaguru Image in the Ancient Period Korea." In *The Cult of the Healing Buddha in East Asia: Donghwasa Temple and Columbia Center for Buddhism and East Asian Religions (C-BEAR) International Conference (May 29–30, 2013)*. Daegu, South Korea: Donghwasa Temple.

Lin, Hsin-Yi. 2017. "Dealing with Childbirth in Medieval Chinese Buddhism: Discourses and Practices." PhD dissertation. Columbia University. https://academiccommons.columbia.edu/doi/10.7916/D8BK1QRX.

Lin, Li-kuang. 1935. "Puṇyodaya (Na-Ti), un propagateur du tantrisme en Chine et au Cambodge, à l'époque de Hiuan-Tsang." *Journal Asiatique* 227: 83–97.

Lipman, Kennard. 2010. *Secret Teachings of Padmasambhava: Essential Instructions on Mastering the Energies of Life*. Boston: Shambhala.

Litis, Linda. 2002. "Knowing All the Gods: Grandmothers, God Families and Women Healers in Nepal." In *Daughters of Haāritiī: Childbirth and Female Healers in South and Southeast Asia*, ed. Santi Rozario and Geoffrey Samuel, 70–89. London: Routledge.

Liu, Michael Shiyung. 2009. *Prescribing Colonization: The Role of Medical Practices and Policies in Japan-Ruled Taiwan 1895–1945*. Ann Arbor, Mich.: Association for Asian Studies.

Liu Shufen. 2006. "Jielü yu yangsheng zhijian—Tang-Song siyuan zhong de wanyao, ruyao he uaojiu." *Zhongyang yanjiuyuan lishi yuyan suo jikan* 77 (3): 357–400.

—. 2008. "Tang-Song shiqi sengren, guojia he yiliao de guanxi: Cong Yaofang Dong dao Huimin Ju." In *Cong yiliao kan Zhongguo shi*, ed. Li Jianmin, 145–202. Taipei: Lianjing chuban gongsi.

Liu Xinru. 1988. *Ancient India and Ancient China: Trade and Religious Exchanges, AD 100–600*. Delhi: Oxford University Press.

Liyanaratne, Jinadasa. 1999. *Buddhism and Traditional Medicine in Sri Lanka*. Kelaniya, Sri Lanka: Kelaniya University Press.

—. 2002–2009. *The Casket of Medicine (Bhesajjamañjūsā)*. 2 vols. Oxford: Pali Text Society.

Lloyd, Geoffrey, and Nathan Sivin. 2002. *The Way and the Word: Science and Medicine in Early China and Greece*. New Haven, Conn.: Yale University Press.

Lo, Vivienne, ed. 2007. Special issue, *Asian Medicine* 3 (2).

Lo, Vivienne, and Christopher Cullen (eds). 2005. *Medieval Chinese medicine: The Dunhuang medical manuscripts*. London: RoutledgeCurzon, 2005.

Lomi, Benedetta. 2014. "Dharanis, Talismans, and Straw-Dolls: Ritual Choreographies and Healing Strategies of the *Rokujikyōhō* in Medieval Japan." *J Jap Rel St* 41 (2): 255–304.

—. 2018. "Ox Bezoars and the Materiality of Heian-Period Therapeutics." *J Jap Rel St* 45 (2): 227–68.

Lopez, Donald S. 2008. *Buddhism and Science: A Guide for the Perplexed*. Chicago: University of Chicago Press.

—. 2012. *The Scientific Buddha: His Short and Happy Life*. New Haven, Conn.: Yale University Press.

—. 2013. *From Stone to Flesh: A Brief History of the Buddha*. Chicago: University of Chicago Press.

Lord, Donald C. 1969. *Mo Bradley and Thailand*. Grand Rapids, Mich.: Eerdmans.

Loseries-Leick, Andrea. 1997. "Psychic Sports: A Living Tradition in Contemporary Tibet?" *Tibetan Studies* 2: 583–94.

Loukota, Diego. 2019. "Made in China? Sourcing the Old Khotanese *Bhaiṣajyaguruvaiḍūryaprab hasūtra*." *JAOS* 139 (1): 67–90.

Lü Jianfu. 2017. "The Terms 'Esoteric Teaching' ('Esoteric Buddhism') and 'Tantra' in Chinese Buddhist Sources." In *Chinese and Tibetan Esoteric Buddhism*, ed. Yael Bentor and Meir Shahar, 72–81. Leiden: Brill.

Lüddeckens, Dorothea, and Monika Schrimpf, eds. 2019. *Medicine—Religion—Spirituality: Global Perspectives on Traditional, Complementary, and Alternative Healing*. Bielefeld: Transcript-Verlag.

Lusthaus, Dan. 2013. "A Note on Medicine and Psychosomatic Relations in the First Two Bhūmis of the Yogācārabhūmi." In *The Foundation for Yoga Practitioners: The Buddhist Yogacarabhumi Treatise and Its Adaptation in India, East Asia, and Tibet*, ed. Ulrich Timme Kragh, 578–95. Cambridge, Mass.: Department of South Asian Studies, Harvard University.

Mabbett, Ian. 1998. "The Problem of Historical Nagarjuna Revisited." *JAOS* 118 (3): 332–46.

MacDonald, Ariane. 1962. *Le Maṇḍala du* Mañjuśrīmūlakalpa. Paris: Adrien-Maisonneuve.

Macdonald, Keith Norman. 1879. *The Practice of Medicine Among the Burmese, Translated from Original Manuscripts, with an Historical Sketch of the Progress of Medicine, from the Earliest Times*. Edinburgh: Maclachlan & Stewart.

Macomber, Andrew. 2018. "Esoteric Moxibustion for Demonic Disease: Efficacy and Ritual Healing in Medieval Japanese Buddhism." PhD dissertation. Columbia University. https://academiccommons.columbia.edu/doi/10.7916/d8-9ear-my71.

Mahasī Sayādaw. 2009 [1976]. *Dhamma Therapy Revisited: Cases of Healing through Vipassanā Meditation*, translated by Aggacitta Bhikkhu. Taiping: Sāsanārakkha Buddhist Sanctuary.

Mai, Cuong T. 2018. "The Guanyin Fertility Cult and Family Religion in Late Imperial China: Repertoires Across Domains in the Practice of Popular Religion." *JAAR* 87 (1): 156–90.

Mair, Victor H. 1990. "[The] File [on the Cosmic] Track [and Individual] Dough[tiness]: Introduction and Notes for a Translation of the Ma-wang-tui Manuscripts of the Lao Tzu [Old Master]." *Sino-Platonic Papers* 20.

—. 2013. *China and Beyond: A Collection of Essays*. Amherst, N.Y.: Cambria.

Majupuria, Trilok Chandra. 2009. *Religious and Useful Plants of Nepal and India: Medicinal Plants and Flowers as Mentioned in Religious Myths and Legends of Hinduism and Buddhism*. New edition revised by D. P. Joshi. Saharanpur: Rohit Kumar.

Mallinson, James. 2019. "Kālavañcana in the Konkan: How a Vajrayāna Haṭhayoga Tradition Cheated Buddhism's Death in India." *Religions* 10.273, doi:10.3390/rel10040273.

Mallinson, James. 2020. "The *Amṛtasiddhi*: Haṭhayoga's Tantric Buddhist Source Text." In *Śaivism and the Tantric Traditions: Essays in Honour of Alexis G. J. S. Sanderson*, ed. Dominic Goodall, Shaman Hatley, Harunaga Isaacson, and Srilata Raman, 409–25. Leiden: Brill.

Mallinson, James, and Mark Singleton, eds. 2017. *Roots of Yoga*. London: Penguin.

Martin, Dan. 2007. "An Early Tibetan History of Indian Medicine." In Schrempf 2007, 305–25.

Martin, Dan. 2010. "Greek and Islamic Medicines' Historical Contact with Tibet: A Reassessment in View of Recently Available but Relatively Early Sources on Tibetan Medical Eclecticism." In Akasoy, Burnett and Yoeli-Tlalim 2008: 117–43.

Mather, Richard B. 1981. "The Bonze's Begging Bowl: Eating Practices in Buddhist Monasteries of Medieval India and China." *Journal of the American Oriental Society* 101 (4): 417–24.

Maue, Dieter. 2008. "An Uighur Version of Vāghaṭa's *Aṣṭāṅgahṛdayasaṃhitā*." *Asian Medicine* 4 (1): 113–73.

Mazars, Sylvain. 2008. *Le bouddhisme et la médecine traditionnelle de l'Inde*. Paris: Springer.

McBride, Richard D. 2005. "Dhāraṇī and Spells in Medieval Sinitic Buddhism." *JIABS* 28 (1): 85–114.

—. 2011. "Esoteric Buddhism and Its Relation to Healing and Demonology." In Orzech, Sørensen, and Payne 2011, 208–14.

McCall, Matthew. 2016. "Mindfulness and Psychotherapy in a Christian Context." PhD dissertation. Divine Mercy University.

McClellan, James E., and Harold Dorn. 2006. *Science and Technology in World History: An Introduction*. Baltimore, Md.: Johns Hopkins University Press.

McDaniel, Justin Thomas. 2011. *The Lovelorn Ghost and the Magical Monk: Practicing Buddhism in Modern Thailand*. New York: Columbia University Press.

McEvilley, Thomas. 2002. *The Shape of Ancient Thought: Comparative Studies in Greek and Indian Philosophies*. New York: Allworth.

McGrath, William A. 2016. "Origin Narratives of the Tibetan Medical Tradition: History, Legend, and Myth." *Asian Medicine* 12 (1/2): 295–316.

—. 2017. "Buddhism and Medicine in Tibet: Origins, Ethics, and Tradition." PhD dissertation. University of Virginia. https://libraetd.lib.virginia.edu/public_view/td96k261g.

—, ed. 2019. *Knowledge and Context in Tibetan Medicine*. Leiden: Brill.

—. 2020a. "On the Very Idea of Buddhist Medicine in Tibet." Unpublished manuscript.

—. 2020b. "Tibetan Medicine Under the Mongols: From Familial Lineages to Monastic Institutions." Unpublished manuscript.

McKay, Alex, and Dorji Wangchuk. 2005. "Traditional Medicine in Bhutan." *Asian Medicine* 1 (1): 204–18.

McMahan, David L. 2008. *The Making of Buddhist Modernism*. New York: Oxford University Press.

—. 2012. *Buddhism in the Modern World*. New York: Routledge.

—. 2017. "Buddhism and Global Secularisms." *J Glo Budd* 18: 122–28.

McMahan, David L., and Erik Braun 2017. *Meditation, Buddhism, and Science*. New York: Oxford University Press.

McNeill, William. 1998 [1976]. *Plagues and People*. New York: Anchor.

Meinert, Carmen. 2015. *Transfer of Buddhism across Central Asian Networks (7th to 13th Centuries)*. Leiden: Brill.

Men-Tsee-Khang, trans. 2011a. *The Basic Tantra and the Explanatory Tantra of Tibetan Medicine*. Dharamsala: Men-Tsee-Khang.

—, trans. 2011b. *The Subsequent Tantra from the Four Tantras of Tibetan Medicine*. Dharamsala: Men-Tsee-Khang.

Messner, Angelika, Geoffrey Samuel, Shizu Sakai, and Judith Farquhar. 2018. "The 2017 Basham Medal Lectures: Revision of the Japanese National Health Insurance in 1976." *Asian Medicine* 13 (1/2): 5–31.

Mettanando Bhikkhu. 1999. *Meditation and Healing in the Theravāda Buddhist Order of Thailand and Laos*. Hamburg, Germany: s.n.

—. 2007. "A Buddhist Model for Health Care Reform." *Journal of the Medical Association of Thailand (Chotmaihet thangphaet)* 90 (10): 2213–21.

Meulenbeld, G. Jan. 1991. "The Constraints of Theory in the Evolution of Nosological Classifications: A Study on the Position of Blood in Indian Medicine (Ayurevda)." In *Medical Literature from India, Sri Lanka and Tibet*, ed. G. Jan Meulenbeld, 91–106. Leiden: Brill.

—. 1992. "The Characteristics of a Doṣa." *Journal of the European Āyurvedic Society* 2: 1–5.

—. 1999–2002. *A History of Indian Medical Literature*. Vols. 1A–3. Groningen: Egbert Forsten.

Meyer, John-Anderson L. 2005. "Buddhism and Death: The Brain-Centered Criteria." *Journal of Buddhist Ethics* 12 https://blogs.dickinson.edu/buddhistethics/files/2010/04/meyer402.pdf.

Millard, Colin. 2007. "Tibetan Medicine and the Classification and Treatment of Mental Illness." In Schrempf 2007, 247–83.

Millward, James A. 2009. *Eurasian Crossroads: A History of Xinjiang*. New York: Columbia University Press.

Misra, R. N. 1981. *Yaksha Cult and Iconography*. Delhi: Munshiram Manoharlal.

Mitchell, Scott A., and Natalie E. F. Quli. 2015. *Buddhism Beyond Borders: New Perspectives on Buddhism in the United States*. Albany, N.Y.: SUNY Press.

Mitra, Jyotir. 1985. *A Critical Appraisal of Ayurvedic Material in Buddhist Literature with Special Reference to Tripitaka*. Varanasi: Jyotiralok Prakashan.

Miyakawa, Hisayuki. 1955. "An Outline of the Naito Hypothesis and Its Effect on Japanese Studies of China." *Far Eastern Quarterly* 14 (4): 533–52.

Miyazaki, Fumiko, and Duncan Williams. 2001. "The Intersection of the Local and the Translocal at a Sacred Site: The Case of Osorezan in Tokugawa Japan." *Japanese Journal of Religious Studies* 28.3/4: 399–440.

Mizuno, Kogen. 1995. *Buddhist Sutras: Origin, Development, Transmission*. Tokyo: Kosei.

Moerman, D. Max. 2015. "The Buddha and the Bathwater: Defilement and Enlightenment in the *Onsenji engi*." *J Jap Rel St* 42 (1): 71–87.

Mollier, Christine. 2008. *Buddhism and Taoism Face to Face: Scripture, Ritual, and Iconographic Exchange in Medieval China*. Honolulu: University of Hawai'i Press.

Monnais, Laurence, C. Michele Thompson, and Ayo Wahlberg. 2012. *Southern Medicine for Southern People: Vietnamese Medicine in the Making*. Newcastle upon Tyne: Cambridge Scholars Publishing.

Monteiro, Lynette M., Frank Musten, and Jane Compson. 2015. "Traditional and Contemporary Mindfulness: Finding the Middle Path in the Tangle of Concerns." *Mindfulness* 6 (1): 1–13.

Mrozik, Susanne. 2007. *Virtuous Bodies: The Physical Dimensions of Morality in Buddhist Ethics*. New York: Oxford University Press.

Muecke, Marjorie A. 1979. "An Explication of 'Wind Illness' in Northern Thailand." *Culture, Medicine and Psychiatry* 3 (3): 267–300.

Mueller-Dietz, Heinz E. 1996. "Stone 'Sarcophagi' and Ancient Hospitals in Sri Lanka." *Medizinhistorisches Journal* 31 (1/2): 49–65.

Muksong, Chatichai, and Komatra Chuengsatiansup. 2011. "Medicine and Public Health in Thai Historiography: From an Elitist View to Counter-Hegemonic Discourse." In *Global Movements, Local Concerns: Medicine and Health in Southeast Asia*, ed. Laurence Monnais and Harold J. Cook, 226–45. Singapore: NUS Press.

Mulholland, Jean. 1979. "Thai Traditional Medicine: Ancient Thought and Practice in a Thai Context." *Journal of the Siam Society* 67 (2): 80–115.

—. 1987. *Medicine, Magic, and Evil Spirits*. Canberra: Australian National University.

—. 1989. *Herbal Medicine in Paediatrics: Translation of a Thai Book of Genesis*. Honolulu: University of Hawai'i Press.

Mullin, Glenn H. 2006. *The Practice of the Six Yogas of Narpoa*. Ithaca, N.Y.: Snow Lion.

Myers, Neely, Sara Lewis, and Mary Ann Dutton. 2015. "Open Mind, Open Heart: An Anthropological Study of the Therapeutics of Meditation Practice in the US." *Culture, Medicine and Psychiatry* 39 (3): 487–504.

Ñāṇamoli, Bhikkhu. 1999. *The Path of Purification (Visuddhimagga) by Bhadantācariya Buddhaghosa*. Seattle, Wash.: BPS Pariyatti.

Ñanamoli, Bhikkhu, and Bhikkhu Bodhi. 1995. *The Middle Length Discourses of the Buddha: A Translation of the Majjhima Nikaya*. Boston: Wisdom.

Nappi, Carla. 2009. "Bolatu's Pharmacy: Theriac in Early Modern China." *Early Science and Medicine* 14 (6): 737–64.

Naqvi, Nasim H. 2011. *A Study of Buddhist Medicine and Surgery in Gandhara*. Delhi: Motilal Banarsidass.

Narain, A. K. 1957. *The Indo-Greeks*. Oxford: Clarendon.

Nattier, Jan. 1990. "Church Language and Vernacular Language in Central Asian Buddhism." *Numen* 37 (2): 195–219.

—. 2000. "*The Teaching of Vimalakīrti (Vimalakīrtinirdeśa)*: A Review of Four English Translations." *Buddhist Literature* 2: 234–58.

Needham, Joseph. 2000. *Science and Civilisation in China*, vol. 6, *Biology and Biological Technology*, part 6, *Medicine*, ed. Nathan Sivin. Cambridge: Cambridge University Press.

Neelis, Jason. 2011. *Early Buddhist Transmission and Trade Networks: Mobility and Exchange Within and Beyond the Northwestern Borderlands of South Asia*. Leiden: Brill.

Nguyen, Duy Hinh. 1990. "Three Legends and Early Buddhism in Vietnam." *Vietnam Forum* 13: 10–23.

Nguyen, Huong. 2014. "Buddhism-Based Exorcism and Spirit-Calling as a Form of Healing for Mental Problems: Stories from Vietnam." *Journal of Religion & Spirituality in Social Work: Social Thought* 33 (1): 33–48.

Nivat, Dhani. 1933. "The Inscriptions of Wat Phra Jetubon." *Journal of the Siam Society* 26 (2): 143–70.

Nobel, Johannes. 1951. "Ein alter Medizinischer Sanskrit-Text und seine Deutung." *JAOS* suppl. 11.

Norbu, Chogyal Namkhai. 2008. *Yantra Yoga: The Tibetan Yoga of Movement*. Ithaca, N.Y.: Snow Lion.

Noree, Thinakorn, Johanna Hanefeld, and Richard Smith. 2016. "Medical Tourism in Thailand: A Cross-Sectional Study." *Bulletin of the World Health Organization* 94 (1): 30–36.

Norman, K. R. 2006. *A Philological Approach to Buddhism: The Bukkyō Dendō Kyōkai Lectures 1994*. 2nd ed. Lancaster, Lancashire, UK: Pali Text Society.

Norov, Batsaikhan. 2019. "Mongolian Buddhist Scholars' Works on Infectious Diseases (Late 17th Century to the Beginning of the 20th Century)" *Religions* 10 (4): 229. https://doi.org/10.3390/rel10040229.

Numrich, P. D. 2005. "Complementary and Alternative Medicine in America's 'Two Buddhisms.'" In *Religion and Healing in America*, ed. Linda L. Barnes and Susan S. Sered, 343–58. Oxford and New York: Oxford University Press.

Obadia, Lionel. 2015. "Buddhism: Modernization or Globalization?" In *Routledge Handbook of Religions in Asia*, ed. Bryan S. Turner and Oscar Salemink, 343–58. Abingdon: Routledge.

Obeyesekere, Gananath. 1969. "The Ritual Drama of the Sanni Demons: Collective Representations of Disease in Ceylon." *Comparative Studies in Society and History* 11 (2): 174–216.

—. 1970. "The Idiom of Demonic Possession." *Social Science & Medicine* 4: 97–111.

O'Brien, Patrick Karl. 2003. *Oxford Atlas of World History*. New York: Oxford University Press.

Ohnuma, Reiko. 2004. "Why the Buddha Had Good Digestion." In *Buddhist Scriptures*, ed. Donald S. Lopez Jr., 136–41. London: Penguin.

Okuda, Jun, Yukio Noro, and Shiro Ito. 2005. "Les pots de médicament de Yakushi Bouddha (Bouddha de la Guérison) au Japon." *Revue d'histoire de la pharmacie* 93 (345): 7–32.

Olivelle, Patrick. 2017. "The Medical Profession in Ancient India: Its Social, Religious, and Legal Status." *eJournal of Indian Medicine* 9: 1–21.

Orzech, Charles. 1998. *Politics and Transcendent Wisdom: The Scripture for Humane Kings in the Creation of Chinese Buddhism*. College Park: Pennsylvania State University Press.

—. 2006. "Looking for Bhairava: Exploring the Circulation of Esoteric Texts Produced by the Song Institute for Canonical Translation." *Pacific World* 8: 139–66.

Orzech, Charles D., and James H. Sanford. 2000. "Worship of the Ladies of the Dipper." In *Tantra in Practice*, ed. David Gordon White. Princeton, N.J.: Princeton University Press.

Orzech, Charles D., Henrik H. Sørensen, and Richard K. Payne, eds. 2011. *Esoteric Buddhism and the Tantras in East Asia*. Leiden and Boston: Brill.

Ovesen, Jan, and Ing-Britt Trankell. 2010. *Cambodians and Their Doctors: A Medical Anthropology of Colonial and Post-colonial Cambodia*. Copenhagen: NIAS.

Ozawa-De Silva, Brendan R., Brooke Dodson-Lavelle, Charles L. Raison, and Lobsang Tenzin Negi. 2012. "Compassion and Ethics: Scientific and Practical Approaches to the Cultivation of Compassion as a Foundation for Ethical Subjectivity and Well-Being." *Journal of Healthcare, Science and the Humanities* 2 (1): 145–61.

Ozawa-De Silva, Chikako, and Brendan R. Ozawa-De Silva. 2011. "Mind/Body Theory and Practice in Tibetan Medicine and Buddhism." *Body & Society* 17 (1): 95–119.

Palmer, David A. 2007. *Qigong Fever: Body, Science, and Utopia in China*. New York: Columbia University Press.

Paonil, Wichit, and Luechai Sringernyuang. 2002. "Buddhist Perspectives on Health and Healing." *Chulalongkorn Journal of Buddhist Studies* 1 (2): 93–105.

Parfionovitch, Yuri, Gyurme Dorje, and Fernand Meyer. 1992. *Tibetan Medical Paintings: Illustrations to the Blue Beryl Treatise of Sangye Gyamtso (1653–1705)*. New York: Abrams.

Patton, Thomas N. 2016. "The Wizard King's Granddaughters: Burmese Buddhist Female Mediums, Healers, and Dreamers." *JAAR* 84 (2): 430–65.

——. 2018. *The Buddha's Wizards: Magic, Protection, and Healing in Burmese Buddhism*. New York: Columbia University Press.

Paul, Diana Y., and John R. McRae. 2005. *The Sutra of Queen Śrīmālā of the Lion's Roar and the Vimalakīrti Sutra*. Berkeley, Calif.: BDK America.

Penny, Benjamin. 2012. *The Religion of Falun Gong*. Chicago: University of Chicago Press.

Peri, Noel. 1917. "Hārītī la mère de demons." *BEFEO* 17: 1–101.

Poceski, Mario. 2014. *The Wiley Blackwell Companion to East and Inner Asian Buddhism*. Chichester, West Sussex, UK: Wiley.

Pols, Hans, Michele Thompson, and John Harley Warner, eds. 2017. *Translating the Body: Medical Education in Southeast Asia*. Singapore: National University of Singapore Press.

Popp, Richard L. 1985. "American Missionaries and the Introduction of Western Science and Medicine in Thailand, 1830–1900." *Missiology: An International Review* 8 (2): 147–57.

Pordié, Laurent. 2003. "The Expression of Religion in Tibetan Medicine: Ideal Conceptions, Contemporary Practices and Political Use." *Pondy Papers in Social Sciences* 29.

——. 2007. "Buddhism in the Everyday Medical Practice of the Ladakhi 'Amchi.' " *Indian Anthropologist* 37 (1): 93–116.

Porter, Roy. 1999. *The Greatest Benefit to Mankind: A Medical History of Humanity*. New York: Norton.

Powers, John. 2016a. *The Buddhist World*. Abingdon: Routledge.

——. 2016b. "Thich Nhat Hanh." In Powers 2016a, 617–28.

——. 2016c. "Tenzin Gyatso, the Fourteenth Dalai Lama." In Powers 2016a, 629–40.

Pranke, Patrick. 1995. "On Becoming a Buddhist Wizard." In *Buddhism in Practice*, ed. Donald S. Lopez Jr., 343–58. Princeton, N.J.: Princeton University Press.

Pratt, Mary Louise. 1991. "Arts of the Contact Zone." *Profession* 91: 33–40.

Prematilleke, L. 1996. "Ancient Monastic Hospital System in Sri Lanka." In *Ancient Trades and Cultural Contacts in Southeast Asia*, ed. A. Srisuchat, 115–26. Bangkok: Office of the National Culture Commission.

Puaksom, Davisakd. 2007. "Of Germs, Public Hygiene, and the Healthy Body: The Making of the Medicalizing State of Thailand." *Journal of Asian Studies* 66 (2): 311–44.

Puente-Ballesteros, Beatriz. 2011. "Jesuit Medicine in the Kangxi Court (1662–1722): Imperial Networks and Patronage." *EASTM* 34: 86–162.

Purser, Ronald. 2019. *McMindfulness.* London: Repeater.

Purser, Ronald E., David Forbes, and Adam Burke, eds. 2016. *Handbook of Mindfulness: Culture, Context, and Social Engagement.* n.p.: Springer.

Pye, Michael. 1978. *Skillful Means: A Concept in Mahāyāna Buddhism.* London: Duckworth.

—. 2002. "Won Buddhism as a Korean New Religion." *Numen* 49.2: 113–41.

Radich, Michael. 2007. "The Somatics of Liberation: Ideas About Embodiment in Buddhism from Its Origins to the Fifth Century C.E." PhD dissertation. Harvard University.

—. 2016. "Perfected Embodiment: A Buddhist-Inspired Challenge to Contemporary Theories of the Body." In *Refiguring the Body: Embodiment in South Asian Religions*, ed. Barbara A. Holdrege and Karen Pechelis, 17–58. Albany, N.Y.: SUNY Press.

Raj, Kapil. 2016. "Go-Betweens, Travelers, and Cultural Translators." In *A Companion to the History of Science*, ed. Bernard Lightman, 39–57. London: Wiley.

Rambelli, Fabio. 2000. "Tantric Buddhism and Chinese Thought in East Asia." In *Tantra in Practice*, ed. David G. White, Princeton, N.J., and Oxford: Princeton University Press.

Ramble, Charles, and Ulrike Roesler. 2015. *Tibetan and Himalayan Healing: An Anthology for Anthony Aris.* Kathmandu: Vajra.

Ratanakul, Pinit. 1999a. "Buddhist Health Care Ethics." In *A Cross-Cultural Dialogue on Health Care Ethics*, ed. Harold G. Coward and Pinit Ratanakul, 119–27. Waterloo, Ont.: Wilfrid Laurier University Press.

—. 1999b. "Buddhism, Health, Disease, and Thai Culture." In *A Cross-Cultural Dialogue on Health Care Ethics*, ed. Harold G. Coward and Pinit Ratanakul, 17–33. Waterloo, Ont.: Wilfrid Laurier University Press.

—. 2004. "The Buddhist Concept of Life, Suffering and Death, and Related Bioethical Issues." *Eubios Journal of Asian and International Bioethics* 14: 141–46.

Ratarasarn, Somchintana Thongthew. 1989. *The Principles and Concepts of Thai Classical Medicine.* Bangkok: Thai Khadi Research Institute, Thammasat University.

Reddy, Subba. 1938. "Glimpses Into the Practice and Principles of Medicine in Buddhistic India in the 7th Century A.D. Gleaned from 'The Records of Buddhist Religion' by the Chinese Monk I-Tsing." *Bulletin of the Indian Institute of History and Medicine* 17: 155–67.

Rees, Gethin, and Fumitaka Yoneda. 2013. "Celibate Monks and Foteus-Stealing Gods: Buddhism and Pregnancy at the Jetavana Monastery, Shravasti, India." *World Archaeology* 45 (2): 252–71.

Rhys Davids, T. W. 1965 [1894]. *The Questions of King Milinda.* New Deli: Motilal Banarsidass.

Richter, Antje. 2020. "Teaching from the Sickbed: Ideas of Illness and Healing in the *Vimalakīrti Sūtra* and Their Reception in Medieval Chinese Literature." In Salguero and Macomber 2020, 57–90.

Ritzinger, Justin. 2017. *Anarchy in the Pure Land: Reinventing the Cult of Maitreya in Modern Chinese Buddhism.* New York: Oxford University Press.

Robinson, Richard H., Williard L. Johnson, and Thanissaro Bhikkhu [Geoffrey DeGraff]. 2011. *Buddhist Religions: A Historical Introduction.* 5th ed. Belmont, Calif.: Thompson Wadsworth.

Robson, James. 2011. "Mediums in Esoteric Buddhism." In Orzech, Sørensen, and Payne 2011: 251–54.

—. 2014. "The Buddha Image Inside-Out: On the Placing of Objects Inside Statues in East Asia." In Sen 2014: 291–308.

Roudometof, Victor. 2016. *Glocalization: A Critical Introduction.* New York: Routledge.

Rozenburg, Guillaume. 2012. "Powerful Yet Powerless, Powerless Yet Powerful: The Burmese Exorcist." *J Burma St* 16 (2): 251–82.

Rozenberg, Guillaume, and George J. Tanabe. 2015. *The Immortals: Faces of the Incredible in Buddhist Burma*, translated by Ward Keeler. Honolulu: University of Hawai'i Press.

Ruegg, David Seyfort. 2008. *The Symbiosis of Buddhism with Brahmanism/Hinduism in South Asia and of Buddhism with "Local Cults" in Tibet and the Himalayan Region.* Vienna: Verlag der Österreichischen Akademie der Wissenschaften.

Ruppert, Brian D. 2000. *Jewel in the Ashes: Buddha Relics and Power in Early Medieval Japan.* Cambridge, Mass.: Harvard University Asia Center.

Sadakata, Akira. 1997. *Buddhist Cosmology: Philosophy and Origins.* Tokyo: Kosei.

Saha, Kshanika. 1985. *Indian Medical Text in Central Asia.* Calcutta: Firma KLM.

Sahni, Pragati. 2008. *Environmental Ethics in Buddhism: A Virtues Approach.* London: Routledge.

Salemink, Oscar. 2015. "Spirit Worship and Possession in Vietnam and Beyond." In *Routledge Handbook of Religions in Asia*, ed. Bryan S. Turner and Oscar Salemink, 231–46. London: Routledge.

Salgado, Nirmala S. 1997. "Sickness, Healing, and Religious Vocation: Alternative Choices at a Theravada Buddhist Nunnery." *Ethnology* 36 (3): 213–27.

Salguero, C. Pierce. 2009. "The Buddhist Medicine King in Literary Context: Reconsidering an Early Medieval Example of Indian Influence on Chinese Medicine and Surgery," *History of Religions* 48 (3): 183–210.

—. 2010–11. "Mixing Metaphors: Translating the Indian Medical Doctrine Tridoṣa in Chinese Buddhist Sources." *Asian Medicine* 6: 55–74.

—. 2013. "Fields of Merit, Harvests of Health: Some Notes on the Role of Medical Karma in the Popularization of Buddhism in Early Medieval China." *Asian Philosophy* 23 (4): 341–49.

—. 2014a. *Translating Buddhist Medicine in Medieval China.* Philadelphia: University of Pennsylvania Press.

—. 2014b. "Medicine." *Oxford Biblio.* https://doi.org/10.1093/obo/9780195393521-0140.

—. 2015a. "Reexamining the Categories and Canons of Chinese Buddhist Healing," *JCBS* 28: 35–66.

—. 2015b. "Toward a Global History of Buddhism and Medicine." *Budd St Rev* 32 (1): 35–61.

—. 2016. *Traditional Thai Medicine: Buddhism, Animism, Yoga, Ayurveda.* Revised ed. Bangkok: White Lotus.

—. 2017. "Honoring the Teachers, Constructing the Tradition: The Role of History and Religion in the Waikrū Ceremony of a Thai Traditional Medicine Hospital." In Pols, Thompson, and Warner 2017, 295–318.

—. 2018a. "Healing and/or Salvation? The Relationship Between Religion and Medicine in Medieval Chinese Buddhism." Working Paper Series of the HCAS: Multiple Secularities—Beyond the West, Beyond Modernities 4.

—. 2018b. "Buddhist Medicine and Its Circulation." In *Oxford Research Encyclopedia of Asian History*, ed. David Ludden. New York: Oxford University Press.

—. 2018c. "'This Fathom-Long Body': Bodily Materiality and Ascetic Ideology in Medieval Chinese Buddhist Scriptures," *Bulletin of the History of Medicine* 92: 237–60.

—. 2018d. "A Missing Link in the History of Chinese Medicine: A Research Note on the Medical Contents in the Chinese Buddhist *Taishō Tripiṭaka.*" *EASTM* 47: 93–119.

—. 2019. "Varieties of Buddhist Healing in Multiethnic Philadelphia," *Religions* 10 (1): 48. https://doi.org/10.3390/rel10010048.

—. 2020a. " 'A Flock of Ghosts Bursting Forth and Scattering': Healing Narratives in a Sixth-Century Chinese Buddhist Hagiography." In Salguero and Macomber 2020, 23–56.

—. 2020b. "Countercurrents and Counterappropriations: Western Mindfulness and Traditional Korean Medicine." *Asian Medicine* 15 (2): 291–300.

Salguero, C. Pierce, and Andrew Macomber, eds. 2020. *Buddhist Healing in Medieval China and Japan*. Honolulu: University of Hawai'i Press.

Salguero, C. Pierce, and William A. McGrath, eds. 2017. "Buddhism and Healing." Special issue, *Asian Medicine* 12 (1–2).

Salguero, C. Pierce, et al. 2017. "Medicine in the Chinese Buddhist Canon: Selected Translations." *Asian Medicine* 12 (1/2): 79–294.

Salomon, Richard. 1999. *Ancient Buddhist Scrolls from Gandhara: The British Library Kharosthi Fragments*. Seattle: University of Washington Press.

Samuel, Geoffrey. 1989. "The Body in Buddhist and Hindu Tantra: Some Notes." *Religion* 19: 197–210.

—. 1999. "Religion, Health and Suffering Among Contemporary Tibetans." In Hinnells and Porter 1999, 85–110.

—. 2001. "Tibetan Medicine in Contemporary India: Theory and Practice." In *Healing Powers and Modernity: Traditional Medicine, Shamanism, and Science in Asian Societies*, ed. Linda H. Connor and Geoffrey Samuel, 247–73. Westport, Conn.: Bergin & Garvey.

—. 2008. *The Origins of Yoga and Tantra: Indic Religions to the Thirteenth Century*. Cambridge: Cambridge University Press.

—. 2010. "A Short History of Indo-Tibetan Alchemy." In *Studies of Medical Pluralism in Tibetan History and Society: Proceedings from the XIth International Association of Tibetan Studies Meetings*, ed. Sienna Craig, Mingji Cuomu, Frances Garrett, and Mona Schrempf, 221–33. Bonn: International Institute for Tibetan and Buddhist Studies.

—. 2012a. "Amitāyus and the Development of Tantric Practices for Longevity and Health in Tibet." In *Transformations and Transfer of Tantra in Asia and Beyond*, ed. István Keul, 263–86. Berlin: De Gruyter.

—. 2012b. *Introducing Tibetan Buddhism*. Oxon: Routledge.

—. 2013. "The Subtle Body in India and Beyond." In Samuel and Johnson 2013: 33–47.

—. 2014a. "Healing in Tibetan Buddhism." In Poceski 2014, 278–96.

—. 2014b. "Between Buddhism and Science, Between Mind and Body." *Religions* 2014 (5): 560–79.

—. 2014c. "Body and Mind in Tibetan Medicine and Tantric Buddhism." In Hofer 2014: 32–45.

—. 2015. "The Contemporary Mindfulness Movement and the Question of Nonself." *Transcultural Psychiatry* 52 (4): 485–500.

—. 2016. "Tibetan Longevity Meditation." In *Asian Traditions of Meditation*, ed. Halvor Eifring, 145–64. Honolulu: University of Hawai'i Press.

Samuel, Geoffrey, and Jay Johnson, eds. 2013. *Religion and the Subtle Body in Asia and the West: Between Mind and Body*. London: Routledge.

Samuels, Jeffrey. 2016. "Buddhist Disaster Relief: Monks, Networks, and the Politics of Religion." *Asian Ethnology* 75 (1): 53–74.

Saowapa, Pornsiripongse. 2010. "Religious Syncretism in Healing Non-communicable Diseases: The Role of Folk Healer Monks." *Mon-Khmer Studies* 39: 167–76.

Schaeffer, Kurtis R. 2003a. "The Attainment of Immortality: From Nathas in India to Buddhists in Tibet." *J Ind Phil* 30: 515–33.

—. 2003b. "Textual Scholarship, Medical Tradition, and Mahayana Buddhist Ideals in Tibet." *J Ind Phil* 31: 621–41.

Schafer, Edward H. 1963. *The Golden Peaches of Samarkand: A Study of T'ang Exotics*. Berkeley, Calif.: University of California Press.

Scharfe, Hartmut. 1999. "The Doctrine of the Three Humors in Traditional Indian Medicine and the Alleged Antiquity of Tamil Siddha Medicine," *JAOS* 119 (4): 609–29.

—. 2002. *Education in Ancient India*. Leiden: Brill.

Scheid, Volker. 2020. "The Neglected Role of Buddhism in the Development of Medicine in Late Imperial China Viewed Through the Life and Work of Yu Chang." *Bulletin of the History of Medicine* 94 (1): 1–28.

Schopen, Gregory. 1978. "The *Bhaiṣajyaguru-Sūtra* and the Buddhism of Gilgit." PhD dissertation. Australian National University. https://openresearch-repository.anu.edu.au/handle/1885/109328.

—. 2004. *Buddhist Monks and Business Matters: Still More Papers on Monastic Buddhism in India*. Honolulu: University of Hawai'i Press.

Schottenhammer, Angela. 2013. "Huihui Medicine and Medicinal Drugs in Yuan China." In *Proceedings of the International Workshop "Eurasian Influences on Yuan China: Cross-Cultural Transmissions in the 13th and 14th Centuries,"* ed. Morris Rossabi, 75–102. Singapore: National University of Singapore Press.

Schrempf, Mona, ed. 2007. *Soundings in Tibetan Medicine: Anthropological and Historical Perspectives*. Leiden: Brill.

Schrempf, Mona, and Nicola Schneider, eds. 2015. Special issue (*Women as Visionaries, Healers and Agents of Social Transformation in the Himalayas, Tibet and Mongolia*), *Revue d'Etudes Tibétaines*, 34.

Schrimpf, Monika. 2019. "Medical Discourses and Practices in Contemporary Japanese Religions." in Lüddeckens and Schrimpf 2019, 57–90.

Sehnalova, Anna. 2017. "Tibetan Bonpo Mendrup: The Precious Formula's Transmission." *Hist Sci SA* 5 (2): 143–80.

Sen, Tansen. 2001. "In Search of Longevity and Good Karma: Chinese Diplomatic Missions to Middle India in the Seventh Century." *Journal of World History* 12 (1): 1–28.

Sen, Tansen. 2003. *Buddhism, Diplomacy, and Trade: The Realignment of Sino-Indian Relations, 600–1400*. Honolulu: Association for Asian Studies and University of Hawai'i Press.

—, ed. 2014. *Buddhism Across Asia: Networks of Material, Intellectual, and Cultural Exchange*. Singapore: Institute of Southeast Asian Studies.

—. 2018. "Yijing and the Buddhist Cosmopolis of the Seventh Century." In *Texts and Transformations: Essays in Honor of the 75th Birthday of Victor H. Mair*, ed. Haun Saussy, 345–68. Amherst, N.Y.: Cambria.

Sengupta, Sukumar. 1989. "Medical Data in the *Milindapañha*." In *Dr. B. M. Barua Birth Centenary Commemoration Volume*, ed. Hemendu Bikash Chowduhury, 111–17. Calcutta: Bengal Buddhist Association.

Shahar, Meir. 2008. *The Shaolin Monastery: History, Religion, and the Chinese Martial Arts*. Honolulu: University of Hawai'i Press.

Sharf, Robert H. 2015. "Is Mindfulness Buddhist? (and Why it Matters)." *Transcultural Psychiatry* 52.4: 470–84.

Sharma, Arvind. 2002. "On Hindu, Hindustān, Hinduism and Hindutva." *Numen* 49 (1): 1–36.

Sharrock, Peter. 2014, July 1. " 'The Grief of Kings Is the Suffering of Their People': The Imperial Mission of the Cambodian Buddha of Medicine." Paper presented at the annual conference of the UK Association of Buddhist Studies, Leeds, Yorkshire, UK, July 1–2, 2014.

Shaw, Miranda. 2005. *Buddhist Goddesses of India*. Princeton, N.J.: Princeton University Press.

Shi Yongxin and Li Liangsong, eds. 2011. *Zhongguo Fojiao yiyao quanshu*, 101 vols. Beijing: Zhongguo shudian.

Shi Zhiru 2020. "Lighting Lamps to Prolong Life: Ritual Healing and the Bhaiṣajyaguru Cult in Fifth- and Sixth-Century China." In Salguero and Macomber 2020, 91–117.

Shinmura Taku. 2013. *Nihon bukkyō no iryōshi*. Tokyo: Hōsei daigaku shuppankyoku.

Shinno, Reiko. 2016. *The Politics of Chinese Medicine Under Mongol Rule*. Oxon: Routledge.

Shinohara, Koichi. 2007. "The Moment of Death in Daoxuan's Vinaya Commentary." In *The Buddhist Dead: Practices, Discourses, Representations*, ed. Bryan J. Cuevas and Jacqueline Stone, 105–33. Honolulu: University of Hawai'i Press.

—. 2014. *Spells, Images, and Mandalas: Tracing the Evolution of Esoteric Buddhist Rituals*. New York: Columbia University Press.

Sik Hin Tak. 2016. "Ancient Indian Medicine in Early Buddhist Literature: A Study Based on the *Bhesajjakkhandhaka* and the Parallels in Other Vinaya Canons." PhD dissertation. University of Hong Kong. http://hub.hku.hk/handle/10722/241256.

Silk, Jonathan A. 2015. *Brill's Encyclopedia of Buddhism*, vol. 1, *Literature and Languages*. Leiden: Brill.

Singleton, Mark. 2010. *Yoga Body: The Origins of Modern Posture Practice*. New York: Oxford University Press.

Sinor, Denis. 1995. "Languages and Cultural Interchange Along the Silk Road." *Diogenes* 43 (171): 1–13.

Sivin, Nathan. 1995. "Emotional Counter-Therapy." In *Medicine, Philosophy and Religion in Ancient China: Researches and Reflections*, section 2, ed. Nathan Sivin, 2–19. Aldershot, UK: Variorum.

Skjaervø, Prods Oktor. 2004. *This Most Excellent Shine of Gold, King of Kings of Sutras: The Khotanese Suvarṇabhāsottamasūtra*. Cambridge, Mass.: Harvard University Department of Near Eastern Languages and Civilizations.

Slouber, Michael. 2017. *Early Tantric Medicine: Snakebite, Mantras, and Healing in the Gāruḍa Tantras*. New York: Oxford University Press.

Smith, Frederick. 2006. *The Self Possessed: Deity and Spirit Possession in South Asian Literature and Civilization*. New York: Columbia University Press.

Smith, Philip Daniel. 2005. *Cultural Theory: An Introduction*. Malden, Mass.: Blackwell.

Snellgrove, D. L. 1959. *The Hevajra Tantra: A Critical Study*. London: Oxford University Press.

Snellgrove, David. 1987. *Indo-Tibetan Buddhism: Indian Buddhists and Their Tibetan Successors*. Boston: Shambhala.

Sodargye, Khenpo, and Dan Smyer Yü. 2017. "Revisioning Buddhism as a Science of the Mind in a Secularized China: A Tibetan Perspective." *J Glo Budd* 18: 91–111.

Somerville, Margaret, and Tony Perkins. 2003. "Border Work in the Contact Zone: Thinking Indigenous/Non-Indigenous Collaboration Spatially." *International Journal of Intercultural Studies* 24 (3): 253–66.

Sopa, Geshe Lhundup. 1983. "An Excursus on the Subtle Body in Tantric Buddhism (Notes Contextualizing the Kālacakra)." *JIABS* 6 (2): 48–66.

Soper, Alexander Coburn, and Seigai Ōmura. 1959. *Literary Evidence for Early Buddhist Art in China.* Ascona: Artibus Asiae.

Souk-Aloum, Phou Ngeum. 2001. *La médecine du bouddhisme théravada au Laos.* Paris: L'Harmattan.

Srivastava, Usha. 2011. *Encyclopaedia of Indian Medicine.* New Delhi: DPS.

Stablein, William G. 1973. "A Medical-Cultural System Among the Tibetan and Newar Buddhists: Ceremonial Medicine." *Kailash* 1 (3): 193–202.

—. 1976a. "The *Mahākālatantra*: A Theory of Ritual Blessings and Tantric Medicine." PhD dissertation. Columbia University.

—. 1976b. "Tibetan Medical-Cultural System." In *An Introduction to Tibetan Medicine*, ed. Dawa Norbu, 39–51. Delhi: Tibetan Review.

—. 1980. "The Medical Soteriology of Karma in the Buddhist Tantric Tradition." In *Karma and Rebirth in Classical Indian Traditions*, ed. Wendy Doniger, 193–216. Berkeley: University of California Press.

Stanley, Philip. 2014. "The Tibetan Buddhist Canon." In Poceski 2014, 383–407.

Stanley, Steven. 2012. "Mindfulness: Towards a Critical Relational Perspective." *Social and Personality Psychology Compass* 6 (9): 631–41.

Stanley-Baker, Michael. 2019a. "Daoing Medicine: Practice Theory for Considering Religion and Medicine in Early Imperial China." *EASTM* 50: 13–59.

—. 2019b. "New Tools to Study Ancient Drugs: At the Crossroads of Medicine, History and Linguistics." *Pushing Frontiers* 15: 22–23.

Starkey, Caroline, and Matt Coward-Gibbs, eds. 2018. Special focus, "Translating Buddhism," *J Glo Budd* 19: 39–125.

Stearns, Cyrus. 2001. *Luminous Lives: The Story of the Early Masters of the Lam 'bras Tradition in Tibet.* Boston: Wisdom.

Steavu, Dominic. 2017. "Buddhism, Medicine, and the Affairs of the Heart: Potency Therapy (Vājīkarana) and the Reappraisal of Aphrodisiacs and Love Philters in Medieval Chinese Sources." *EASTM* 45: 9–48.

Stein, Justin B. 2017. "Hawayo Takata and the Circulatory Development of Reiki in the Twentieth Century North Pacific." PhD dissertation. University of Toronto. https://tspace.library.utoronto.ca/handle/1807/98803.

Stone, Jacqueline I. 2008. "With the Help of 'Good Friends': Deathbed Ritual Practices in Early Medieval Japan." In *Death and the Afterlife in Japanese Buddhism*, ed. Jacqueline I. Stone and Mariko Namba Walter, 61–101. Honolulu: University of Hawai'i Press.

—. 2016. *Right Thoughts at the Last Moment: Buddhism and Deathbed Practices in Early Medieval Japan.* Honolulu: Kuroda Institute, University of Hawai'i Press.

Storch, Tanya. 2014. *The History of Chinese Buddhist Bibliography: Censorship and Transformation of the Tripitaka.* Amherst, N.Y.: Cambria.

Streicher, Ruth, and Adrian Hermann. 2019. "'Religion' in Thailand in the 19th Century." In *Companion to the Study of Secularity*, ed. the Humanities Centre for Advanced Studies, Leipzig University. http://www.multiple-secularities.de/publications/companion/religion-in-thailand-in-the-19th-century/.

Strickmann, Michel. 1996. *Mantras et mandarins: Le bouddhisme tantrique en Chine.* Paris: Gallimard.

—. 2002. *Chinese Magical Medicine*, ed. Bernard Faure. Stanford, Calif.: Stanford University Press.

Strong, John S. 1979. "The Legend of the Lion-Roarer: A Study of the Buddhist Arhat Piṇḍola Bharadvaja." *Numen* 26 (1): 50–88.

—. 1983. *The Legend of King Aśoka: A Study and Translation of the Aśokāvadāna.* Princeton, N.J.: Princeton University Press.

—. 2012. "Explicating the Buddha's Final Illness in the Context of His Other Ailments: The Making and Unmaking of Some *Jātaka* Tales." *Budd St Rev* 29 (1): 17–33.

Stuart, Daniel M. 2017. "Insight Transformed: Coming to Terms with Mindfulness in South Asian and Global Frames." *Religions of South Asia* 11 (2/3): 158–81.

—. 2020. *S. N. Goenka: Emissary of Insight.* Boulder, Colo.: Shambhala.

Sudarshan, S. R., ed. 2005. *Encyclopaedia of Indian Medicine*, vol. 4, *Materia Medica—Herbal Drugs.* Bangalore: Popular Prakashan.

Sulek, Emilia. 2006. "Imagining Tibet in Poland: A Contribution to Anthropology of Imagined Countries." *Tibet Journal* 31 (2): 49–68.

Suzuki, Yui. 2012. *Medicine Master Buddha: The Iconic Worship of Yakushi in Heian Japan.* Leiden: Brill.

Swanson, Paul. 2017. *Clear Serenity, Quiet Insight: T'ien-T'ai Chih-I's Mo-Ho Chih-Kuan.* 3 vols. Honolulu: University of Hawai'i Press.

Swartz, David. 2009. *Culture and Power: The Sociology of Pierre Bourdieu.* Chicago: University of Chicago Press.

Taee, Jonathan. 2017. *The Patient Multiple: An Ethnography of Healthcare and Decision-Making in Bhutan.* New York: Berghahn.

Takakusu Junjirō. 1966 [1896]. *A Record of the Buddhist Religion as Practiced in India and the Malay Archipelago (AD 671–695) by I-Tsing.* Delhi: Munshiram Manoharlal.

Takakusu, Junjirō, and Watanabe Kaikyoku (eds.) (1924-1935), *Taishō shinshū daizōkyō*, 85 vols., Tokyo: Issaikyō kankōkai.

Tambiah, Stanley J. 1984. *The Buddhist Saints of the Forest and the Cult of Amulets.* Cambridge: Cambridge University Press.

Taylor, G. 1887. "Chinese Folk Lore." *The China Review, or, Notes and Queries on the Far East* 16: 163–77.

Taylor, Kim. 2005. *Chinese Medicine in Early Communist China, 1945–63: A Medicine of Revolution.* London and New York: RoutledgeCurzon.

Teiser, Stephen F. 2009. "Ornamenting the Departed: Notes on the Language of Chinese Buddhist Ritual Texts." *Asia Major* 22 (1): 201–37.

Ṭhānissaro Bhikkhu [Geoffrey DeGraff]. 2007. *The Buddhist Monastic Code II: The Khandhaka Training Rules Translated and Explained.* Valley Center, Calif.: Metta Forest Monastery.

Thompson, Ashley. 2004. "The Suffering of Kings: Substitute Bodies, Healing, and Justice in Cambodia." In *History, Buddhism and New Religious Movements in Cambodia*, ed. John Marston and Elizabeth Guthrie, Elizabeth, 91–112. Honolulu: University of Hawai'i Press.

Thompson, C. Michele. 2014, March 29. "The Travels and Travails of Tuệ Tĩnh, a Gift from the Royal Court of the Trần to the Royal Court of the Ming." Paper presented at the annual conference of the Association for Asian Studies, Philadelphia, Pa., March 27–30, 2014.

Thurman, Robert A. F. 2003. *The Holy Teaching of Vimalakīrti: A Mahāyāna Scripture.* University Park, Pa.: Penn State University Press.

Tidwell, Tawni. 2020. "The Role of Blood and Chuser in How Biomedical Cancer Maps Into Tibetan Medical Nosology: Facilitating Collaborative Research Foundations." *Asian Medicine* 15 (2): 209–50.

Tomecko, Denise. 2009. *Buddhist Healing in Laos: Plants of the Fragrant Forest.* Bangkok: Orchid.

Toneatto, Tony. 2018. "Re-contextualizing Mindfulness Meditation: Integrating Traditional Buddhist and Contemporary Approaches to Healing and Well-Being." *International Journal of Traditional Healing & Critical Mental Health* 1 (1): 34–47.

Triplett, Katja. 2010. "Esoteric Buddhist Eye-Healing Rituals in Japan and the Promotion of Benefits." In *Grammars and Morphologies of Ritual Practices in Asia*, section 2, ed. Lucia Dole, Gil Raz, and Katja Triplett, 485–97. Wiesbaden: Harrassowitz.

—. 2012. "Magical Medicine? Japanese Buddhist Medical Knowledge and Ritual Instruction for Healing the Physical Body." In Kleine and Triplett 2012: 63–92.

—. 2013. "Healing Rituals in Contemporary Japanese Esoteric Buddhism as Acts of Individual and Collective Purification." In *Purification: Religious Transformations of Body and Mind*, ed. Gerhard Marcel Martin and Katja Triplett, 107–17. London: Bloomsbury.

—. 2014a. "For Mothers and Sisters: Care of the Reproductive Female Body in the Medico-Ritual World of Early and Medieval Japan." *Dynamis* 34 (2): 337–56.

—. 2014b. "Magische Medizin? Kulturund religionswissenschaftliche Perspektiven auf die tibetische Heilkunde." In *Tote Objekte—lebendige Geschichten. Exponate aus den Sammlungen der Philipps-Universität Marburg*, ed. Irmtraut Sahmland and Kornelia Grundmann, 189–205. Petersberg: Imhof.

—. 2019a. "Pediatric Care and Buddhism in Premodern Japan: A Case of Applied 'Demonology'?" *Asian Medicine* 14 (2): 313–41.

—. 2019b. *Buddhism and Medicine in Japan: A Topical Survey (500–1600 CE) of a Complex Relationship.* Berlin: De Gruyter.

—. 2019c. "Potency by Name? 'Medicine Buddha Plant' and Other Herbs in the Japanese *Scroll of Equine Medicine (Ba'i sōshi emaki*, 1267)." Special issue (*Approaching Potent Substances in Medicine and Ritual Across Asia*, ed. Barbara Gerke and Jan van der Valk), *Himalaya* 39 (1): 189–207.

Unschuld, Paul U. 2006. "The Limits of Individualism and the Advantages of Modular Therapy: Concepts of Illness in Chinese Medicine." *Asian Medicine* 2 (1): 14–37.

—. 2010 [1985]. *Medicine in China: A History of Ideas.* Berkeley: University of California Press.

Upasak, C. S. 1977. *Nalanda Past and Present, Silver Jubilee Souvenir.* Baragaon, India: Nava Nalanda Mahavihara.

Van Vleet, Stacy. 2015. "Medicine, Monasteries and Empire: Tibetan Buddhism and the Politics of Learning in Qing China." PhD dissertation. Columbia University. https://academiccommons.columbia.edu/doi/10.7916/D8J38RDJ.

—. 2016. "Medicine as Impartial Knowledge: The Fifth Dalai Lama, the Tsarong School, and Debates of Tibetan Medical Orthodoxy." In *The Tenth Karmapa and Tibet's Turbulent Seventeenth Century*, ed. Karl Debreczeny and Gray Tuttle, 263–91. Chicago: Serindia.

Vargas-O'Bryan, Ivette. 2010. "Legitimizing Demon Diseases in Tibetan Medicine: The Conjoining of Religion, Medicine and Ecology." In *Studies of Medical Pluralism in Tibetan History and*

*Society*, ed. Sienna Craig, Mingji Cuomu, Frances Garrett, and Mona Schrempf, 397–404. Leiden: Brill.

—. 2011. "Disease, the Demons and the Buddhas: A Study of Tibetan Conceptions of Disease and Religious Practice." In *Health and Religious Rituals in South Asia: Disease, Possession and Healing*, ed. Fabrizio M. Ferrari, 81–99. New York: Routledge.

Vaziri, Mostafa. 2012. *Buddhism in Iran: An Anthropological Approach to Traces and Influences*. London: Palgrave Macmillan.

Veidlinger, Daniel. 2010. "History of the Buddhist Canon." *Oxford Biblio*. https://doi.org/10.1093/OBO/9780195393521-0036.

Vogel, Claus. 1965. *Vāgbhaṭa's Aṣṭāngahṛdayasaṃhitā: The First Five Chapters of Its Tibetan Version*. Wiesbaden: Franz Steiner.

von Schiefner, F. Anton. 1906. *Tibetan Tales Derived from Indian Sources: Translated from the Tibetan of the Kah-Gyur*. London: Kegan Paul.

Wallace, Alan. 2003. *Buddhism and Science: Breaking New Ground*. New York: Columbia University Press.

Wallace, Vesna, trans. 2001. *The Inner Kālacakratantra: A Buddhist Tantric View of the Individual*. New York: Oxford University Press.

—. 2004. *The Kālacakratantra: The Chapter on the Individual Together with the Vimalaprabhā*. New York: Columbia University Press.

—. 2008. "A Convergence of Medical and Astro-Sciences in Indian Tantric Buddhism: A Case of the *Kālacakratantra*." In Akasoy, Burnett, and Yoeli-Tlalim 2008.

—. 2012. "The Method-and-Wisdom Model of the Medical Body in Traditional Mongolian Medicine." *Arc* 40: 1–22.

—. 2019. "Buddhist Medicine in India, Tibet, and Mongolia." Special issue, *Religions*.

Wallis, Glenn. 2002. *Mediating the Power of Buddhas: Ritual in the Mañjuśrīmūlakalpa*. Albany, N.Y.: SUNY Press.

Walser, Joseph. 2016. "Nāgārjuna." In Powers 2016a, 496–511.

Walshe, Maurice. 1995. *The Long Discourses of the Buddha: A Translation of the Digha Nikaya*. Boston: Wisdom.

Walter, Michael L. 1980. "The Role of Alchemy and Medicine in Into-Tibetan Tantrism." PhD dissertation. Indiana University.

Walter, Michael. 1992. "Jābir, the Buddhist Yogi." *J Ind Phil* 20: 425–38.

Wangchuk, Phurpa, Dorji Wangchuk, and Jens Aagaard-Hansen. 2007. "Traditional Bhutanese Medicine (gSo-BA Rig-PA): An Integrated Part of the Formal Health Care Services." *Southeast Asian Journal of Tropical Medicine and Public Health* 38 (1): 161–67.

Wangmo, Tashi, and John Valk. 2012. "Under the Influence of Buddhism: The Psychological Well-Being Indicators of GNH." *Journal of Bhutan Studies* 26: 53–81.

Wasson, R. Gordon, and Wendy Doniger O'Flaherty. 1982. "The Last Meal of the Buddha." *JAOS* 102 (4): 591–603.

Watson, Burton, trans. 1993. *The Lotus Sutra*. New York: Columbia University Press.

—, trans. 1997. *The Vimalakirti Sutra*. New York: Columbia University Press.

Wattanagun, Kanya. 2017. "Karma Versus Magic: Dissonance and Syncretism in Vernacular Thai Buddhism." *Southeast Asian Studies* 6 (1): 115–37.

Wayman, Alex. 1957. "The Concept of Poison in Buddhism." *Oriens* 10 (1): 107–9.

Weaver, Andrew J., Adam Vane, and Kevin J. Flannelly. 2008. "A Review of Research on Buddhism and Health: 1980–2003." *Journal of Health Care Chaplaincy* 14 (2): 118–32.

Wedemeyer, Christian K. 2007. *Āryadeva's Lamp that Integrates the Practices (Caryāmelāpakapradīpa): The Gradual Path of Vajrayāna Buddhism According to the Esoteric Community Noble Tradition.* New York: American Institute of Buddhist Studies.

Weiss, Mitchell G. 1980. "Caraka Saṃhitā on the Doctrine of Karma." In *Karma and Rebirth in Classical Indian Traditions*, ed. Wendy Doniger, 90–115. Berkeley: University of California Press.

Wezler, Albrecht. 1984. "On the Quadruple Division of the Yogaśāstra, the Caturvyūhatva of the Cikitasāśāstra and the 'Four Noble Truths' of the Buddha." *Indologica Taurinensia* 12: 291–337.

White, David Gordon. 1996. *The Alchemical Body: Siddha Traditions in Medieval India.* Chicago and London: University of Chicago Press.

—. 2003. *Kiss of the Yogini: 'Tantric Sex' in Its South Asian Contexts.* Chicago: University of Chicago Press.

Wibulbolprasert, Suwit, ed. 2005. *Thailand Health Profile 2001–2004.* Nonthaburi: Bureau of Policy and Strategy, Ministry of Public Health.

Williams, Duncan Ryūken. 2004a. "Edo-Period Tales of the Healing Jizō Bodhisattva: A Translation of *Enmei Jizōson Inkō Riyakuki.*" *Monumenta Nipponica* 59 (4): 493–524.

—. 2004b. "Esoteric Waters: Meritorious Bathing, Kōbō Daishi, and Legends of Hot Spring Foundings." Special issue (*Matrices and Weavings: Expressions of Shingon Buddhism in Japanese Culture and Society*), *Bulletin of the Research Institute of Esoteric Buddhist Culture* (October): 195–216.

—. 2005. *The Other Side of Zen: A Social History of Sōtō Zen: Buddhism in Tokugawa Japan.* Princeton, N. J.: Princeton University Press.

Williams, J. Mark G., and Jon Kabat-Zinn, eds. 2011. Special issue (*Mindfulness: Diverse Perspectives on Its Meaning, Origins, and Multiple Applications at the Intersection of Science and Dharma*), *Contemporary Buddhism* 12 (1).

Williamson, Laila, and Serinity Young. 2009. *Body and Spirit: Tibetan Medical Paintings.* New York: American Museum of Natural History and University of Washington Press.

Wilson, Jeff. 2014. *Mindful America: The Mutual Transformation of Buddhist Meditation and American Culture.* New York: Oxford University Press.

Wilson, Liz. 1995. "The Female Body as a Source of Horror and Insight in Post-Ashokan Indian Buddhism." In *Religious Reflections on the Human Body*, ed. Jane Marie Law, 76–99. Bloomington: Indiana University Press.

—. 2004. "Perspectives on the Body." In Buswell 2004: 63–66.

Winfield, Pamela D. 2005. "Curing with Kaji: Healing and Esoteric Empowerment in Japan." *J Jap Rel St* 32 (1): 107–30.

Winternitz, M. 1898. "Folk-Medicine in Ancient India." *Nature* 58 (1497): 233–35.

Wirz, Paul. 1954. *Exorcism and the Art of Healing in Ceylon.* Leiden: Brill.

Wong, Dorothy C., and Gustav Heldt. 2014. *China and Beyond in the Mediaeval Period: Cultural Crossings and Inter-regional Connections.* New Delhi: Manohar.

Wood, Frances, and Mark Barnard. 2010. *The Diamond Sutra: The Story of the World's Earliest Dated Printed Book.* London: British Library.

Woodward, F. L., and Caroline A. F. Rhys Davids. 2003. *Manual of a Mystic: Being a Translation from the Pali and Sinhalese Work Entitled The Yogāvachara's Manual.* Oxford: Pali Text Society.

Woodward, Hiram. 2011. "Cambodian Images of Bhaiṣajyaguru." In *Khmer Bronzes: New Interpretations of the Past*, ed. Emma C. Bunker and Douglas Latchford, 497–502. Chicago: Art Media Resources.

World Health Organization. 2008. "China's Village Doctors Take Great Strides." *Bulletin of the World Health Organization* 86 (12): 909–88. http://www.who.int/bulletin/volumes/86/12/08-021208/en/.

Wright, Arthur F. 1948. "Fo-tu-têng: A Biography." *HJAS* 11 (3/4): 312–71.

Wu, Hongyu. 2002. "Buddhism, Health, and Healing in a Chinese Community." *The Pluralism Project*. Harvard University. http://www.pluralism.org/affiliates/sered/Wu.pdf.

Wu, Jiang, and Lucille Chia, eds. 2015. *Spreading Buddha's Word in East Asia: The Formation and Transformation of the Chinese Buddhist Canon*. New York: Columbia University Press.

Wu, Yi-Li. 2000. "The Bamboo Grove Monastery and Popular Gynecology in Qing China." *Late Imperial China* 21 (1): 41–76.

Wu, Yu-Chuan. 2012. "A Disorder of Ki: Alternative Treatments for Neurasthenia in Japan, 1890–1945." PhD dissertation. University College London. https://core.ac.uk/download/pdf/8772487.pdf.

Wujastyk, Dominik. 1998a. "Miscarriages of Justice: Demonic Vengeance in Classical Indian Medicine." In *Religion, Health and Suffering*, ed. John R. Hinnells and Roy Porter, 256–75. London and New York: Routledge.

—. 1998b. "Medical Demonology in the Kasyapasamhita." In *Holistic Life and Medicine*, ed. T. S. Murali, C. Ramankutty, K. V. Ramachandran, and P. K. Warrier, 153–59. Kottakal: Arya Vaidya Sala.

—. 2003. *The Roots of Ayurveda*. London: Penguin.

—. 2009a. "Interpreting the Image of the Human Body in Premodern India." *Hindu Studies* 13 (2): 189–228.

—. 2009b. "'The Nurses Should Be Able to Sing and Play Instruments': The Evidence for Early Hospitals in South Asia." Unpublished manuscript. http://univie.academia.edu/DominikWujastyk/Talks.

—. 2016. "From Balkh to Baghdad: Indian Science and the Birth of the Islamic Golden Age in the Eighth Century." *Indian Journal of History of Science* 51.4: 679–90.

—. 2017. "Indian Medicine." *Oxford Biblio*. https://doi.org/10.1093/OBO/9780195399318-0035.

Wynne, Alexander. 2019. "Did the Buddha Exist?" *Journal of the Oxford Centre for Buddhist Studies* 16: 98–148.

Yalman, Nur. 1964. "The Structure of Sinhalese Healing Rituals." *Journal of Asian Studies* 23: 115–50.

Yang, Dolly. 2018. "Prescribing 'Guiding and Pulling': The Institutionalisation of Therapeutic Exercise in Sui China (581–618 CE)." PhD dissertation. University College London. https://discovery.ucl.ac.uk/id/eprint/10061324/.

Yang Ga. 2010. "The Sources for the Writing of the *Rgyud bzhi*, Tibetan Medical Classic." PhD dissertation. Harvard University.

—. 2014. "The Origins of *The Four Tantras* and an Account of Its Author, Yuthong Yonten Gonpo." In Hofer 2014, 154–77.

—. 2019. "A Preliminary Study on the Biography of Yutok Yönten Gönpo the Elder: Reflections on the Origins of Tibetan Medicine." In McGrath 2019, 59–84.

Yao, Yu-Shuang. 2012. *Taiwan's Tzu Chi as Engaged Buddhism: Origins, Organization, Appeal and Social Impact*. Leiden: Brill.

Yeh, Hui-Yuan, Ruilin Mao, Hui Wang, Wuyun Qi, and Piers D. Mitchell. 2016. "Early Evidence for Travel with Infectious Diseases Along the Silk Road: Intestinal Parasites from 2000-Year-Old Personal Hygiene Sticks in a Latrine at Xuanquanzhi Relay Station in China." *Journal of Archaeological Science: Reports* 9: 758–64.

Yoeli-Tlalim, Ronit. 2010. "Tibetan 'Wind' and 'Wind' Illnesses: Towards a Multicultural Approach to Health and Illness." *Studies in History and Philosophy of Biological and Biomedical Sciences* 41: 318–24.

—. 2012. "Re-visiting 'Galen in Tibet.'" *Medical History* 56 (3): 355–65.

—. 2013. "Central Asian Mélange: Early Tibetan Medicine from Dunhunag." In *Scribes, Texts, and Rituals in Early Tibet and Dunhuang*, ed. Brandon Dotson, 53–60. Wiesbaden: Reichert-Verlag.

—. 2015. "Between Medicine and Ritual: Tibetan 'Medical Rituals' from Dunhuang." In Ramble and Roesler 2015: 749–55.

—. 2019. "Galen in Asia." In *Brill's Companion to the Reception of Galen*, ed. Petros Bouras-Vallianatos and Barbara Zipser, 594–608. Leiden: Brill.

—. 2021. *ReOrienting Histories of Medicine: Encounters Along the Silk Roads*. London: Bloomsbury.

Young, Stuart. 2014. *Conceiving the Indian Buddhist Patriarchs in China*. Honolulu: Kuroda Institute, University of Hawai'i Press.

Yü, Chün-fang. 2001. *Kuan-yin: The Chinese Transformation of Avalokiteśvara*. New York: Columbia University Press.

Zhang, Daqing, and Paul U. Unschuld. 2008. "China's Barefoot Doctor: Past, Present, and Future." *Lancet* 372 (9653): 1865–67.

Zhao, Dong. 2016. "Power-Laden Words: Taoist and Buddhist Healing Mantras in Jinzhuang Village." In *Religious Diversity Today: Experiencing Religion in the Contemporary World*, vol. 1., *Suffering and Misfortune*, ed. Liam D. Murphy and Jean-Guy A. Goulet, 113–29. Santa Barbara, Calif.: Praeger.

Zieme, Peter. 2007. "Notes on Uighur Medicine, Especially on the Uighur Siddhasāra Tradition." *Asian Medicine* 3 (2): 308–22.

Žižek, Slavoj. 2001. "From Western Marxism to Western Buddhism." *Cabinet Magazine*, 2 (Spring). http://www.cabinetmagazine.org/issues/2/western.php.

Zürcher, Erik. 2012 [1999]. "Buddhism Across Boundaries: The Foreign Input." *Sino-Platonic Papers* 222: 1–25.

Zysk, Kenneth G. 1998. *Asceticism and Healing in Ancient India: Medicine in the Buddhist Monastery*. Delhi: Motilal Banarsidass.

—. 1999. "Mythology and the Brāhmanization of Indian Medicine: Transforming Heterodoxy into Orthodoxy." In *Categorisation and Interpretation: Indological and Comparative Studies from an International Indological Meeting at the Department of Comparative Philology, Göteborg University*, ed. Folke Josephson, 125–45. Göteborg: Adoptionscentrum.

—. 2007. "The Bodily Winds in Ancient India Revisited." *Journal of the Royal Anthropological Institute* 13 (S1): S105–15.

—. 2016. *The Indian System of Human Marks*. 2 vols. Leiden: Brill.

# Index


acupuncture, 52, 115, 130, 157, 169–70
Afghanistan, 18, 19, 90, 125
alchemy, 41, 127, 136, 161; inner, 57–58, 73, 151
Alexander the Great, 91
Alma-Ata Declaration (WHO; 1978), 156
American Institute of Buddhist Studies (Columbia University), 112
Amitābha (Amitāyus), 40–41, 50, 58, 152
Anagārika Dharmapāla, 153
Ānanda, 30, 31
*Angulimāla sutta* (*Discourse to Angulimāla*), 30
An Shigao, 125
anthologization, 115
antibiotics, 150
apocrypha, 113
Arabic language, 94, 121, 127–28, 173
*āsana*, 63, 64, 142
Asian medicine, 3, 11, 151; and Buddhism, 159–63; and globalization, 166–70; revitalization of, 154–57, 159, 168
Aśoka, King, 83, 90, 95–96, 99, 192n2
*Aṣṭāṅgahṛdaya saṃhitā* (*Compendium of the Essence of the Eight Branches*), 92, 93, 94, 97, 120, 136, 140
*Aṣṭāṅga saṃgraha* (*Treatise on the Eight Branches*), 92
astrology, 61, 135, 155, 161
Ātreya, 92
*avadānas* (Buddhist narratives), 28, 49, 120
Avalokiteśvara, 39–40, 43, 46, 50, 53, 74, 133, 171; and modern medicine, 163, 166; official patronage of, 100
Awakening Factors, 30, 80
Āyurvedic medicine, 24–26, 32, 59, 155; in China, 125, 130–31; contemporary forms of, 161, 173; and Islamic medicine, 126, 127; and Mahāyāna Buddhism, 36–38; and Nikāya Buddhism, 47; spread of, 90–92, 131, 135, 136, 140; and Tantric Buddhism, 55; texts of, 37, 38, 110, 114, 120. *See also* particular texts and doctrines

Bactria, 127
Bamiyan, 92
Bangladesh, 128
bathhouses, 35, 77
*Bathhouse Sūtra* (*Wenshi jing*), 77
*Beryl Mirror* (*Vaidurya melong*; Desi Sangyé Gyatso), 121
Bhaiṣajyaguru (Medicine Buddha), 6, 7, 41–43, 46, 78, 192n11; in contemporary era, 155, 162; in Japan, 97; in Korea, 131, 133; official support for, 99, 100; in Tantric Buddhism, 50, 53, 54, 96, 136
*Bhaiṣajyaguru Sūtra*, 43, 46, 92, 102, 108, 117, 118
Bhaiṣajyaraja (Medicine King), 40, 119
Bharadhaja, 127

*Bhesajjamañjūsā* (*Casket of Medicine*), 121, 140
Bhutan, 3, 139, 146, 162, 197n46
Bīmāristān hospital (Baghdad), 127
*Binding of the Wheels Tantra* (*Cakrasaṃvara tantra*), 53–54, 60, 118
*Blue Beryl* (*Baidurya ngönpo*; Desi Sangyé Gyatso), 121, 138
*bodhicitta* (thought of awakening), 63–64, 65
body, physical, 68–74, 79; detachment from, 69, 70; and enlightenment, 66–67, 72, 73, 74, 76; and environment, 83; female, 71–72, 190n11; and modern science, 151; pollution of, 70–71; and suffering, 69–70; in Tantric Buddhism, 72–73. *See also* Elements, Four Great; mind-body relationship; subtle body
Borobudur, 93, 126
*Bower Manuscript*, 121
*Brahmā's Net Sūtra* (*Fanwang jing*), 35
brain scans, 1, 6, 8
breathing exercises, 31, 63, 65, 152
British Empire, 145–46, 155
Buddha, the (Siddhārtha Gautama; Śākyamuni Buddha), 17–18, 92; death of, 18, 73–74, 186n44; and demons, 26–28; and germs, 150–51; in healing narratives, 20–22, 24; healing power of, 6, 25, 28–31; illnesses of, 30, 73, 76–77; in Islam, 196n11; in Nikāya Buddhism, 34; past lives of, 28–30, 35, 49, 120; as proto-scientist, 150, 157
*Buddhakapāla tantra* (*Tantra of the Buddha's Skull*), 52
buddhas and bodhisattvas, 34–40, 43, 47, 53, 118, 180; female, 50, 137; multiple bodies of, 74. *See also* deities; *particular deities*
Buddhism: and art, 4–6; hybrids of, 1, 98–99, 135, 156, 173; morality in, 78, 81–85, 106, 140, 152; official patronage of, 99–102, 133, 155, 156, 159, 180; and science, 11, 12, 149–51, 163–66; sectarian divisions (vehicle, *yānas*) of, 18; and secular medical institutions, 159; suppression of, 103, 129, 146–47, 148; transmission of, 89–93. *See also* Mahāyāna Buddhism; Nikāya Buddhism; Tantric (Esoteric, Vajrayāna) Buddhism
Buddhist Digital Resource Centre, 112
Buddhist medicine, 1–7; circulation of, 89–123, 170–74; contemporary, 159–76; continuities in, 48, 50–55, 142, 158; diversity of, 1–2, 3, 6, 38, 84–85; doctrinal themes in, 68–85; as general term, 3–7, 183nn5–6; lineages of, 6, 49–50, 54, 56–57, 63, 135, 138; localization of, 89, 91, 124–43, 144; modernization of, 144–58, 159, 161, 162; and modern scientific medicine, 4, 12, 144, 146–47, 150, 151, 155–57, 158, 161–62; official regulation of, 98, 102, 159–63, 170; outlawing of, 147, 149, 156; popularization of, 1, 11, 130, 144, 152–53, 157–58, 164, 166–68, 171–73; revival of, 154–57, 159, 167–68; scholarship on, 7–11, 174–75, 181; secularization of, 70, 164–65, 166, 168, 181; as superstition, 75, 144, 146–48, 150, 151, 155, 156, 157, 180; suppression of, 103, 147–49; syncreticism of, 171, 173
Buddhist modernism, 151–52
Burma. *See* Myanmar

*Cakrasaṃvara tantra* (*Binding of the Wheels Tantra*), 53–54, 60, 118
Cambodia, 90, 93, 97, 103, 110, 139, 140
Caṇḍālī, 65
*Caraka's Compendium* (*Caraka saṃhitā*; Ātreya), 25, 92
*Casket of Medicine* (*Bhesajjamañjūsā*), 121, 140
Central Asia, 4, 41, 100, 135; Mahāyāna Buddhism in, 33, 52; medical texts in, 59, 94; Silk Road across, 4, 46, 59, 90, 125, 131, 174; spread of Buddhism in, 90, 124; trade in, 96, 127. *See also particular kingdoms*
Ceylon Religious Tract Society, 146
Chagpori monastic medical college, 102, 155
chakras (*cakra*), 61, 62, 63

Chakri dynasty (Thailand), 140
Chan (Zen) Buddhism, 130, 152, 153, 171
Chang'an (China), 93, 98, 128
chanting, 48, 53, 118, 128, 131, 140, 178; of *sūtras*, 30, 41, 43, 46, 109, 111, 135, 144
chaplaincy, 163–64, 171
charity, medical, 6, 35, 133, 145, 170; and COVID-19 pandemic, 2, 177–79; organizations for, 6, 84, 99–100, 108, 163; and Won Buddhism, 169
Chenla, 103
Chiang Mai (Thailand), 140
China: Buddhism in, 33, 39, 40, 43, 50, 53, 90, 94, 99–100, 103, 124, 128–30, 142, 163; Buddhist medicine in, 8, 20, 125, 132–33, 171; cross-cultural exchange with, 93, 129, 130; health care system in, 155, 162; Islamic medicine in, 127; medicinal substances in, 95, 96, 129, 131; modernity in, 150, 151, 155, 198n1; official patronage of Buddhism in, 99–100; suppression of Buddhism in, 103, 129; Tibetan medicine in, 102, 139, 162; and Vietnam, 97; Western missionaries in, 145, 146; women and health care in, 56, 133
Chinese Buddhist Electronic Texts Association, 112
Chinese language: digital sources in, 173; excavated texts in, 108; medical terminology in, 130; medical texts in, 94, 121; received texts in, 110; translations of texts into, 19, 33–34, 52, 94, 115, 117, 129
Chinese medicine, classical, 128–30, 135, 136, 155, 156, 173
Chopra, Deepak, 203n59
Chögyam Trungpa, 153
Christianity, 1, 108, 144–46, 150, 168–69, 196n11
Christian Science, 153
Chulalongkorn, King (Rama V; Thailand), 148–49
*Classified Collection of Medical Prescriptions* (*Ŭibangyuch'wi*), 122
colonialism, 12, 145–49, 152, 154–55, 167, 174, 180; and modernity, 144, 199n8
compassion, 2; and bodhisattvas, 34, 39, 50, 82; and COVID-19 pandemic, 177, 178; and healing, 28, 34, 82–83; in Mahāyāna Buddhism, 33, 36, 47, 50, 63, 130; in modern medicine, 83, 163, 164
Confucianism, 108
consciousness (*vijñāna*), 24, 61
corpse-vector disease, 115
COVID-19 pandemic, 2, 12, 177–79, 181, 182
cross-cultural exchange, 9, 10, 180–81; with China, 93, 129, 130; and digital technology, 171–74; of disease, 90; and diversity of medical practices, 98–99; and globalization, 12, 166–70; and Islam, 125, 126; and Japan, 8, 93, 97, 132, 171; and local politics, 99–102; of material objects, 94–99; of medical knowledge, 89, 91, 94, 98, 117, 121, 122, 131, 134, 135, 174; of medicinal substances, 95–96; modern, 150, 174; networks and nodes of, 12, 89–95; and non-Buddhist travelers, 98; of people, 96–99; of texts, 94, 105–6, 113–16, 122; and translocation, 135–42

*ḍākinī* (female spirits), 50, 65
Dalai Lama: fifth, 102, 138, 141; thirteenth, 155; fourteenth (Tenzin Gyatso), 75, 82–83, 171–72, 178, 203n59
Daoism, 59, 94, 96, 108, 115, 133, 151
Daoshi, 115
Daoxuan, 116, 117
death: Buddhist view of, 68, 69, 72, 74, 76; and infectious disease, 157; in Japan, 40, 164; signs of, 37, 55
deities: and COVID-19, 178, 179; female, 51; and karma, 78; and local traditions, 135; in Mahāyāna Buddhism, 33, 38–42, 45, 47, 50, 55–56, 130; in Nikāya Buddhism, 47; protective, 41, 44, 51; in Southeast Asia, 139, 160; in Tantric Buddhism, 48, 50, 53, 55–56, 138; and texts, 118, 120, 139. *See*

deities (*continued*)
*also* buddhas and bodhisattvas; *particular deities*
deity yoga (*devatāyoga*), 55–56, 58, 73
Demiéville, Paul, 8
demons: converted, 26–28, 29, 41, 52; female, 27, 28, 43, 44, 52, 72; in Mahāyāna Buddhism, 33, 41, 43, 44, 45; in Nikāya Buddhism, 26–28, 29, 31; vs. science, 146; in Tantric Buddhism, 49, 52, 56; and texts, 94, 115, 117, 118, 121, 146
Dhammakaya (organization), 178
*dhāraṇī* (incantations), 43–45, 92, 118; in local traditions, 126, 128, 131, 133, 135, 167; pronunciation of, 44; and Tantric Buddhism, 48, 53
diagnosis: in local traditions, 133, 140, 160; in Mahāyāna Buddhism, 37, 46; in Nikāya Buddhism, 22, 31; in Tibetan medicine, 55, 127, 139
*Diamond Sūtra*, 109, 111
diasporic communities, 8, 9, 162–63
digital technology, 12, 112, 159, 171–74
Ding Fubao, 151
*Discourse to Girimānanda* (*Girimānanda sutta*), 31, 119
*Dorjé lükyi beshé* (*Hidden Description of the Vajra Body*), 65, 118
Dunhuang, 93, 98, 108, 109, 112, 136

Earth Treasury (Kṣitigarbha), 40, 133
Elements, Four Great (*mahābhūta*): in Āyurvedic medicine, 24, 38; and the environment, 83; and Islamic medicine, 126; in local traditions, 125, 129, 131, 133, 136, 139, 140, 142, 160; in Mahāyāna Buddhism, 36, 38; and meditation, 69; in Nikāya Buddhism, 24–25, 31; and subtle body, 59, 60; in Tantric Buddhism, 52, 58, 189n50; texts on, 110, 117, 120. See also *tridoṣa*; Winds
elites: and Buddhist medicine, 97, 110, 135, 139; global, 1, 150; local, 99, 146–47; Tang Chinese, 129
emptiness (*śunyatā*), 37, 73, 74, 117, 120
environment, 83–84, 181
essence, vital (*rasa*), 57–58, 63
*Essence of the Eight Branches, Compendium of the* (*Aṣṭāṅgahṛdaya saṃhitā*), 92, 93, 94, 97, 120, 136, 140
exorcism, 56, 118, 135, 146, 160. *See also* demons

Falun Gong, 1
*Fanwang jing* (*Brahmā's Net Sūtra*), 35
Faxian, 97, 129
Five Phases (*wuxing*; *gogyō*), 83, 133, 139
Five Sciences (*paṇcavidyā*), 36, 92
flavors (*rasa*), 36, 37, 38, 125, 140, 142, 160
Fotucheng, 72
Foundation for a Mindful Society, 164
*Four Tantras* (*Gyushi*; *Secret Essence of Ambrosia in Eight Branches: An Intructional Tantra*), 121, 136–38
Funan (Cambodia), 93, 97
*Fundamental Spell Book of Mañjuśrī* (*Mañjuśrī[ya]mūlakalpa* ), 52, 54, 118

Galen, 127
*Gaṇḍavyūha sūtra* (*Sūtra of the Entry Into the Realm of Reality*), 35, 37, 129
Gandhāra, 19, 91–92, 108
Gāndhāri language, 108
*Garbhāvakrānti sūtra* (*Sūtra of the Descent of the Embryo*), 121
Garuḍa, 26, 52
gender, 8, 39, 65, 98; and pollution, 71–72; and Tantric Buddhism, 57, 65. *See also* women
genres, 106–7
Gilgit, 92, 93, 108
*Girimānanda sutta* (*Discourse to Girimānanda*), 31, 119
globalization, 8, 12, 85, 159, 166–71
Goenka, Satya Narayan, 153
Göttingen Register of Electronic Texts in Indian Languages, 112

*Great Compassion Dhāraṇī Sūtra of Avalokitesvara*, 40, 43, 115, 118
*Great Elephant Footprint Simile* (*Mahāhatthipadopama sutta*), 120
*Great Exhortation to Rāhula* (*Mahārāhulovāda sutta*), 120
Great Peahen Wisdom Queen (Mahāmāyūri Vidyārājñi), 51–52
Greco-Roman medicine, 24, 126, 127, 136
*Guhyasamāja tantra* (*Tantra of the Secret Community*), 60, 79
Gyalwa Yangönpa Gyaltsen Palzang, 118
*Gyushi* (*Four Tantras*; *Secret Essence of Ambrosia in Eight Branches: An Intructional Tantra*), 121, 136–38

Hara Tanzan, 151
Hāritī, demoness, 27, 28, 43, 44
Harṣavardhana, King, 95, 99, 193n47
*haṭhayoga*, 63, 64, 142
Headspace (meditation app), 179
health care systems, 159–63; in China, 155, 162; and COVID-19 pandemic, 179; in Myanmar, 161–62; in Thailand, 149, 159–61, 167, 180; in United Kingdom, 164–65
health insurance, 156
*Heart Essence of Yutok* (*Yutok nyingthig*), 138
Hellenistic culture, 91
herbs, 1, 35, 45, 95, 115
*Hevajra Tantra*, 60, 118
*Hidden Description of the Vajra Body* (*Dorjé lükyi beshé*), 65, 118
Hīnayāna Buddhism. *See* Nikāya Buddhism
Hinduism, 48, 60, 153, 187n2; and Buddhist medicine, 127–28; displacement of Buddhism by, 103, 124, 125
*homa* (fire sacrifice), 55–56
hospices, monastic, 40, 98, 99, 115
hospitals, 6, 21, 35, 108, 127, 163; and Buddhism, 165, 180; in China, 99, 100; in India, 129; in Southeast Asia, 139–40; in Thailand, 75, 149; and Western missionaries, 145
Huichang Persecution (China; 842–845), 129
Hyetong, 96

illness: of the Buddha, 30, 73, 76–77; categorization of, 31; causes of, 26, 31, 36–38, 76–77, 79, 80; cross-cultural exchange of, 90; cures for, 69–70; emptiness of, 69, 117; and enlightenment, 73–75; eradication of, 69–70, 157; and karma, 76–79; and microorganisms, 149, 150–51, 157; and mind-body relationship, 17, 79–81; and suffering, 34, 68–70; and vegetarianism, 84. *See also* mental illness; *tridoṣa*
India: displacement of Buddhism in, 125, 126; hospitals in, 129; mandalas in, 53–54; medicinal substances from, 96, 131; national health-care system of, 162; non-Buddhist traditions in, 52, 59, 69; spread of Buddhism from, 89–90, 103; subtle body system in, 59, 66; Tantra in, 52, 55, 59; Tantric Buddhism in, 48, 49; texts from, 33–34, 94, 108, 118; Tibetan medicine in, 139, 162; tsunami in (2004), 163; Western missionaries in, 145; women's health care in, 132
Indian medicine. *See* Āyurvedic medicine
Indian Ocean, 90, 174
Indonesia, 90, 126, 128
Information Age, 12
institutions, Buddhist, 6–7, 130, 147, 150, 155; and local rulers, 99–102, 149; in Southeast Asia, 139, 142, 160. *See also* hospices, monastic; hospitals; temples
International Dunhuang Project (IDP), 112
Iran, 125, 128
*Ishinpō* (*Prescriptions at the Heart of Medicine*), 122, 131
Islam, 103, 127–28, 135, 196n11; displacement of Buddhism by, 124, 125, 126
Islamic medicine (*yūnānī tibb*), 126–27, 135, 136

Jainism, 30, 48, 69, 185n9
Jalavāhana, 35, 82

Jāṅgulī, 52
Japan: birth rituals in, 46, 52; Chinese medicine in, 131, 133; and COVID-19 pandemic, 178, 179; and cross-cultural exchange, 8, 93, 97, 132, 171; death rituals in, 40, 164; Islamic medicine in, 127; localization of Buddhism in, 90, 130–33; Mahāyāna Buddhism in, 33; March 11 (2011) earthquake and tsunami in, 163; and meditation, 152, 168; Meiji reforms in, 147; New Religions in, 1; Tantric Buddhism in, 50, 52, 90; temples in, 1, 131, 132; texts from, 94, 115, 116, 118, 119, 131; traditional medicine in, 156; Western missionaries in, 145; women in, 56, 133
*jātakas* (stories about the Buddha's past lives), 28, 49, 120
Jayavarman VII (Khmer king), 100, 101, 140, 141
Jesuits, 145
*Jialouluo ji zhutian miyan jing* (*Sūtra on the Mantras of Garuḍa and Other Gods*), 52
Jiankang (China), 129
*Jinapañjara gāthā* (*Verses on the Victor's Armor*), 140
Jīvaka Kumārabhṛta, 6, 121; biographies of, 22–23, 31, 119–20; ethics of, 81–82, 191n40; long-distance travel by, 96; in mandalas, 54; in Taxila, 91–92; in Thailand, 75, 142, 160, 167; translated versions of, 114–15
*Jīvakapustaka* (*Book of Jīvaka*), 121
Jōdō Shinshū sect, 152
Judaism, 108

Kabat-Zinn, Jon, 154, 165
Kajiwara Shōzen, 116, 133
*Kālacakra tantra* (*Wheel of Time Tantra*), 55, 57, 60, 61, 63, 65, 118, 126
*Kangyur* (Tibetan canon), 107
karma, 31, 60, 120; boomerang, 77, 79; and healing, 28–29, 35, 76–79; in Mahāyāna Buddhism, 33, 37, 78; in Tantric Buddhism, 58; and vegetarianism, 84
karmic merit, 28, 35, 46, 76–77, 82–83, 96, 99
*Kāśyapa's Compendium*, 121
Khitans, 100
Khmer empire, 100, 101, 140, 141, 180
Khmer language, 94
Khotan, 52, 93, 94, 98, 119, 125
Khotanese language, 117, 121
Khruba Siwichai, 148–49
Kokan Shiren, 116
Kōmyō, Queen Consort (Japan), 131
Korea: Buddhism in, 33, 50, 90; Buddhist medicine in, 9, 131, 133, 147; Christian missionaries in, 168–69; and cross-cultural exchange, 90, 93, 96, 131; temples in, 42, 44, 111, 131; texts from, 111, 119; Won Buddhist order in, 168, 202n50
Kornfield, Jack, 153
Koryŏ kingdom (Korea), 131
Kṣitigarbha (Earth Treasury), 40, 133
Kuchean language, 121
Kūkai, 97, 100, 133
Kuṇḍalinī, 65
*kuṣṭha* (leprosy), 78

Laos, 9, 110, 139, 140
Ledi Sayadaw, 152
leprosy (*kuṣṭha*), 78
Lhasa (Tibet), 93, 98
Liao dynasty, 100
Lokottaravādin nuns, 116
longevity: elixirs for, 41, 58; healing rituals for, 1, 43, 50; and subtle body, 63
Longmen grottoes (Henan Province), 83, 111
*Lotus Sūtra* (*Saddharmapuṇḍarīka sūtra*), 39–40, 43, 46, 117
Luoyang (China), 128

Macdonald, Keith Norman, 146
Magadha (India), 93
*mahābhūta*. *See* Elements, Four Great
*Mahāhatthipadopama sutta* (*Great Elephant Footprint Simile*), 120
Mahāmāyūri Vidyārājñi (Great Peahen Wisdom Queen), 51–52

*Mahāparinibhāṇa sutta* (*Sūtra on the Great Liberation*), 73–74, 117–18
*Mahārāhulovāda sutta* (*Great Exhortation to Rāhula*), 120
Mahasi Sayadaw, 153
*Mahāvairocana tantra* (*Tantra of the Great Vairocana*), 53
Mahāyāna Buddhism, 11, 18, 33–47, 68; and Āyurvedic medicine, 36–38; and Chinese medicine, 130; compassion in, 33, 36, 47, 50, 63, 82, 130; deities in, 33, 38–42, 45, 47, 50, 55–56, 130; healing in, 34–36, 41, 43–46, 47, 180; hybridization of, 173; on illness, 69–70, 74–75; on karma, 33, 37, 78; on merit, 82–83; vs. Nikāya Buddhism, 33, 34, 36, 40, 41, 46–47; and physical body, 70, 72, 74, 180; rituals in, 33, 35, 41, 43–46; and rulers, 99; spread of, 33, 52, 90; and Tantric Buddhism, 33, 48, 50–55, 58, 66, 69, 180; texts of, 33, 35–38, 109, 117, 119, 180; vegetarianism in, 84
Mahīśāsaka school, 116
Maitreya, 100
Manchu language, 110
Manchuria, 102
mandalas, 48, 53–54, 55, 56, 58, 63
Manichaeism, 108
Mañjuśri, 133
*Mañjuśrī[ya]mūlakalpa* (*Fundamental Spell Book of Mañjuśrī*), 52, 54, 118
mantras, 52, 55, 74, 119, 135, 136, 171; in contemporary Myanmar, 162; and COVID-19 pandemic, 178; in Tantric Buddhism, 48, 53, 58, 63
Mao Zedong, 155
massage, 142, 167, 168, 202n49
material objects: in cross-cultural exchange, 94–99; medical, 141; ritual, 63
MBCT (mindfulness-based cognitive therapy), 154
MBSR (mindfulness-based stress reduction), 154
medical ethics, 81–85
medicinal substances, 20–22; and bodhisattvas, 35, 40; and the Buddha, 28; in China, 83, 95, 96, 129, 131; cross-cultural exchange of, 95–96; efficacy of, 23, 38; essences of, 58; Indian, 96, 131; and Islamic medicine, 126, 127; in Japan, 131; methods of using, 46–47; precious pills (*rinchen rilbu*), 58, 162; in rituals, 45, 46; stories about, 95–96; in Tantric Buddhism, 52, 53, 55, 57; texts on, 31, 41, 45; in Thailand, 160; Tibetan, 95, 96, 127, 162; Vietnamese, 97; *vinayas* on, 21–22, 31, 106, 116. *See also* antibiotics; herbs; tea
Medicine Buddha. *See* Bhaiṣajyaguru
Medicine King. *See* Bhaiṣajyaraja
*Medicine of the Moon King* (*Menché dawé gyelpo*), 136
meditation: and bodily transformation, 72–73; compassion, 164; in contemporary Southeast Asia, 162, 167; and COVID-19 pandemic, 178, 179; in India, 153; in Japan, 152, 168; in Mahāyāna Buddhism, 34, 40; and mental health, 69, 80–81, 152–53, 165, 172; mindfulness, 1, 7–8, 70, 83, 154, 164–65, 168, 177, 180; modernization of, 1, 151–54; Naikan, 152–53; popular media on, 1, 11, 164; scientific research on, 1, 6, 7–8, 10–11, 81, 154, 164; secularization of, 164–65, 168; and sexuality, 65; in Tantric Buddhism, 49, 63–64, 119; texts on, 30–31, 106, 116, 119; therapeutic, 2, 8, 144, 164–65; in U.S., 153, 164, 171, 179, 180; and visualization, 40, 59, 119. *See also* Transcendental Meditation
meditation illness (*chanbing*), 80–81, 119, 165
Meiji reforms (Japan), 147
*Menché dawé gyelpo* (*Medicine of the Moon King*), 136
mental health: and Buddhism, 1, 151, 152; and meditation, 69, 80–81, 152–53, 165, 172
mental illness, 25, 76, 151; and meditation, 80–81, 119, 165; and physical illness, 30–31, 37, 79–81
Men-Tsee-Khang (Dharamshala, India), 162

Mentsikhang medical college, 155, 162
Michigan (U.S.), 179, 180
Mihintale (Sri Lanka), 139
Mind and Life Institute, 172
mind-body relationship, 24, 32, 49, 59, 106, 120, 181; and physical illness, 17, 79–81; and Winds, 60, 80
Mind Cure movement, 153
mindfulness, 1, 7–8, 70, 83, 154, 164–65, 168, 177, 180. *See also* meditation
Mindfulness Initiative, 164
Mindfulness in Schools Project, 164
Minoru Harada, 178
*Miraculous Drugs of the South* (*Nam d'ọ'c thần hiệu*), 97
missionaries, 144–47, 150; Catholic, 145; Protestant, 145–46, 168–69; Won Buddhist, 168, 169–70
modernization, 85, 144–58; and colonialism, 145–49, 152, 154, 155; and defense of Buddhism, 149–51; of meditation, 151–54; push and pull models of, 199n8; and racism, 150; and revitalization of Asian medicine, 154–57; and Thai medicine, 159–61, 167
Mogao Caves (Dunhuang), 46
Mongkut, King (Rama IV; Thailand), 148
Mongol Empire, 100, 102, 127
Mongolia, 33, 118, 135, 139, 147, 163
Mongolian language, 110, 115
moxibustion, 115, 130
*mudrās* (hand gestures), 55
Myanmar (Burma), 75, 110, 140, 146, 152; contemporary health care system in, 161–62; Western missionaries in, 145, 146

*nāḍīs* (channels of subtle body), 60–62
Nāgārjuna, 41, 49, 79, 121, 131
*nāga* (serpent spirits), 26, 28, 52
Naigamesha, 28
Naikan, 152–53
Naitō Torjirō, 198n1
Nālandā (monastic university; Bihar), 36, 92, 93, 98, 125, 126
*Nam d'ọ'c thần hiệu* (*Miraculous Drugs of the South*), 97
Nara (Japan), 93, 98
Naropa, Six Teachings of, 118
narratives, 117, 129, 160; English translations of, 119–20; of healing, 20–22, 24
neo-Confucianism, 129, 131
Nepal, 9, 139, 146, 163, 178
Nestorian Christianity, 108
Netherlands, 145
Nida Chenagtsang, 171, 178, 198n54, 203n59
Nikāya Buddhism, 11, 17–32, 68, 173; demons in, 26–28, 29, 31; healing in, 19–24, 26, 28–31, 32; on illness and enlightenment, 73–74; and Indian medical knowledge, 24–26; on karma, 78; vs. Mahāyāna Buddhism, 33, 34, 36, 40, 41, 46–47, 82, 90; monastic disciplinary codes (*vinayas*) of, 18–24; physical body in, 58, 70; physicians in, 47, 69, 81–82; vs. Tantric Buddhism, 50, 72; texts of, 18–24, 25, 26, 30, 31, 32, 119; and Theravāda Buddhism, 50; vegetarianism in, 84
*nirvāṇa*: and bodhisattvas, 34; Factors of, 19; and illness, 73–75; and physical body, 66–67, 72, 73, 74, 76; scientific model for, 151
Norbu, Khyenrap, 155

Obama, Barack, 172
"On the Difference Between the Brain and the Spinal Cord" (Hara Tanzan), 151
ophthalmology, 41, 131, 163
orality, 18, 105, 107, 109, 149

Padmasambhava, 65, 74
Pakistan, 19, 90, 108, 125, 128
Pāla dynasty (India), 125
Pāli Canon, 73, 76, 109–10, 180, 191n40; digitized, 112
Pāli language, 82, 109, 114, 116, 119; earliest texts in, 18, 19; medical texts in, 121, 140
Pali Text Society, 153
*paṇcavidyā* (Five Sciences), 36, 92

*parittas* (recitations), 30, 43, 69
Parthian empire, 125
Patañjali, 187n13
Philadelphia, Pennsylvania (U.S.), 169–70, 171, 202n50
physicians, 22–23, 32, 35, 131; idealized, 81–82; Japanese 131, 133; monastic 97, 108, 131, 133, 138–39; in Nikāya Buddhism, 47, 69, 81–82; official regulation of, 102; Tibetan, 138–39. *See also* Jīvaka Kumārabhṛta
pollution, 26, 57, 70–71, 72
Portugal, 145
*prāṇa*. *See* Winds
*prāṇāyāma*. *See* breathing exercises
*Prescriptions at the Heart of Medicine* (*Ishinpō*), 122, 131
*Prescriptions Worth a Thousand in Gold* (*Qinjin yaofang*), 122
printing, 111–12
Protestantism, 145–46, 168–69
Puṇyodaya, 97
Pure Land, 40–41, 171

*qi* (*ki*), 59, 83, 133
Qing dynasty (China), 102
*Qinjin yaofang* (*Prescriptions Worth a Thousand in Gold*), 122

racism, 146–47, 150, 181
*rasa* (flavors), 36, 37, 38, 125, 140, 142, 160
*rasa* (vital essence), 57–58, 63
Rattanakosin kingdom (Thailand), 141, 147–49
Reiki, 1
Rikpé Yeshé Yilekyé, 136
Rinchen Zangpo, 97
rituals, 32, 55, 70; birth, 28, 30, 39, 46, 52, 66, 121; black magic, 56–57; and COVID-19 pandemic, 178; death, 40, 164; empowerment, 45, 97, 100, 133, 135, 147, 167; healing, 30, 41, 43–47, 50, 55, 56, 58, 73, 95–98, 100, 102–3, 118, 130, 133–34, 156, 160, 167; *homa* fire sacrifice, 55–56; *kaji* empowerment, 97, 133; of Mahāyāna Buddhism, 33, 35, 41, 43–46; manuals for, 118; in Mongolia, 139; protective, 26–31, 32, 35, 41, 44, 51; protocols for, 45–46, 53; and science, 166; sexual, 65; Tantric, 48–49, 65, 97, 102, 118, 133, 136; in Thailand, 160, 161
*ruesi* (Buddhist yogi), 64, 142, 161
*ruesi dat ton* (stretching of the sages), 63, 64, 167
rulers, 99–102, 111; Dharma kings, 99; and sangha, 103, 149. *See also particular individuals*
Russia, 139

*Saddharmapuṇḍarīka sūtra* (*Lotus Sūtra*), 39–40, 43, 46, 117
Saichō, 97
Śaivism, 59, 193n47
Sakya Monastery, 138
Sakya Paṇḍita, 102
Samantanetra, 35
*Samantapāsādikā*, 117
Sangermano, Father, 146
sangha (ordained monastics), 19–24; bodies of, 72; and cross-cultural exchange, 103, 139; donations to, 82, 95–96; and exorcisms, 56; female (*bhikṣuṇī*), 19, 35, 116; as healers, 19, 31, 35–36, 120, 130, 131, 135, 156; long-distance travel by, 97–98, 103; medical care for, 40, 69, 77, 84, 98; modern, 156, 168; and rulers, 103, 149; and women's health, 132–33
Sangyé Gyatso, Desi, 138
Sanskrit language: in Indonesia, 126; in Japan, 133; terms from, 114, 130, 135; texts in, 18, 94, 108, 121; in Thailand, 142; translations of texts into, 117
Sarasvatī, 45, 118
*śāstras* (treatises; commentaries), 107, 116, 120–21
SAT Daizōkyō Text Database, 112
science: and Buddhism, 149–51; in contemporary Myanmar, 161–62; and modern medicine, 4, 12, 144–47, 150, 151, 155–58, 161–62; vs. religion, 166

scientific research, 157, 159, 172, 174, 181; on meditation, 1, 6, 7–8, 10–11, 81, 154, 164
*Secret Essence of Ambrosia in Eight Branches: An Instructional Tantra* (*Four Tantras*; *Gyushi*), 121, 136–38
*Secret Essential Methods for Curing Meditation Sickness* (*Zhi chanbing miyao fa*), 52, 59
self-cultivation (*yangsheng*), 59, 130, 133, 138
*Seminal Heart Essence in Four Parts* (*Nyingthig yazhi*), 65
Seung Sahn, 154
sexual cultivation, 65, 66, 73
sexuality, 56–57, 64–66, 72, 81–82, 190n11
shamanism, 5, 135, 173
Shambhala, 126, 127
Shaolin Temple (Henan), 112, 130
Shintō, 133, 152
*Siddhasāra*, 120
Silk Road, 4, 46, 59, 90, 125, 131, 174
Silla kingdom (Korea), 7, 131
singing bowl therapy, Tibetan, 1
skillful (expedient) means (*upāyakauśalya*), 61, 64; healing as, 34–35, 36, 82, 180; illness as, 70, 74; in Mahāyāna Buddhism, 47, 50, 180; meditation as, 165; in Nikāya Buddhism, 47; in Tantric Buddhism, 50, 56, 57, 66, 180
social Darwinism, 150
Sogdian language, 108, 117
Soka Gakkai International, 177–78
Southeast Asia: Buddhism in, 41, 50, 90; Buddhist institutions in, 139, 142, 160; colonization of, 145; cross-cultural exchange in, 93, 94, 95, 96, 119; translocation of Buddhism in, 124, 135, 139–42. *See also particular countries*
Sowa Rigpa (Tibetan medical tradition), 96, 102, 136, 138–39, 171; and COVID-19 pandemic, 178; modernization of, 155, 162; in U.S., 163
spirits, 26–27 *See also ḍākinī*; deities; demons; *nāga*
spiritualism, 153, 155
Sri Lanka: and COVID-19 pandemic, 179; cross-cultural exchange with, 93, 97; and Pāli Canon, 109–10; spread of Buddhism to, 90; texts from, 18, 94, 109, 121, 140; translocation of Buddhism in, 135, 139; and the West, 145, 146
Srivijaya (Sumatra, Indonesia), 93, 126
subtle body, 6, 49, 52, 58–66, 94, 118, 152; channels (*nāḍīs*) of, 60–62
*Sukhāvatī* (Land of Bliss), 40
Sun Simiao, 82, 129
*śunyatā* (emptiness), 37, 73, 74, 117, 120
Supreme Medicine (Bhaiṣajyasamudgata), 40, 119
Supreme Yoga (*anuttarayoga*) *tantras*, 49, 50, 53–54, 55, 58
*Suśruta's Compendium* (*Suśruta saṃhitā*), 25, 41
*Sūtra of Golden Light* (*Suvarṇaprabhāsa sūtra*), 35, 37, 45, 82, 117, 118, 129
*Sūtra of the Descent of the Embryo* (*Garbhāvakrānti sūtra*), 121
*Sūtra of the Entry Into the Realm of Reality* (*Gaṇḍavyūha sūtra*), 35, 37, 129
*Sūtra of the Great Compassion Dhāraṇī of Avalokiteśvara*, 115
*Sūtra on the Great Liberation* (*Mahāparinibhāṇa sutta*), 73–74, 117–18
*Sūtra on the Mantras of Garuḍa and Other Gods* (*Jialouluo ji zhutian miyan jing*), 52
*sūtras* (*sutta*), 24, 36, 94, 106–7, 113, 136; chanting of, 30, 41, 43, 46, 109, 111, 135, 144; in Korea, 131; vs. *tantras*, 49; translations of, 115, 117–18. *See also particular titles*
Sutta Central, 112
*Suvarṇaprabhāsa sūtra* (*Sūtra of Golden Light*), 35, 37, 45, 82, 117, 118, 129
Suzuki, D. T., 152, 153
Suzuki, Shunryu, 153
Swedenborgianism, 153
Syriac language, 108

Taiwan, 102, 147, 168, 171
Taixu, 150–51
Taizong (Tang emperor), 95

Tajikistan, 90
talismans, 1, 40, 41, 75, 135; in Arabic language, 127–28; in Chinese language, 44, 45; in Korea, 131; texts as, 43
Tamil language, 94
Tanba no Yasuyori, 131
Tangut language, 110
Tanguts, 100
*Tantra of Rāvaṇakumāra*, 94, 121
*Tantra of the Buddha's Skull* (*Buddhakapāla tantra*), 52
*Tantra of the Great Vairocana* (*Mahāvairocana tantra*), 53
*Tantra of the Secret Community* (*Guhyasamāja tantra*), 60, 79
*tantras*, 106–7; English translations of, 117–18; Supreme Yoga (*anuttarayoga*), 49, 50, 53–55, 58; vs. *sūtras*, 49. *See also particular titles*
Tantric (Esoteric, Vajrayāna) Buddhism, 11, 18, 48–67, 68; *bodhicitta* in, 63–64, 65; in contemporary era, 171–72; and COVID-19 pandemic, 178; and Daoism, 94; Elements in, 52, 58, 189n50; healing in, 50, 52–56, 58, 69–70, 73, 74–75; hybridization of, 173; in Japan, 90, 133; lineages of, 49–50, 54, 56–57, 63; and Mahāyāna Buddhism, 33, 48, 50–55, 58, 66, 69, 180; meditation in, 49, 63–64, 119; and modern medicine, 155; vs. Nikāya Buddhism, 50, 72; official patronage of, 100; and physical body, 72–73; practitioners of (*tāntrikas*), 49, 55–56, 74–75, 78–79; rituals of, 48–49, 65, 97, 102, 118, 133, 136; Sakya order of, 102; secrecy in, 48–49; sexuality in, 56–57, 64–66, 73; spritual weapons in, 49; subtle body in, 58–66; and Theravāda, 50; texts of, 99, 118, 136; unique features of, 55–58; women in, 55, 56, 57, 65; worldly vs. otherworldly in, 66–67
Tārā, 50, 51, 53, 58
tattoos, empowered, 167
Taxila (Takṣaśilā, Pakistan), 91–92, 93, 96, 98
tea, 96
temples, 6, 46; in China, 112, 130; in Japan, 1, 131, 132; in Korea, 42, 44, 111, 131; in Taiwan, 39; in Thailand, 23, 29, 64, 140–42, 147, 160, 167; in U.S., 169, 170
*Tengyur* (Tibetan canon), 107, 120
*terma* (treasure texts), 113
texts: adaptations of, 113–16; chanting of, 30, 41, 43, 46, 109, 111, 135, 144; cross-cultural exchange of, 12, 94, 105–6; earliest, 18, 108; excavated, 107–9, 121; extracanonical, 121–22; in Japan, 94, 115, 116, 118, 119, 131; Mahāyāna, 33, 35–38, 109, 117, 119, 180; modern availability of, 112–13; monolingual, 115–16; protective, 32, 44; received, 109–10; recitation of, 30, 43, 69; on stone, 110–11; as talismans, 43. *See also* anthologies; apocrypha; *avadānas*; digital technology; genres; *jātakas*; narratives; *sūtras*; *tantras*; *terma*; texts, medicinal; *vinayas*; *particular titles*
texts, medical: adaptations of, 113; Āyurvedic, 37, 38, 110, 114, 120; in Chinese language, 94, 121; on Elements, 110, 117, 120; Mahāyāna, 37, 38; on medicinal substances, 31, 41, 45; in Pāli language, 121, 140; Sino-Tibetan, 136; in Tibet, 102, 138; in Tibetan language, 94, 121; treatises (*śāstras*; commentaries), 107, 116, 120–21; Western, 145. *See also* translations
Thailand (Siam): Buddhist humanitarian aid in, 178; Buddhist medicine in, 140–42; and COVID-19 pandemic, 179; health care system in, 159–61, 167, 180; licensing of practitioners in, 160–61; mindfulness courses in, 168; and Pāli Canon, 110; suppression of Buddhist medicine in, 147–49; temples in, 23, 29, 64, 140–42, 147, 160, 167; translocation of Buddhism in, 75, 139–42, 180; Western missionaries in, 145; yoga in, 63, 94
Thai Traditional Medicine (TTM), 155, 156, 159–61, 167–68
Theosophical Society, 153

Theravāda Buddhism, 50, 110, 139. *See also* Nikāya Buddhism
Thesaurus Literaturae Buddhicae, 112
Thích Nhất Hạnh, 69, 154
Tibet, 6, 9, 197n46; alchemy in, 57; and cross-cultural exchange, 93, 96, 98; and globalization, 8, 171; Islamic medicine in, 127; Mahāyāna Buddhism in, 33; medicinal substances in, 95, 96, 127, 162; and Mongols, 102; official health care system in, 180; physicians in, 138–39; subtle body system in, 59, 63; suppression of Buddhism in, 103; texts in, 94, 102, 113, 138; translocation of Buddhism in, 90, 135–39; vegetarianism in, 84; Western missionaries in, 145.
Tibetan language: texts in, 94, 108, 110, 114, 121; texts translated from, 119; translations of texts into, 19, 34, 115, 117, 136
Tibetan medicine: in China, 102, 139, 162; diagnosis in, 55, 127, 139; in India, 139, 162; and modern medicine, 155. *See also* Sowa Rigpa
Tocharian language, 108
Tōdaiji temple (Nara, Japan), 131
tourism, 167, 168, 170
trade routes, 90, 95, 98–99, 126. *See also* Silk Road
Traditional Chinese Medicine (TCM), 156. *See also* Chinese medicine, classical
Transcendental Meditation (TM), 153, 173, 200n37
translations, 105–23, 144; into Chinese language, 19, 33–34, 52, 94, 115, 117, 129; cross-cultural circulation of, 94; and local terminology, 114; of narratives, 119–20; pseudo-, 113; of *sūtras*, 115, 117–18; into Tibetan language, 19, 34, 115, 117, 136; of treatises, 120–21; of *vinayas*, 116–17; into Western languages, 116–22
translocation, 12; in Southeast Asia, 124, 135, 139–42; in Thailand, 75, 139–42, 180; in Tibet, 135–39
travelogues, 97, 115, 129
*Treatise on the Eight Branches* (*Aṣṭāṅga saṃgraha*), 92
treatises (*śāstras*; commentaries), 107, 116, 120–21
*tridoṣa* (disease factors), 25–26, 60, 185n29; in Japan, 133; and mind-body connection, 80; in Mongolia, 139; in Pāli Canon, 110; in Parthia, 125; and sexuality, 65; in *sūtras*, 117; in Tang China, 129; texts on, 25, 31, 36, 37, 38, 120, 136; in Thailand, 142, 160. *See also* Elements, Four Great; Winds
*Tripiṭaka* (Buddhist canon), 106, 110, 111, 115
Tuệ Tĩnh, 97, 134
Turfan, 93, 115
*tummo* (yogic heat), 63
Tzu Chi Foundation (Taiwan), 163, 171, 177, 201n19

Uighur language, 108, 117, 121
UNESCO (United Nations Educational, Scientific, and Cultural Organization), 162
United Kingdom, 164–65. *See also* British Empire
United States (U.S.): Buddhist humanitarian aid in, 163, 178; infant mortality in, 199n18; infectious disease in, 157; meditation in, 153, 164, 165, 171, 179, 180; Sowa Rigpa in, 163; texts available in, 112; Won missionaries in, 169–70
universities, monastic, 36, 92, 93, 98, 100, 102, 125, 126
*Upaniṣads*, 59
*upāyakauśalya*. *See* skilfull (expedient) means
Uṣṇīṣavijaya, 50
Uzbekistan, 90

Vāgbhaṭa, 92, 94, 97, 120, 136, 140
*Vaidurya melong* (*Beryl Mirror*; Desi Sangyé Gyatso), 121
Vairocana Buddha, 53, 131
Vajrayāna Buddhism. *See* Tantric (Esoteric, Vajrayāna) Buddhism
*vāta*. *See* Winds

*vāyu*. *See* Winds
vegetarianism, 2, 78, 84, 130, 177
*Verses on the Victor's Armor* (*Jinapañjara gāthā*), 140
veterinary medicine, 133
Vietnam, 9, 97, 134, 155; Buddhism in, 33, 90; Western missionaries in, 145
Vikramaśilā, 93
Vimalakīrti, 74
*Vimalakīrti Sūtra* (*Vimalakīrti-nirdeśa sūtra*), 74, 117
*Vimuttimagga*, 120
*vinayas* (monastic disciplinary codes), 18–24, 35, 36, 106–7; English translations of, 116–17; on medicinal substances, 21–22, 31, 106, 116; vs. *tantras*, 49
Vipassana Research Institute (VRI), 112
visualization: and *bodhicitta*, 64–65; medicinal substances in, 96; and meditation, 40, 59, 119; and mental health, 80; of microorganisms, 70, 150; and modern medicine, 164, 166; and sexuality, 65–66; and subtle body, 59, 63, 73; in Tantric Buddhism, 48, 52–55, 58; in Tibetan medicine, 136
*Visuddhimagga*, 120
Vivekananda, 153
votive plaques (*ema*), 132

Wat Phra Chetuphon Temple (Bangkok), 29, 64, 140–42, 147, 160, 167
*Weber Manuscript*, 121
*weikza* (Buddhist wizard), 75, 161
Weil, Andrew, 203n59
Wen, Emperor (Chen dynasty), 46, 99
*Wenshi jing* (*Bathhouse Sūtra*), 77
West, the: Asian medicine in, 157, 163, 171; Buddhist modernism in, 151; missionaries from, 145–47; racism in, 150; religio-medical tourists from, 167–68; trade with, 95, 127. *See also* British Empire; colonialism; United Kingdom; United States
Western languages, 116–22, 173
*Wheel of Time Tantra* (*Kālacakra tantra*), 55, 57, 60, 61, 63, 65, 118, 126
Winds (*vāyu*; *vāta*; *prāṇa*), 24, 38, 189n50; as cause of disease, 25, 37, 76, 80; and essence extraction, 58; and mind-body relationship, 60, 80; and subtle body, 59–61, 63; in Thailand, 142; in Tibet, 63, 65, 136. *See also* Elements, Four Great; *tridoṣa*
women: demonic, 52; as healers, 56, 98; lack of texts by, 105; and long-distance travel, 98; medical issues of, 8, 36, 55, 94, 121, 130, 132–33; as mediums, 56; as monastics, 19, 35, 116; polluted bodies of, 71–72; as rulers, 100; and Tantric Buddhism, 55, 56, 57, 65. *See also* gender
Won Buddhism, 168, 202n50
Won Institute of Graduate Studies (Philadelphia, U.S.), 169
Wonkwang University (Iksan, South Korea), 168, 170
World Health Organization (WHO), 155–56, 160
*wuxing* (*gogyō*; Five Phases), 83, 133, 139
Wu Zetian, Empress, 100

Xavier, Francis, 145
Xinjiang, 125, 128
Xixia dynasty, 100
Xuanzang, 97, 129, 193n47

*yangsheng* (self-cultivation), 59, 130, 133, 138
*yantra* yoga. *See* yoga
Yellow Emperor, 127
Yijing, 92–93, 97, 126, 129
*yin-yang* (*onmyō*), 83, 133, 139
yoga, 153, 157, 173; deity (*devatāyoga*), 55–56, 58, 73; *haṭha*, 63, 64, 142; in Thailand, 63, 64, 142, 167; Tibetan, 94, 142; *yantra*, 63, 64, 142, 162, 164
*Yogācārabhūmi*, 120
*Yogaśataka* (Nāgārjuna), 41, 121
*Yoga Sūtras* (Patañjali), 187n13
*Yogāvacara's Manual*, 119

Yoshimoto Ishin, 152–53
Yuan dynasty (China), 127
*yūnānī tibb* (Islamic medicine), 126–27, 135, 136
*Yutok nyingthig* (*Heart Essence of Yutok*), 138
Yutok Yönten Gonpo, 6, 54, 96, 116, 137, 138
Zen (Chan) Buddhism, 130, 152, 153, 171
*Zhi chanbing miyao fa* (*Secret Essential Methods for Curing Meditation Sickness*), 52, 59
Zhiyi, 116, 119
Zoroastrianism, 108

GPSR Authorized Representative: Easy Access System Europe, Mustamäe tee 50, 10621 Tallinn, Estonia, gpsr.requests@easproject.com

www.ingramcontent.com/pod-product-compliance
Lightning Source LLC
Chambersburg PA
CBHW021939290426
44108CB00012B/901
* 9 7 8 0 2 3 1 1 8 5 2 7 1 *